# RESILIENCE IN ACTION:
# WORKING WITH YOUTH ACROSS CULTURES AND CONTEXTS

Edited by Linda Liebenberg and Michael Ungar

*Resilience* ... ng people's
vulnerabil... , and access
to resourc... e to foster
resilience. ... in the field,
this collab... e and qualitative stud... , including
social wor... c health, as
well as on ...

The boo... a different
aspect of v... dual health
and the w... en personal
resources. ... ons in relation to spe... izing holistic approac... f resilience.
The book c... o resources
that encou... s explore a
range of to... sed youth,
understanc... rategies for
survival, i... help frontline worke... nd the role
of commur...

Featurin... ic and cul-
tural back... conceptual
and practic... o fostering
healthy, po... th.

LINDA LIEB... e Research
Centre in t... y.

MICHAEL UNGAR is a professor in the School of Social Work at Dalhousie University and principal investigator of the International Resilience Project.

# Resilience in Action

## Working with Youth across Cultures and Contexts

EDITED BY
LINDA LIEBENBERG AND MICHAEL UNGAR

UNIVERSITY OF TORONTO PRESS
Toronto   Buffalo   London

© University of Toronto Press Incorporated 2008
Toronto Buffalo London
www.utppublishing.com
Printed in Canada

ISBN 978-0-8020-9269-4 (cloth)
ISBN 978-0-8020-9471-1 (paper)

∞

Printed on acid-free paper

---

**Library and Archives Canada Cataloguing in Publication**

Resilience in action : working with youth across cultures and contexts /
edited by Linda Liebenberg and Michael Ungar.

ISBN 978-0-8020-9269-4 (bound).  ISBN 978-0-8020-9471-1 (pbk.)

1. Resilience (Personality trait) in adolescence.   2. Resilience (Personality
trait).   3. Youth – mental health.   I. Liebenberg, Linda   II. Ungar, Michael,
1963–

BF724.3.R47R46  2008      155.5'1824      C2008-902166-5

---

This book has been published with the help of a grant from the Canadian
Federation for the Humanities and Social Sciences, through the Aid to
Scholarly Publications Programme, using funds provided by the Social
Sciences and Humanities Research Council of Canada.

University of Toronto Press acknowledges the financial assistance to its
publishing program of the Canada Council for the Arts and the Ontario
Arts Council.

University of Toronto Press acknowledges the financial support for its
publishing activities of the Government of Canada through the
Book Publishing Industry Development Program (BPIDP).

# Contents

# Acknowledgments

This book wouldn't exist without the inspiration of youth around the world. They never fail to remind us of what it is to live with dignity amidst adversity. This publication recognizes the life lessons they have to share with us.

More practically, though, this book owes much to those who work with these youth daily, exploring the intricacies of their lives and how we can best use this information to improve what we as adults have to offer young people. Some of these individuals are the authors of the work presented here.

We would also like to acknowledge those who contributed to the conceptualization and realization of this work and the 2005 International Pathways to Resilience conference in Halifax, Canada, upon which it is based. Special thanks are extended to Nora Didkowsky, conference organizer, and Nicholas Graham, who painstakingly helped to copyedit each of the chapters, as well as Amy Hum, Lisa Davies, and Chris Hurst for their assistance in preparing the manuscript. We are also indebted to the editorial staff at the University of Toronto Press for their invaluable assistance, most notably senior editor Virgil Duff and managing editor Anne Laughlin, who have worked so patiently with us on this project.

Bringing this work to completion has also been greatly assisted by our families. Janus, who has spent endless and very selfless hours providing moral and practical support, never questioning ventures into the unknown, and providing an ever-present critical ear. Cathy, Scott, and Meg, who have always been there, even when commitments to writing have meant time away from them.

Lastly, this work would never have appeared without the financial support of various granting agencies, including the Canadian Federation for the Humanities and Social Sciences, which funded the publication of this book, as well as the Social Sciences and Humanities Research Council of Canada and the Nova Scotia Health Research Foundation, which supported the research upon which it is conceptually based. Well-funded research enables the luxury of our collaborations and research. We are indebted to those who contribute their time and leadership to those agencies.

RESILIENCE IN ACTION

Working with Youth across Cultures and Contexts

# Introduction: Understanding Youth Resilience in Action: The Way Forward

LINDA LIEBENBERG AND MICHAEL UNGAR

> There will be something solid for you to stand upon, or, you will be
> taught how to fly.
>> Patrick Overton (1975), Community arts developer and educator

This book was born out of the *Pathways to Resilience* conference hosted
in Halifax, Canada, in June 2005. The aim of the conference was to
bring together researchers, professionals working with youth, policy
advocates, and policy makers from around the world (and others), to
share ideas concerning critical issues in understanding youth
resilience. The fascinating, innovative, and diverse topics and studies
discussed at the event underscored both the growth of knowledge in
the field of resilience, and the extent of what remains to be understood.

Attending the event with 320 delegates from twenty-two countries,
we were reminded of Suniya Luthar's (1993) early call to move
forward from questions regarding 'what makes for resilience' to ones
concerning 'what are the types of processes via which a particular
attribute might moderate the effects of risk, with reference to a specific
aspect of competence' (p. 451). In the past decade or so, leading
authors have made substantial contributions to addressing Luthar's
question (see, for example, Fraser, 1997; Glantz & Johnson, 1999;
Luthar, 2003; Ungar, 2005; Werner & Smith, 1998). Such answers
appear to be of increasing importance as global demographics change.
Reports such as he UN's *World Economic and Social Survey* (2006), for
example, consistently point to a growing disparity between the rich
and poor, with incomes in the poorest communities of the world
declining substantially in recent decades. Within this context of

growing inequality, Fussell and Greene (2002) remind us that by 'October 1999 the world's population reached 6 billion, with children under the age of 15 constituting one-third of the population in developing countries and nearly half in sub-Saharan Africa' (p. 22), one of the poorest regions in the world. And yet, in spite of this, other research demonstrates that in many ways youth are doing better than ever before (see Brown, Larson, & Saraswathi, 2002; Lerner & Benson, 2003).

It is within the intersection of these three phenomena that we turn our attention to resilience, a term that will be defined by each of the contributors to this volume. Their plurality of perspectives speaks to the emerging nature of this field of practice. All, however, argue that resilience is indicative of personal characteristics together with access to social resources and engagement in interactive processes that predict positive growth and development despite exposure to significant amounts of risk. All highlight the need for sensitivity to individual, relational, community, and cultural forces at play in the lives of youth challenged by adversity. The resilience of individuals is closely linked to the resilience of young people's families and communities.

As we gain understanding of the dynamics of resilience, however, questions begin to arise concerning how we implement this knowledge in practice with youth. It was to this issue that many of the presentations at the conference spoke. It made sense, given the wealth of knowledge shared, to create a forum to continue the process of dialogue begun during those three days in Halifax and to build upon the many conversations that have emerged since.

## Diversity and Complexity in Resilience-Oriented Interventions

The contents of this book highlight the diversity and complexity of both understanding and promoting healthy outcomes in youth confronted by adversity. From the confounding nature of self-mutilation as an attempt at exercising agency (chapter 2) to the engagement of youth in overseas learning expeditions so as to strengthen personal resources (chapter 10), the authors of this volume collectively underscore the importance of a holistic approach to the exciting and developing notion of the 'ordinary magic' (Masten, 2001) that is at the heart of resilience.

As youth around the world continue to teach us, we realize with increasing confidence that in spite of cultural variations, all youth rely on the resources of an 'ecological model' (Bronfenbrenner, 1979). While Canadian middle-class white urban youth may draw more on their relationships with peers, for example, than youth in China, whose culture values personal and family resources, all youth rely to varying degrees on the multifaceted components of themselves, their relationships with others, their culture, and their environment to negotiate the best outcomes possible in spite of the challenges and limitations they face. Simultaneously, however, many of these chapters support the growing literature emphasizing cultural and contextual relevance in the study of resilience and the interventions that follow (see, for example, Glantz & Johnson, 1999; Johnson-Powell & Yamamoto, 1997; McCubbin, Thomson, Thompson, & Fromer, 1998; Ungar, 2005; Werner & Smith, 2001). Together, the components of this book suggest ways in which, we as members of the communities in which youth find themselves, can enhance resources and outcomes. Reflecting on a variety of studies, theories, and conceptual models, these chapters come together to create a patchwork of components to be drawn on and integrated into successful programs, interventions, and work with youth and those around them. A veritable array of 'patches' are presented from which suggestions can be taken, new ideas stimulated, and, perhaps, entire interventions and programs replicated in ways that are meaningful to the populations being served.

At the very least, these chapters offer those already entangled in the complexities of work with youth empathy for the enormity of what is to be dealt with in the face of limited resources and burdened staff. Furthermore, these chapters reflect the long line of authors who have advocated a more holistic, action-orientated, constructionist approach to working with youth (Dallape, 1996; Donald & Dawes, 1994; Luthar, 1999; Tyler, Tyler, Tommasello, & Connolly, 1992; Ungar, 2003, 2004). Such an approach would enable an identification of root causes of problems to be addressed in meaningful ways, as opposed to merely dealing with symptoms. Furthermore, an approach that accounts for the interaction of micro- and macro-structures has the potential to enhance successes (see, for example, Gilmour & Soudien, 1994), moving discourses on outcomes further away from a tendency to 'blame the victim' for his or her shortcomings (Ungar, 2005).

## A Need for Research

The chapters in this volume demonstrate the struggle to make use of available research tools within strictures of scientific rigour and a lack of measures applicable to youth in this young theoretical field. More often than not, youth who participate in studies of resilience live within a 'matrix of domination' (Collins, 1991), where their marginalized position as youth is compounded by race, class, and geographic location. How exactly do we ensure then that we are indeed hearing issues of central importance to the youth with whom we work (Liebenberg, 2005, 2006)? Such questions point to concerns about voice and social constructions within and around communities that share common experiences. If we are going to understand whether, and why, our interventions work, we will have to continue to address the need for research methods tailored to the study of well-being instead of those better suited to documenting illness.

Furthermore, research into something as challenging to define as resilience must necessarily attend to the complexity of *who* is defining positive outcomes and who has the power to say *what* a sign of health is. In this regard, the notions of *construction* and *social construction* (Berger & Luckmann, 1966) in particular have come to hold important meaning to resilience researchers, who work with many different populations of young people. Working from a view of resilience that demonstrates awareness of the dynamics of social constructionism allows us to better understand the manner in which labels such as 'successful,' 'healthy,' and 'resilient' attach to individual lives and experiences. This is not a wholly academic exercise. The nature of these labels affects our experience of the world and our self-definitions. The label 'resilient,' or its opposite, 'vulnerable,' are constructions, highly dependent on our interactions with others for validation. Consequently, the meaning that grows from these classifications has an impact on society in its entirety – its institutions, practices, and so forth. These classifications and their meanings represent 'how the world is' and often inform our so-called 'facts.' The problem for researchers, then, is: how do we ensure that what we hear from participants is their reality, and not the dominant discourse that fashions their realities as other than the norm, and therefore of lesser importance? This question reflects both what we ask as researchers and how participants respond to our questions. Accordingly, how do we know if the numerous programs aimed at youth are in fact effective if we don't use research methods that are sensitive to the context in which people cope? It is a challenge resilience researchers are particularly concerned with, as positive outcomes change according to context and culture. Adaptation, in the face of contextual adversity, is always the result of a dynamic interplay of individual and social forces. Documenting resilience and demonstrating the success of programs promoting it are daunting tasks once we accept claims of relative truth. While this volume focuses on creating the conditions for resilience to be realized, many of the authors also address issues of research and the effectiveness of their interventions. This theme of research is to be taken up further in a companion volume to this one (Liebenberg & Ungar, in press).

Though we have gathered papers from around the world and demonstrated the plurality of perspectives on positive growth and development, this volume will not succeed in offering a definitive understanding of what works or doesn't work when it comes to helping youth grow up well. It can only start the debate, waiting for the next group of frontline professionals to use what they glean from this volume in their own local attempts to help youth cope with adversity.

This exercise in replication, adaptation, and research on outcomes from programming is going to require communication. Researchers and participants are rarely from the same context. Even more rarely do we see a volume such as this that brings together academics and practitioners from around the globe. Many of the authors who attended the meeting in Halifax found it both challenging and invigorating to build bridges of understanding across language and cultural barriers. Our hope is this volume sets the same tone. Still, we struggled to understand what resilience means both around the world and across the street in our neighbours' more proximal worlds. The chapters in this volume are a collective effort to disentangle the complexities of working with youth, providing services, intervention, and assistance. We seek to create new pathways to meaningful interventions with youth living in adversity that take into account the realities of different communities and how both youth and those with whom they live are situated within a global context that either promotes or inhibits their achievement of resilience.

## A Chapter-by-Chapter Summary

In chapter 1, Michael Ungar provides an extension to this Introduction, linking theory and intervention – the core of this publication. Ungar integrates five aspects of the study of resilience to practical interventions with youth. Specifically, he looks at resilience as an ecologically based construct, focusing on strengths of both individuals and their contexts that manifest through a variety of pathways. Furthermore, he highlights the growing importance of social justice in meaningful programs aimed at youth as well as the fundamental requirement of contextual relevance in such programs. These five aspects are demonstrated through the integration of a reflection on Phoenix Youth Programs, a frontline organization serving at-risk and homeless youth in Halifax, Nova Scotia. This first chapter establishes the framework for the structure of this book and the ideas and research contained therein. Specifically, the chapters in this publication address various components of an ecological understanding of resilience. Together, they point to a variety of pathways used to achieve healthy outcomes, and how we can better understand the positive resources and strengths available in youths' contexts. Numerous authors also reflect on the emphasis on social justice and contextual relevance that are necessary to this work.

To better highlight the specific focus and contribution brought to the discussion of resilience within each of the chapters, the remainder of the collection has been divided into four sections. Each of these reflect the ecological model of resilience theory, namely intrapersonal traits connected to resilience, community factors in the form of schools and programs available to youth, cultural dynamics related to healthy outcomes, and, finally, policy components that affect youth. All chapters review efforts made to enhance resilient outcomes. The structure of each chapter and the section in which it is placed allow us to explore in more detail how specific factors relating to positive development can be understood and facilitated.

In the first section,'Promoting Individual Well-Being,' authors bring together an array of strategies used by youth to manage their often traumatic experiences. In spite of this focus on the individual, discussions are anchored to contexts, always pointing to the relevance of social and structural supports in how individual youth negotiate outcomes. Nancy Heath, Jessica Toste, and Lana Zinck (chapter 2) focus on behaviour that more often than not is labelled as unhealthy: self-injury, or SI. As a form of maladaptive coping, SI is gaining increased public attention. Interpretations of SI as a precursor to deleterious behaviours such as suicide often prevent meaningful supports from being provided to youth who self-injure. The authors challenge these interpretations and present SI as a coping tool used by those who do not ordinarily appear to be struggling, in an effort to regulate extreme emotions. After situating SI within a resilience framework and presenting a variety of contextual manifestations of the behaviour, the authors offer approaches to working with these youth.

Exploring a wider collection of resilience resources, Kim Anderson (chapter 3) presents findings from her work with women who have survived childhood incest. Focusing on strategies used by these women in their youth, Anderson presents a conceptual model of resilience encompassing the resourcefulness of these women as young girls. The reflective process involved in her study, where participants speak as adults on childhood experiences, further underscores the longevity of these processes. The narratives of women in this study also demonstrate the importance of social supports in healthy outcomes, deflecting attention away from narrowly defined notions of resilience as comprising individual traits. Anderson, too, channels her findings into recommendations for professionals working with victimized youth. Together these two chapters exemplify the many routes to many good ends found amongst youth who thrive.

Placing the emphasis on the professional, the following two chapters of this section explore specific therapeutic approaches with youth. First, Roni Berger (chapter 4) discusses meaningful ways of fostering post-traumatic growth in adolescent immigrants. Explaining the stress experienced by youth at the intersection of new positions in life as young adults as well as new roles as members of a foreign culture, Berger reflects on useful tools that cross age and cultural boundaries that frontline workers can incorporate into work with youth. Used appropriately, these tools may create safe spaces for youth to make sense of and thereby manage their experiences. Commenting on the role of families and communities in this process, Berger's work hints at what is to come in the next section of this volume and also provides a link to the work of Sanders and Munford (chapter 15). Both chapters reflect on the importance of social justice to successful outcomes.

Continuing the challenge to how we approach therapeutic interventions with youth, Normand Carrey reflects on the place of both the *Diagnostic and Statistical Manual of Mental Disorders* (DSM) and resilience theory in the practice of psychiatry (chapter 5). His discussion seeks to engage frontline workers in a critique of the DSM, arguing for a need for contextualization while reflecting on its historical development. Reminding readers of the document's original intention and the principles of effective use of the DSM, Carrey underscores the importance of understanding youth who present with mental health issues within their context, exploring both risks and resources. Working on a case-by-case approach to diagnosis then allows clinicians to apply and use diagnoses in constructive ways that integrate meaningful treatment where it is necessary, thereby enhancing and strengthening available supports for youth.

Bringing this initial section to a close, but connecting it with those to follow, Linda Smith and Sandra Drower present understandings of resilience as well as contextual risk and protective factors among South African social work students (chapter 6). This chapter offers an interesting reflection on both contextual understandings of thriving as well as the need for enhanced resilience in social workers themselves when living and working in adverse contexts.

The sections 'Structuring Services for Youth' and 'Cultural Relevance' connect the preceding focus on youth themselves to the contexts in which they exist. These communities originate with families and extend to schools, services, and cultures. As highlighted previously, in this text as well as in other collections (Glantz & Johnson, 1999; Luthar, 2003; Ungar, 2005), we can no longer afford to see resilient outcomes as solely dependent on individuals themselves. It is the combination of personal, social, and structural resources available to youth and how youth call upon and integrate these resources into their actions that affects how they will fare. Furthermore, approaches to program design need to bear in mind that while there is much to be learned from the existing resilience literature, cultural relevance is crucial to meaningful interventions. In this regard, whilst 'Structuring Services for Youth' focuses on programs tailored to enhance healthy outcomes in youth, 'Cultural Relevance' reflects on culture and cultural variation in risk and protective factors.

Working from the understanding that oftentimes services meant to be available to youth are structured in ways that are, in fact, irrelevant, Nicole Letourneau, Miriam Stewart, Linda Reutter, and Krista Hungler discuss research aimed at highlighting the needs of youth living on the street (chapter 7). Accounting for the dynamic background against which youth who live on the streets function, the authors point out the complexity of service provision. Their study incorporates perspectives of youth and service providers into a peer and adult mentor support program for street youth in Edmonton, Canada. Linking outcomes with factors identified in the literature as being central to youth well-being when living on the street, findings from a program evaluation point to the relevance of the work to the well-being of vulnerable youth.

Many of the issues pushing youth towards a life on the street are also prevalent in the lives of youth who leave school prematurely. Providing youth with a meaningful connection to their education and a concrete set of career goals may in some instances buffer against dropping out of school and perhaps even leaving home. Targeting younger, academically at-risk youth, Katherine Levine and Dawn Sutherland review Career Trek (chapter 8), the primary aim of which is to direct youth to post-secondary education in ways that enhance successful graduation, minimizing children's future risk of living in poverty. Given such long-term outcomes in the face of contextual risks, the program draws on powerful community resources such as universities and local industry to build understanding among youth of how to navigate their way to careers that oftentimes seem beyond their reach. Activities in which youth engage allow future career options to take on a realistic meaning in their lives, as well as helping to link the youth with academic programs. Parents are also integral to the program. Their participation means that misconceptions around university education, for example, can be clarified and financial paths for youth's attainment of a tertiary qualification set in motion.

Staying with youth at increased risk of leaving school early, Linda Theron examines an intervention for youth with learning disabilities attending a specialized school in South Africa (chapter 9). Set against the previous chapter, we realize the diversity required when working with youth in educational settings who present with alternative risk factors. Building on the work of Kumpfer (1999), this multidisciplinary pilot intervention targeted personal protective factors of participating youth in a directed yet flexible manner. The value of this discussion lies in the lessons to be learned from a pilot intervention, highlighting benefits, issues, and potential pitfalls to be borne in mind when establishing interventions of this nature.

Lee Mah-Ngee and Tay-Koay Siew-Luan review an evaluation of the overseas Youth Expedition service learning project in Singapore, and its impact on factors contributing to the development of tenacity and resilience in participating youth (chapter 10). The study included 347 participants engaged in service learning opportunities in various

Asian countries. In this preliminary analysis, youth were classified into resilient and non-resilient types, based on self-reported assessments, and data were analysed in terms of problem-focused coping strategies, goal mastery, levels of self-esteem and self-efficacy. Findings suggest that participation in community service learning opportunities may enhance these features in youth. In addition to identifying prominent features in resilient youth, the study links civic attitudes to adaptive coping and positive development, pointing to future studies that might connect citizenship and resilience.

Lisbeth Pike, Lynne Cohen, and Julie Ann Pooley end this section. They outline Australian approaches to providing marginalized youth a more stable base from which to engage in both educational and social development (chapter 11). Focusing on the TALK program, the authors argue that improving communication skills of students, along with fostering self-esteem and a sense of belonging, will improve interaction between youth and others in their families and communities, lowering rates of violence and other disruptive behaviours as well as increasing their sense of community and interpersonal responsibility. Discussion of the TALK evaluation points to success of the program's goals as well as the value of providing youth a space in which they feel secure enough to voice their opinions and experiences, as well as respected and heard. Reflection on the evaluation process also points to the dearth of measures available for assessing positive outcomes in youth.

As suggested in chapters such as those by Smith and Drower, Berger, and Lee and Tay-Koay, as well as the previously mentioned writings of Glantz and Johnson (1999), Johnson-Powell and Yamamoto (1997), McCubbin et al., (1998), and Werner and Smith (2001), cultural considerations constitute a critical component of ecological understandings of resilience. The three chapters dealing with cultural relevance position culture within our approach to working with youth confronted by adversity. Jean Lafrance, Ralph Bodor, and Betty Bastien begin this section with a discussion of the relationship between resilience theory and aboriginal world views and philosophies (chapter 12). Situating current challenges of aboriginal communities within a historical context of aboriginal communities in Canada under white governance, Lefrance and his colleagues reflect on the root causes of risks facing aboriginal youth today. Building on this, they situate community-driven attempts at reclaiming culture and health outcomes, in previously oppressed aboriginal communities within Westernized theories of resilience. Highlighting the importance of social justice in research as well as contextual sensitivity, their main argument of the centrality of traditional culture to healthy youth outcomes is driven by strong inclusion of community voice in the form of interview transcripts.

In chapter 13, Julie Haddow unpacks the meaning of resilience among Japanese youth. Conducting research with a representative sample of 802 Japanese students aged eighteen to twenty-two, she explores the relevance and positioning of established Western risk and protective factors as they relate to Japanese youth. She also investigates previously unexplored Japanese risk and protective factors. Importantly, Haddow's research reviews risk and resilience factors found in both Western and Japanese cultures along gender lines. Her analysis includes the complexity of absent protective factors, as well as the potential risk inherent in certain 'protective factors' when present in the lives of either young men or women, pointing to the danger of interventions that fail to appreciate the subtleties of cultural influence on youth.

The Understanding the Adolescent Project (UAP) is an initiative aimed at promoting healthy outcomes in youth. Exploring Chinese understandings of resilience, Francis Wing-lin Lee and Kennedy Kwong-hung Ng look at how resilience is fostered and enhanced by means of the UAP in at-risk youth living in Hong Kong (chapter 14). In line with cultural interpretations of resilience, the program targets internal aspects of youth within cultural contexts. As with Theron's chapter, Lee and Ng provide the reader with very practical considerations in the implementation of a program, reflecting on obstacles they encountered. This final chapter of 'Cultural Relevance' also creates an interesting bridge to the last section, 'Government Policy and Service Provision.' Although the program was built on culturally relevant understandings of resilience, its implementation through government organizations introduced the tensions and dynamics that exist between these more formal structures and the realities of frontline work.

The final section of the book, then, speaks to policy and services. Without meaningful support in the form of legalizing policies, the disconnect currently characterizing so many resources for youth will never truly dissipate. As seen in the lives of youth such as William (see Ungar, this volume), silo effects thrive on limited and often mismanaged resources operating within compartmentalized sectors of the 'service industry.'

Jackie Sanders and Robyn Munford (chapter 15) discuss how, by centralizing youth voices in decision making, we can begin to move away from such 'silo-ed' service provision. Stemming from research on the experiences of young women in a community well-being study, the authors found themselves engaged in two public decision-making processes that occurred almost simultaneously in the community concerned. As they show, youth participation now provides a unique opportunity to reflect on the interpretation imposed by outsiders on youth behaviour and the effects of the resulting decisions on youth themselves, and how incorporating youth in these processes can, in fact, lead to healthier outcomes for both youth and communities.

Finally, Anne Marshal and Bonnie Leadbeater situate policy within ecological resilience models (chapter 16). They emphasize the importance of considering the cultural and familial contexts in which youth function and how these align with policy and program development and implementation. Integrating examples from their own work, the authors explore responses to the tensions found in efforts to bridge cultural and contextual divides. They also reflect on efforts to overcome the established focus on pathological outcomes and risk as opposed to strengths-based foci and positive outcomes, sectioned and separated responses rather than interdisciplinary and collaborative approaches, and the position of research and training in meaningful responses.

## Multiple Perspectives on Resilience in Action

Importantly, these chapters point to continuing concerns within the field of resilience. First, this collection of papers demonstrates the continuing dominance of North American and western European literature in a field of importance to youth in non-Western settings as well. Second, they underscore the need to continue our investigations and understanding of how ecological components can best be brought together to enhance the quality of young people's lives. As Dallape (1996) argued a decade ago, 'we need to look at children in their communities and consider their development within their own living conditions' (p. 290). Doing so permits us to understand their realities, making services relevant and appropriate. Given current consensus on the contextual relevance of risk, resources, and health in youth outcomes (Ungar & Liebenberg, 2005), the onus is on us to make use of available research and exemplary interventions that enable us as researchers, frontline workers, and policy advocates to respond to youth in ways that they say honour their truth.

# REFERENCES

Berger, P., & Luckmann, T. (1966). *The social construction of reality.* New York: Penguin.

Bronfenbrenner, U. (1979). *Ecology of human development.* Cambridge, MA: Harvard University Press.

Brown, B.B., Larson, R.W., & Saraswathi, T.S. (Eds.). (2002). *The world's youth: Adolescence in eight regions of the globe.* New York: Cambridge University Press.

Collins, P.H. (1991). *Black feminist thought: Knowledge, consciousness and the politics of empowerment.* New York: Routledge.

Dallape, F. (1996). Urban children: A challenge and an opportunity. *Childhood,* 3, 131–45.

Donald, D., & Dawes, A. (1994). The way forward: Developmental research and intervention in contexts of adversity. In A. Dawes & D. Donald (Eds.), *Childhood and adversity: Psychological perspectives from South African research* (pp. 261–71). Cape Town: David Philip.

Fraser, M.W. (Ed.). (1997). *Risk and resilience in childhood: An ecological perspective.* Washington, DC: NASW Press.

Fussell, E., & Greene, M.E. (2002). Demographic trends affecting youth around the world. In B. Bradford Brown, R.W. Larson, & T.S. Saraswathi (Eds.), *The world's youth: Adolescence in eight regions of the globe* (pp. 21–60). Cambridge: Cambridge University Press.

Gilmour, D., & Soudien, C. (1994). Disadvantage in South African education: The issue of transformative policy and research. In A. Dawes & D. Donald (Eds.), *Childhood and adversity: Psychological perspectives from South African research* (pp. 122–35). Cape Town: David Philip.

Glantz, M.D., & Johnson, J.L. (Eds.). (1999). *Resilience and development: Positive life adaptations.* New York: Kluwer Academic/Plenum.

Johnson-Powell, G., & Yamamoto, J. (Eds.). (1997). *Transcultural child development: Psychological assessment and treatment.* New York: John Wiley.

Kumpfer, K.L. (1999). Factors and processes contributing to resilience. In M.D. Glantz & J.L. Johnson (Eds.), *Resilience and development: Positive life adaptations* (pp. 179–224). New York: Kluwer Academic/Plenum.

Lerner, R.M., & Benson, P.L. (Eds.). (2003). *Developmental assets and asset-building communities: Implications for research, policy, and practice.* New York: Kluwer Academic/Plenum.

Liebenberg, L. (2005). The use of visual research methods in the South African research context. Unpublished doctoral dissertation. Stellenbosch: Stellenbosch University.

Liebenberg, L. (2006). The 'us' and 'them' in research: Can we get around it? *Qualitative research in organizations and management,* 1(2), 138–40.

Liebenberg, L., & Ungar, M. (in press). *Researching youth resilience*. Toronto: University of Toronto Press.

Luthar, S.S. (1993). Annotation: Methodological and conceptual issues in research on childhood resilience. *Journal of Child Psychology and Psychiatry, 34*(4), 441–53.

Luthar, S.S. (1999). *Poverty and children's adjustment*. Thousand Oaks, CA: Sage.

Luthar, S.S. (Ed.). (2003). *Resilience and vulnerability: Adaptation in the context of childhood adversities*. Cambridge: Cambridge University Press.

Masten, A. (2001). Ordinary magic: Resilience processes in development. *American Psychologist, 56*(3), 227–38.

McCubbin, H.I., Thomson, E.A., Thompson, A.I., & Fromer, J.E. (1998). *Resiliency in Native American and immigrant families*. Thousand Oaks, CA: Sage.

Overton, P. (1975). *The leaning tree*. Bloomington, MN: Bethany Press.

Tyler, F.B., Tyler, S.L., Tommasello, A., & Connolly, M.R. (1992). Huckleberry Finn and street youth everywhere: An approach to primary prevention. In G.W. Albee, L.A. Bans, & T.V.C. Monsey (Eds.), *Improving children's lives: Global perspectives on prevention* (pp. 200–12). Newbury Park, CA: Sage.

Ungar, M. (2003). Qualitative contributions to resilience research. *Qualitative Social Work, 2*(1), 85–102.

Ungar, M. (2004). A constructionist discourse on resilience: Multiple contexts, multiple realities among at-risk children and youth. *Youth and Society, 35*(3), 341–65.

Ungar, M. (2005). Introduction: Resilience across cultures and contexts. In M. Ungar (Ed.), *Handbook for working with children and youth: Pathways to resilience across cultures and contexts* (pp. xv–xxxix). Thousand Oaks, CA: Sage.

Ungar, M., & Liebenberg, L. (2005). The International Resilience Project: A mixed methods approach to the study of resilience across cultures. In M. Ungar (Ed.), *Handbook for working with children and youth: Pathways to Resilience across cultures and contexts* (pp. 211–26). Thousand Oaks, CA: Sage.

United Nations (2006). *World Economic and social survey: Diverging growth and development*. Economic and Social Affairs, United Nations. Retrieved 15 October 2006 from http://www.un.org/esa/policy/wess/wess2006files/wess2006.pdf.

Werner, E., & Smith, R. (1998). *Vulnerable but invincible: A longitudinal study of resilient children and youth*. New York: Adams, Bannister, Cox.

Werner, E., & Smith, R. (2001). *Journeys from childhood to midlife: Risk, resilience and recovery*. Ithaca, NY: Cornell University Press.

# 1 Putting Resilience Theory into Action: Five Principles for Intervention*

MICHAEL UNGAR

This volume owes a debt to Kurt Lewin (1890–1947). A social psychologist, Lewin in his prolific work stressed the importance of linking personal characteristics and the environments in which we live. That work preceded studies of resilience by several decades, and yet would find a comfortable place among the growing body of literature seeking to understand children's successful development when growing up exposed to chronic and acute problems. By the very nature of its perspective, the field of resilience research has positioned individuals in their environments. It is hard to believe that we could think of concepts like resilience isolated from the context in which such positive development takes place. And yet, though this point is now taken for granted in the fields of social psychology, social work, child and youth care, nursing, and other allied professions, it was a novel idea in its time. Lewin, and later his students such as Urie Bronfenbrenner (1979), helped us to develop a more ecological understanding of people and problems. Their work was a response to the increasingly intra-psychic Freudian-inspired perspective of well-being that de-emphasized social interventions that were so evidently at the root of dysfunction. It would take time, but with the advent of research on resilience, we came to understand that people's physical and social ecologies were also responsible for their capacity to overcome the same adversity that predisposed them to breakdown and disorder (Seccombe, 2002; Wolkow & Ferguson, 2001).

* The author wishes to thank Tim Crooks, Executive Director of Phoenix Youth Programs, for his helpful comments on an earlier draft of this paper. The author also gratefully acknowledges the Social Sciences and Humanities Research Council of Canada and the Nova Scotia Health Research Foundation for their financial support of this work.

As indebted as I am to Lewin for his contribution to theory, it is his practicality that guides me. Lewin is famous for saying, 'There is nothing so practical as a good theory' (Stivers & Wheelan, 1986). Unfortunately, that injunction to use theory to inform practice has often been overlooked by those who build theory. The grunt work of bringing about change is left to lay community members, frontline professionals, policy developers or, worse, politicians. Busy schedules and client demands often prevent these people from delving deep into the academic literature of outcome studies and theory-driven discussions of what should work and why. As ideal as it would be to ensure that robust theories inform interventions and policies, more often they remain disconnected. That is unfortunate, as Lewin also tells us, 'If you want truly to understand something, try to change it' (Stivers & Wheelan, 1986). There is much to be said for putting theory into action.

In this chapter I will discuss the theory of resilience as it relates to interventions with child populations under stress. These may be children in families experiencing divorce, homeless youth, youth who have grown up exposed to war, or recent immigrants coping with their displacement. Though the study of resilience has produced many insights into the ontogeny, or step-by-step progression, of positive development among at-risk populations, this chapter, like others in this volume, will demonstrate the synergy between how resilience is understood and the principles of intervention it informs. Specifically, I will discuss five aspects of the study of resilience as they relate to practice: (1) the emphasis in studies of resilience on the generation of ecological, multilevel theory; (2) the focus of resilience researchers on processes that build upon strengths; (3) the multifinality, or many routes to many good ends, of processes associated with resilience; (4) the focus on movement towards social justice as foundational to successful development; and (5) culturally and contextually sensitive appreciation for heterogeneity in how resilience is understood. To demonstrate these five aspects of resilience as they relate to what we actually do as professionals, I will discuss Phoenix Youth Programs, a multiservice non-profit organization that provides primary prevention services, secondary interventions, and tertiary-level long-term support for at-risk and homeless youth in Halifax, Nova Scotia, Canada. This example, like the practice examples in the chapters that follow, heeds Lewin's injunction to make theory practical.

## Thriving Dangerously?

It is easy to be afraid of Cyndi and her friends. They have the piercings and tattoos of the urban street youth. Their clothes and attitude invoke fear. On warm afternoons, Cyndi sits with her friends on the grass next to a busy intersection. She doesn't like to squeegee car windows, or beg, but values the feeling of comfort she finds on the street, where she doesn't feel herself threatened. This public space is so much better than the conflict-ridden home from which she comes. Her mother and younger sister live in a subsidized housing development. Her mother has always told Cyndi to keep to herself and made arrangements for her to attend school away from the other Project kids. She wanted her daughter to do more than just get by; she wanted her to make something of herself. Unfortunately, her mother also refused to let her daughter grow up. The life preserver she strapped to her when they arrived in the city eight years ago was meant to keep Cyndi safe. It did for a time, until the girl in the jacket outgrew the protection her mother could provide. Halfway through grade 10, Cyndi dropped out of school. She began to smoke and experiment a little with drinking and drugs. She is sexually active, though she says she doesn't like to talk much about it. She hesitates when asked if she practices safe sex. 'You mean always?' is the way she answers.

Since she turned fifteen, Cyndi has been drifting more and more to the street, couch surfing the basement rooms of friends who are still at home with their parents. However, when her friends are themselves on the street, and it's too cold to camp outdoors, Cyndi goes to the emergency youth shelter run by Phoenix. The shelter gives her and her mother a respite. Cyndi keeps hoping her relationship with her mother will improve, but each time Cyndi returns home the arguments start again, and with them the locked doors shutting the girl back out onto the street.

## Phoenix Youth Programs, Halifax, Canada

By 1984, a group of concerned professionals and volunteers had recognized the need in the Halifax region for a coordinated response to youth aged sixteen to twenty-four who lived on the street and were in need of shelter and support. In 1987 Phoenix opened its first group living facility. It was at the time the only residential service available for youth in this age group in a community of over three hundred thousand people.

The youth served by Phoenix come from family and community contexts where they are commonly exposed to a number of risks. Many show signs of stress related to physical and sexual abuse. Many have been witnesses to, or participated in, patterns of family conflict. They also bring with them to programming problems with addictions, truancy and school conflict, learning difficulties, and threatened self-concepts resulting from their living situations. These also tend to be youth who have experienced high amounts of racism, homophobia, and other forms of discrimination related to poverty and violence. Youth frequently report experiences of being bullied, of depression, and of self-harming behaviours that include suicidality and eating disorders.

In response to the growing community intolerance for having these youth on the streets of Halifax and underserviced, Phoenix grew rapidly starting in the late 1990s. In the new millennium, Phoenix initiated a follow-up care program for youth who had been in conflict with their families; a supervised apartment program for youth ready to transition to independent living; and a drop-in centre staffed with a nurse and youth workers, that also provides laundry facilities, showers, and advocacy to secure financial and educational resources. Furthermore, in collaboration with its federal funder, the Phoenix Learning and Employment Centre supports youth with academic upgrading and life skills training. The centre also provides career counselling and employment-related services to youth, helping them become independent financially. To these core services have been added other special initiatives that promote youth development through creative expression such as art and music. The Phoenix Prevention Program provides community outreach services in schools, a youth speakers bureau to sensitize the community to youth issues, and individual and family therapeutic services for youth served by Phoenix and those at risk of becoming homeless in the greater Halifax region. In 2003 a major expansion to Phoenix programs included the addition of a twenty-bed emergency shelter.

Phoenix is now staffed by over seventy child and youth care workers, social workers, case managers, psychologists, educators, health care professionals, and therapists. The target population has grown from youth on the street to those at risk of becoming homeless, providing service to those aged twelve to twenty-four. The youth using the service are most often those who fall beyond the mandate of Child Protection Services, which rarely deal with youth at risk after their sixteenth birthday. Recently, Phoenix management have sought to create greater integration and improve case management functions across the organization in order to facilitate the seamless delivery of services to youth. This has also meant creating a service network with other community care providers such as Child Welfare, the local Children's Health Centre, and the regional school board. Funding for the programs now includes both private donations solicited through a diversity of fund-raising activities and government core funding.

## Resilience as Applied Theory

Resilience is a theory that can inform action. It is a concept that changes our focus from the breakdown and disorder attributed to exposure to stressful environments, to the individual characteristics and social processes associated with either normal or unexpectedly positive psychosocial development. By way of illustration, we can look at Greene, Anderson, Hetherington, Forgatch, and DeGarmo's (2003) meta-analysis of studies of children's experiences of the divorce of their parents. Findings show that only 20% of children from divorced families demonstrate signs of mental health problems. In families where there has not been a divorce, only 10% of children will show overt signs of mental illness. While a child in a family where a divorce has occurred is twice as likely to require a mental health intervention, we often overlook the fact that 80% of children in these families remain healthy. This doubling of the incidence of disorder is certainly worrisome and cause for intervention, but we should not ignore the fact that, metaphorically speaking, the glass is far from empty. Greene et al. show through their meta-analysis of the research that four-fifths of children will navigate through a divorce without breakdown. It is the capacities and environmental resources that sustain these 80% of children that are the focus of those who study resilience.

As Crawford, Wright, and Masten (2005) explain, the study of resilience is 'a search for knowledge about the processes that could account for positive adaptation and development in the context of adversity and disadvantage' (p. 355). Clearly, then, a child's resilience is dependent upon the environment in which he or she grows up. That environment must necessarily include services that seek to meet the needs of children and families at risk (see, for related discussions, Barber, 2006; Boyden & Mann, 2005; Leadbeater, Dodgen, & Solarz, 2005; Wyman, 2003). As a contextually relevant field of research, the study of resilience is becoming increasingly focused on understanding what resilience looks like in many profoundly different cultures and contexts. Arguably, there are highly specific protective processes in each community and culture that contribute to positive development. While we know many of these processes are shared, there remains a tension in the resilience literature accounting for *both* homogeneity and heterogeneity in the way resilience is manifested among different populations. This is to be expected if resilience is a function of a child's or family's interaction with their physical and social ecologies. Our physical ecology includes tangible aspects of our environment such as the quality of the water we drink, our housing, the safety of our streets, and the level of pollutants in the air. Social ecologies can range from informal personal attachments and opportunities to experience rites of passage, to structural supports like schools, transportation, and medical care, many of which are culturally determined (i.e., whether boys and girls have equal educational opportunities, and how medical care is provided). Combined, these dual ecologies provide a context in which individuals can realize resilience. It is this emphasis on person in environment that reminds us of Lewin's point that how people behave is a function of their interaction with their environments. Change those environments and it would be expected that strategies for survival will also need to change.

Those studying resilience and resilience-related concepts like Positive Youth Development are looking at these constructs as clusters of assets, both individual and environmental (Benson, 2003; Lerner, Brentano, Dowling, & Anderson, 2002). This dual focus is important. A more individualized understanding of resilience is less informing of practical solutions. An individualized understanding quietly places the burden of growth, of adaptation, solely on the child. A more ecological perspective implicates those mandated to help (social workers, child and youth care workers, nurses, psychologists, and others) in the process of intervening to provide an opportunity structure for a child to realize his or her potential. It is with this broad perspective in mind that I define resilience as follows:

First, resilience is the capacity of individuals to navigate their way to resources that sustain well-being;
Second, resilience is the capacity of individuals' physical and social ecologies to provide these resources; and
Third, resilience is the capacity of individuals and their families and

communities to negotiate culturally meaningful ways for resources to be shared.

This broad definition of resilience emphasizes the need for individuals to exercise enough personal agency to make their way (navigate) to the many resources they require to meet their developmental needs. These resources must be both available and accessible. They range from psychological resources like feelings of self-esteem and a sense of attachment, to accessing health care, schooling, and opportunities to display one's talents to others. Combined, individual, family, community, and cultural resources need to be there for children if they are to succeed following exposure to adversity. Organizations like Phoenix Youth Programs concretely address this need for resources on the front lines of service.

The definition also makes clear that resilience only exists to the extent that a child's physical and social ecology are within reach of the child. Those ecologies include the vast matrix of care providers and community resources that support well-being. The phrase 'he is resilient' is inaccurate because it individualizes what is a condition of both individuals and their contexts. One need only think of the person with a disability who succeeds because of some innovation (a prosthesis, medications, or Braille) to realize that our capacity to achieve success is dependent on resources to activate opportunities for us to show ourselves as competent. Studies of lives lived well frequently point to special relationships with educators or other extra-familial adults that mentor at-risk children and shelter them from adversity (see, for example, Ungar & Teram, 2000; Werner & Smith, 2001).

Finally, the definition reminds us of the importance of culture and the meaning culture informs. Understanding which aspects of our physical and social ecologies will most influence resilience depends upon an appreciation for how these aspects of resilience are valued by our culture. In other words, a resource such as medical care, education, or a foster parent may be perfectly adequate as a buffer against risk, but of little use to a particular child if what is offered is not understood as helpful. As a case in point, one need only think of aboriginal youth offered non-aboriginal foster placements. Foster placements that are kin based are far more likely to produce positive developmental gains even if they are with less stable families challenged by multiple risks (Blackstock & Trocmé, 2005). Similarly, studies of marginalized youth from cultural groups where post-secondary education is seen as unattainable or irrelevant (Dei, Massuca, McIsaac, & Zine, 1997) have shown that in such cases youth may drop out of school and put themselves at risk (at least in the judgment of cultural outsiders). This pattern of 'resistance' is not necessarily a sign of disorder, but likely a message that the service being offered lacks cultural relevance.

Thus, the study of resilience can be reflexive. Research with resilient individuals about their physical and social ecologies helps to provide a depth of understanding of both the characteristics and processes that are associated population-wide with successful development (Kirby & Fraser, 1997; Rutter, 2005). If, for example, children who are the most successful despite exposure to risk show a particular constellation of factors that predict their positive development, then it would be reasonable to ensure these same resources are made available in culturally relevant ways for other children similarly at risk. We might imagine having a million dollars to invest in our community, and a wish to efficaciously assist the most vulnerable. It would seem prudent to investigate factors most relevant and useful to those who are already successfully coping with adversity. It is this potential for reflexivity that makes resilience research well positioned to inform practice.

Caution is, however, required when translating research into practice. Children, like Cyndi, have complex interactions with their physical and social ecologies. Findings from studies of resilience do not tend to be uniform across populations. For example, in a study of Positive Youth Development (PYD), a term synonymous with aspects of resilience, Phelps and her colleagues (2007) studied 1,122 children in grades 5, 6, and 7 looking for patterns of change over time associated with both PYD and risk/problem behaviours. Though it was reasonable to expect the coupling of increases in PYD with decreases in children's exposure to risks and manifestations of behaviour problems, this relationship held for only one-sixth of the children studied. Others remained stable over time, showed increases in both PYD and the level of risk they experienced, or a decline in PYD from one grade to another regardless of their level of exposure to risk. The child's socio-economic status, gender, and grade level all influenced the findings. What then are we to make of such multiplicity of patterns in the development of resilience for a population under stress? Furthermore, what does such complexity in the growth trajectories of children tell us about the design of programs and interventions to keep them safe? Examining how we might help a youth like Cyndi through exemplary programming like Phoenix can help answer these questions.

## Seeing Resilience beneath Problem Behaviours

Though from the outside it looks like Cyndi is a danger to herself and others, while getting to know her one discovers a different story. She may have left school, but she is committed to completing her high-school education. Only, she'd prefer to do this in the less structured environment of an alternative education setting, a place where she doesn't have to spend six hours a day listening to teachers tell her what she has to do. She's also happy to hold down a job. She'd worked as a cashier for almost a year, being fired only when her living situation changed and she found her life in too much chaos to make her shifts. Getting to know Cyndi, one quickly realizes the girl we see from our car window at rush hour sitting on the grass with her friends near a busy intersection is only a snapshot of a life that is far more complex than we might assume.

It's this multidimensional young woman whom workers at Phoenix meet when they provide Cyndi with a seamless continuum of services. By integrating a number of programs, Phoenix has been able to meet Cyndi's needs in ways that have allowed her to nurture the building blocks for survival. While many of the qualities that Cyndi builds upon were already latent in her prior to her attachment to service, it is the context Phoenix provides that helps to facilitate Cyndi's development. Informing these interventions with a theory like resilience provides a basis for intentional practice. Phoenix provides a continuum of care that is theoretically sound and reflects the five principles that research on resilience teaches us.

## Five Principles of Resilience Relevant to Practice

*Resilience is nurtured by an ecological, multilevelled approach to intervention.*
Large epidemiological studies that formed the basis for early studies of resilience demonstrated the cumulative effect of risk in a child's life and the constellation of factors and processes that protect them. Werner and Smith's (2001) study of a birth cohort on the island of Kuaii, for example, examined hundreds of factors over the forty-plus years of the study. Such efforts show that resilience, the capacity to overcome, was complex in its dimensions. Cyndi's efforts to thrive are

similarly complex and multilayered. Shelter workers have offered Cyndi not only the primary care of shelter and access to education. Phoenix staff have also married these instrumental resources with access to mentors and emotional supports, formal counselling (if requested), and plans for family reunification (when appropriate). If youth like Cyndi attach to service, it is most likely because the service is by design intentionally structured to be multidimensional. As Phoenix has grown, their challenge has been to continue to integrate case management functions. Like the disparate services in the community at large, there tends to be a silo mentality among service providers who are mandated to provide for youth like Cyndi. The schools may try to speak to social services about housing, but their role in these negotiations is vague and the linkages are only informal. Phoenix, by bringing a number of services together, provides a seamless emergency response to youth at risk. The problem, however, becomes one of reintegrating these youth back into mainstream services. Youth workers must create continuity with a youth's care providers by partnering with them and other agencies that will follow youth after Phoenix's involvement ends. Recent efforts at the level of local administrators to coordinate services for the most vulnerable youth in the Halifax community are addressing this problem.

*The study of resilience shifts our focus to the strengths of individuals and communities.*

The study of resilience helped to move researchers away from examining psychological distress and related problems among populations under stress. It opened the possibility of studying strengths, and of designing programs that build capacity rather than addressing risk (Chazin, Kaplan, & Terio, 2000; Norman, 2000). However, this capacity to cope is contextually referent. What is taken to be adaptive in one context may be maladaptive in another, a fact that perplexes refugees, survivors of sexual abuse, and anyone else who has learned to cope under adverse circumstances. Patterns of violence, dissociation, mistrust, and even suicidality may be symbolic of adaptive behaviours to survive when living under difficult circumstances. Seen in context, even problem behaviours may demonstrate the plasticity (Lerner, Alberts, Anderson, & Dowling, 2006) required of individuals who have few, if any, options. For example, Jobin and Mandeville (2005), like other positive psychologists concerned with aspects of coping, argue that when we hit either a crisis or period of discontent, even suicide may be used as a problem-solving strategy. Taken out of context, and viewed only through the lens of psychopathology, such behaviour is seldom understood as a solution to a situation in which no other resolution appears possible. Frequently, when their lives are decontextualized, children and youth may be seen as maladaptive in their behaviour rather than well adjusted to the demands placed upon them. The more disordered their environments, the more likely children are to accommodate themselves to that disorder with antisocial behaviours. Research with youth in gangs, for example, has demonstrated this trend. Gang behaviour is not always emblematic of a desire to be bad, but is more often a response to threats from others. In the case of immigrant and other youth who experience systemic prejudice because of race, ethnicity, or class, gang membership may actually resolve some of the tensions caused by their marginalization (Solis, 2003).

Resilience researchers, notably Rutter (1987), have named several clusters of protective processes evident in the actions of children who develop well. These include processes that reduce the impact of risk on a child (as in when a perceived danger like foster placement is made to seem less frightening); reducing negative chain reactions such that one problem, like time spent on the street, doesn't lead to other problems, like addiction or risky sexual behaviour; improving self-esteem and self-efficacy, or the ability to like one's self and change one's world; and opening up opportunities, as when the student who leaves school takes advantage of alternative educational pathways. If one thinks of making practice intentional (guided by theory) then promoting each of these four protective processes becomes crucial to positive development. Arguably, for Cyndi and others like her, experience with Phoenix provides opportunities for each of these four processes to occur.

*Research on resilience shows that multifinality, or many routes to many good ends, is characteristic of populations of children who succeed.*

Our tendency as those intervening with at-risk children and families might be to acknowledge many paths to the same ends. However, in practice we tend to ignore the evidence that children demonstrate a great deal of difference in how they define and experience success. For example, programs may seek to reintegrate youth who leave school through a variety of means such as the provision of alternative educational settings, individualized education plans, one-on-one workers, streaming, or even the fining of parents and forced education of children who otherwise resist intervention. What these efforts share in common is the goal of educating children in the formal system in the belief that education leads to future employment security. It is a difficult argument to refute. But it is not the only argument. If we were to broaden our perspective to another context, such as Tanzania, or Nepal, we would find evidence that education may be valued almost universally, but that it is seen as less practical for some of the most vulnerable children to pursue. In Tanzania, for example, where fewer than 50% of girls advance past grade 6, families may emphasize entrepreneurship as an alternative (Gupta & Mahy, 2003). In Nepal, child labourers are more likely to attend school when they can continue to work half-days (International Union of Anthropological and Ethnological Sciences, 2002). Similarly, in Canada, we might explore the need for less academic solutions to children who leave school early. Vocational apprenticeships are thankfully gaining greater popularity, with some recognition that not every student needs to complete his or her formal education inside the school system. In all three cases, careful collection of children's own accounts of their experiences show that there are many manifestations of resilience, and many paths to achieving the well-being associated with resilience. To argue for a single set of outcomes is culturally naive.

Other research supports this same multifinality. A study from Israel shows that when children are exposed to trauma associated with war and conflict they may increase their risk-taking behaviour as a way to cope (Pat-Horenczyk, Doppelt, Meiron, Baum, & Brom, 2004). The study's authors speculate that even though this adaptive behaviour places children at greater risk of harm, it may in fact help them to confront the stress they experience, alleviating symptoms of distress. The children labelled clinically depressed following exposure to trauma were those who were the least likely to take risks. The question such findings raise is whether it is better to adapt to stress by taking risks or becoming depressed. The findings suggest that both are adaptive strategies. Both make use of the resources at hand to self-soothe and deal with the after-effects of exposure to the conditions of war. Can we, therefore, really say that one is any better than the other?

Though Phoenix holds to specific objectives, recent innovation in its programming has resulted in a more narrative approach to intervention, in which greater emphasis is being placed on each youth's own construction of successful development (see Ungar, 2004). Dangerous and delinquent behaviours are discussed as part of adaptive stories of personal survival that may not have achieved conventional expressions of success, like attachment to school or employment. This approach fits well with harm-reduction models now gaining popularity in the fields of addictions and suicide prevention.

*The study of resilience has shown that a focus on social justice is foundational to successful development.*

Each of the above three points emphasizes the need for young people to participate in the design of interventions meant for them. Making complex multilevel interventions responsive, ensuring the strengths a child values are given space for expression, and respecting the divergent paths to well-being children may follow, are aspects of programming congruent with a concern for children's rights (Chan, Carlson, Trickett, & Earls, 2003). In a number of international contexts, the rights of the child to supportive and healthy physical and social ecologies are understood as important contributors to children's well-being (McAdam-Crisp, 2004). At the level of individual service, such as that provided by Phoenix to youth like Cyndi, social justice means maintaining the young person's voice in the process of service. Interventions that help children achieve resilience are more likely to succeed when this voice is present, a point demonstrated well by Hjörne (2005) in regard to negotiations concerning a child's identity as a 'problem' child in a public school in Sweden. Hjörne spent two years examining the way in which parents and schools negotiate a child's identity as a child with Attention Deficit Hyperactivity Disorder (ADHD). She notes that the labelling process and negotiation for control of labels are not neutral: 'A critical element in this process is that the institutional representatives determine the allocation of services and resources through their categorizing practices. And this has profound implications for the individual and the organization' (p. 490). In other words, the process of negotiating identity brings with it concretely the provision of resources necessary to ensure a child succeeds. This is more than a case of good or bad case management. There are fundamental issues of rights and 'voice' lurking within these negotiations, and their outcomes concern appropriate response to a child in need. What Hjörne shows is that within people-processing organizations 'diverse arguments and accounts are used by the participants when negotiating meaning and providing explanations' (p. 492). In these negotiations, very different agendas can be represented. The schools will provide service that fits with their view of the child, in this case a boy named William. The diagnosis of ADHD is, however, a double-edged sword for educators. On the one hand it can be used to coerce parents into medicating the child to make him more manageable in the classroom. On the other hand, it can obligate the school to provide expensive services. Meanwhile, the child's parents seek to maintain their child in the everyday world of their community and with a definition of normal, making it likely they resist the label of ADHD. Needless to say, the school wins, but only after making the rather vacuous promise to 'still "see William as William"' (p. 503). In this example we can see that services shape outcomes for children, with the definition of both a child's problems and strengths the result of negotiations that determine how a child's behaviour is understood and responded to.

While the term 'social justice' conjures up images of macro-level interventions to address social inequities, a social justice perspective may also inform interventions that create opportunities for resilience to be realized. In William's case, as in Cyndi's, the provision of resources that fit the child and his or her family's definition of the problem is an issue of equity and access to justice. Arguably, interventions that are top down, unaccountable to those served, and inflexible are less likely to develop the conditions necessary for resilience to manifest.

*Resilience research focuses on cultural and contextual heterogeneity related to children's thriving.*

What we now know about resilience is beginning to inform a rich tapestry of interventions that must be tailored to the specific cultures and contexts in which they are used. Thus, the benchmarks associated with success are no longer fixed, but fluid (see McGoldrick, 2003; Ungar, in press). Culture and context (the community's geographic location, the economic status of the child's family, the level of safety in the child's family, school, or community) will influence the quality of the indicators of success the child and his or her family seek to attain.

For example, a streetfront coffee shop in Toronto, the Ground Level Café, provides street youth with employment and training to help them migrate from the street. Such an initiative makes sense in a community populated with Starbucks and its competitors. It makes less sense in Digby Neck, Nova Scotia, or Hudson's Bay, Saskatchewan, where the coffee shop itself would become the one and only employer of barristas. In an edited volume of international examples of resilience promotion strategies, contributors from around the world showed how interventions need to be tailored to the requirements of local populations, helping individuals set personal development goals that are relevant to a community's definition of resilience (Ungar, 2005).

Such initiatives show that children and youth at risk thrive in ways that make sense to them and their communities. Furthermore, the antecedents of that success are found across a community and reflect how well people's complex needs are met. An interesting illustration of this comes from Lalonde's (2006) study of 196 First Nations communities in British Columbia. Lalonde found that a small number of community factors, such as women in local government, a dedicated space for cultural events, and a fire hall, could distinguish communities who have experienced both high and low rates of youth suicide from those which have not had any episodes over a fourteen-year period. In summarizing his findings Lalonde argues for an understanding of successful growth that takes into account the individual in context:

> The surprising outcomes – the transcendence – are not found in the single 'hardy' or 'invulnerable' child who manages to rise above adversity, but in the existence of whole communities that demonstrate the power of culture as a protective factor. When communities succeed in promoting their cultural heritage and in securing control of their own collective future – in claiming ownership over their past and future – the positive effects reverberate across many measures of youth health and well-being. Suicide rates fall, fewer children are taken into care, school completion rates rise, and rates of intentional and unintentional injury decrease. (p. 67)

Lalonde's work could erroneously lead to the assumption that a single model of community organization (one that promotes cultural adherence and pride of place) always predicts better mental health outcomes for youth under stress. However, culture will only affect youth if cultural adherence is meaningful to children in their particular context. It is doubtful, for example, that Cyndi, a white youth living in a predominantly white urban environment, considers her whiteness as a cultural force in her life. The presence of a fire hall or space for cultural events is far less likely to be significantly correlated with her negative or positive outcomes. It is not that Cyndi doesn't have a culture: it is that her culture, as the dominant culture, is invisible in its ubiquity. It would be just as problematic to assume that all individuals from cultural minorities would necessarily view cultural adherence as positive. While in the case of British Columbia's First Nations communities, the broad trend is to link resilience and culture, this is not always the case.

One can see this distinction among participants in a research project carried out by the Aspen Family and Community Network Society in Alberta. The Youth Matters Multicultural Project sought to examine issues of access to services for Calgary youth from different minority cultural backgrounds (Taylor, 2005). Documenting the stories of youth, they found that young people are far from homogeneous even if they are from the same ethnic or racial minority group: 'It is important to note that immigrant youth do not place a common value on their cultural heritage. Some express a distance from what they consider their parents' culture, while others have a great deal of pride in their diverse background and see it as a benefit in their lives. This challenges adults working with immigrant or visible minority youth to be sensitive to this variation' (p. 22). In understanding resilience as related to cultural adherence, we need also to be open to culture being resisted, or rejected, and an alternate culture being adopted as a pathway to successful development.

### Interventions as Expressions of the Five Principles

Throughout this volume there are many examples of interventions that focus on one or more of the five principles discussed here. In the chapters that follow, the authors detail research relevant to practice and interventions with at-risk children and youth that helps them to find structural solutions leading to personal growth and healthy development. These interventions tend to exemplify the five principles in action. All show the promise of being ecological in their focus, affecting more than just the individual child. All appear by their design to be attuned to the complexity involved in nurturing and maintaining resilience. All are strengths based, building on capacities of individuals and their communities. A great many focus on changing the meaning attached to the behaviours of youth, and in the process appreciating their definitions of successful development (the multifinality of their ways of manifesting resilience). Many others seek, like Phoenix, to represent the concerns of youth and uphold principles of social justice. Finally, all are in one way or another sensitive to the culture and context in which they are implemented.

With the bringing together of such a diverse collection of papers, there is cause to be optimistic that a focus on successful outcomes is seeding a new generation of interventions. There was a time not long ago when interventions were exclusively focused on combating disorder. The shift to building resilience at the level of both individuals and communities is more than just semantic. When we study resilience and design interventions to build strengths, we are challenging funders to finance interventions that reflect what we know is already helping children thrive. The five principles discussed in this chapter are meant to guide the design of these interventions. If they work, it is because they are grounded in the experiences of those young people already demonstrating resilience, even when that resilience is hidden behind problem behaviours that are chosen in resource-challenged environments.

## REFERENCES

Barber, J.G. (2006). A synthesis of research findings and practice and policy suggestions for promoting resilient development among young people in crisis. In R.J. Flynn, P.M. Dudding, & J.G. Barber (Eds.), *Promoting resilience in child welfare* (pp. 418–29). Ottawa: University of Ottawa Press.

Benson, P.L. (2003). Developmental assets and asset-building community: Conceptual and empirical foundations. In R.M. Lerner & P.L. Benson (Eds.), *Developmental assets and asset-building communities: Implications for research, policy, and practice* (pp. 19–46). New York: Kluwer Academic/Plenum.

Blackstock, C., & Trocmé, N. (2005). Community-based child welfare for aboriginal children: Supporting resilience through structural change. In M. Ungar (Ed.), *Handbook for working with children and youth: Pathways to resilience across cultures and contexts* (pp. 105–20). Thousand Oaks, CA: Sage.

Boyden, J., & Mann, G. (2005). Children's risk, resilience, and coping in extreme situations. In M. Ungar (Ed.), *Handbook for working with children and youth: Pathways to resilience across cultures and contexts* (pp. 3–26). Thousand Oaks, CA: Sage.

Bronfenbrenner, U. (1979). *The ecology of human development: Experiments by nature and design.* Cambridge, MA: Harvard University Press.

Chan, B., Carlson, M., Trickett, B., & Earls, F. (2003). Youth participation: A critical element of research on child well-being. In R.M. Lerner & P.L. Benson (Eds.), *Developmental assets and asset-building communities: Implications for research, policy, and practice* (pp. 65–96). New York: Kluwer Academic/Plenum.

Chazin, R., Kaplan, S., & Terio, S. (2000). Introducing a strengths/resiliency model in mental health organizations. In E. Norman (Ed.), *Resiliency enhancement: Putting the strengths perspective into social work practice* (pp. 192–210). New York: Colombia University Press.

Crawford, E., Wright, M.O., & Masten, A. (2005). Resilience and spirituality in youth. In E.C. Roehlkepartain, P.E. King, L. Wagener, & P.L. Benson (Eds.), *The handbook of spiritual development in childhood and adolescence* (pp. 355–70). Thousand Oaks, CA: Sage.

Dei, G.J.S., Massuca, J., McIsaac, E., & Zine, J. (1997). *Reconstructing 'drop-out': A critical ethnography of the dynamics of black students' disengagement from school.* Toronto: University of Toronto Press.

Greene, S.M., Anderson, E.R., Hetherington, E.M., Forgatch, M.S., & DeGarmo, D.S. (2003). Risk and resilience after divorce. In F. Walsh (Ed.), *Normal family processes* (3rd ed., pp. 96–120). New York: Guilford.

Gupta, N., & Mahy, M. (2003). Adolescent childbearing in sub-Saharan Africa: Can increased schooling alone raise ages at first birth? *Demographic Research, 8*(4). (Available online http://www.demographic-research.org).

Hjörne, E. (2005). Negotiating the 'problem-child' in school: Child identity, parenting and institutional agendas. *Qualitative Social Work, 4*(4), 489–507.

International Union of Anthropological and Ethnological Sciences. (2002). *Studies of integrated holistic programmes with children and youth: Child labour in Nepal.* New York: IUAES.

Jobin, S., & Mandeville, L. (2005). Une vision positive du precessus suicidaire: Pour comprendre et intervenir différemment. *Revue Québécoise de Psychologie, 26*(1), 111–30.

Kirby, L.D., & Fraser, M.W. (1997). Risk and resilience in childhood. In M. Fraser (Ed.), *Risk and resilience in childhood: An ecological perspective* (pp. 10–33). Washington, DC: NASW Press.

Lalonde, C.E. (2006). Identity formation and cultural resilience in aboriginal communities. In R.J. Flynn, P.M. Dudding, & J.G. Barber (Eds.), *Promoting resilience in child welfare* (pp. 52–71). Ottawa: University of Ottawa Press.

Leadbeater, B., Dodgen, D., & Solarz, A. (2005). The resilience revolution: A paradigm shift for research and policy. In R.D. Peters, B. Leadbeater, & R.J. McMahon (Eds.), *Resilience in children, families, and communities: Linking context to practice and policy* (pp. 47–63). New York: Kluwer.

Lerner, R.M., Alberts, A.E., Anderson, P.M., & Dowling, E.M. (2006). On making humans human: Spirituality and the promotion of positive youth development. In E.C. Roehlkepartain, P.E. King, L. Wagener, & P.L. Benson (Eds.), *The handbook of spiritual development in childhood and adolescence* (pp. 60–72). Thousand Oaks, CA: Sage.

Lerner, R.M., Brentano, C., Dowling, E.M., & Anderson, P.M. (2002). Postive youth development: Thriving as the basis of personhood and civil society. In R.M. Lerner, C.S. Taylor, & A. Von Eye (Eds.), *Pathways to positive development among diverse youth* (pp. 11–34). New York: Jossey-Bass.

McAdam-Crisp, J. (2004). Cross-cultural research with children: A relationship of integrity. *Relational Child and Youth Care Practice, 17*(3), 47-54.

McGoldrick, M. (2003). Culture: A challenge to concepts of normality. In F. Walsh (Ed.), *Normal family processes* (3rd ed., pp. 61–95). New York: Guilford.

Norman, E. (2000). Introduction: The strengths perspective and resiliency enhancement – A natural partnership. In E. Norman (Ed.), *Resiliency enhancement: Putting the strengths perspective into social work practice* (pp. 1–16). New York: Colombia University Press.

Pat-Horenczyk, R., Doppelt, O., Meiron, T., Baum, N., & Brom, D. (2004, November). *Risk-taking behaviors in Israeli adolescents living under the continuous threat of terrorism.* Paper presented at the ISTSS Annual Meeting, New Orleans, LA.

Phelps, E., Balsano, A.B., Fay, K., Peltz, J.S., Zimmerman, S.M., Lerner, R.M., & Lerner, J.V. (2007). Nuances in early adolescent developmental trajectories of positive and of problematic/risk behaviors: Findings from the 4-H study of positive youth development. *Child and Adolescent Psychiatric Clinics of North America, 16*(2), 473–96.

Rutter, M. (1987). Psychosocial resilience and protective mechanisms. *American Journal of Orthopsychiatry, 57,* 316-31.

Rutter, M. (2005). Environmentally mediated risks for pyschopathology: Research strategies and findings. *Journal of the American Academy of Child and Adolescent Psychiatry, 44*(1), 3–18.

Seccombe, K. (2002). 'Beating the odds' versus 'Changing the odds': Poverty, resilience, and family policy. *Journal of Marriage and Family, 64*(2), 384–94.

Solis, J. (2003). Re-thinking illegality as a violence *against*, not *by* Mexican immigrants, children, and youth. *Journal of Social Issues, 59*(1), 15–33.

Stivers, E., & Wheelan, S. (Eds.). (1986). *The Lewin legacy: Field theory in current practice.* New York: Springer-Verlag.

Taylor, C. (2005). *All kids have dreams: Immigrant youth in Greater Forest Lawn.* Calgary: Aspen Family & Community Network Society.

Ungar, M. (2004). A constructionist discourse on resilience: Multiple contexts, multiple realities among at-risk children and youth. *Youth and Society,* *35*(3), 341–65.

Ungar, M. (2005). Introduction: Resilience across cultures and contexts. In M. Ungar (Ed.), *Handbook for working with children and youth: Pathways to resilience across cultures and contexts* (pp. xv–xxxix). Thousand Oaks, CA: Sage.

Ungar, M. (in press). Resilience across cultures. *British Journal of Social Work.*

Ungar, M., & Teram, E. (2000). Drifting towards mental health: High-risk adolescents and the process of empowerment. *Youth and Society 32*(2), 228–52.

Werner, E.E., & Smith, R.S. (2001). *Journeys from childhood to midlife: Risk, resilience, and recovery.* Ithaca, NY: Cornell University Press.

Wolkow, K.E., & Ferguson, H.B. (2001). Community factors in the development of resiliency: Considerations and future directions. *Community Mental Health Journal, 37*(6), 489–98.

Wyman, P.A. (2003). Emerging perspectives on context specificity of children's adaptation and resilience: Evidence from a decade of research with urban children in adversity. In S.S. Luthar (Ed.), *Resilience and vulnerability: Adaptation in the context of childhood adversities* (pp. 293–317). Cambridge: Cambridge University Press.

# PART ONE

## Promoting Individual Well-Being

# 2 Understanding Adolescent Self-Injury from a Resilience Perspective: A Model for International Interpretation

NANCY L. HEATH, JESSICA R. TOSTE, AND LANA C. ZINCK

Self-injury (SI) is a growing concern amongst professionals working with youth. Some would even argue that it is the epidemic of the new millennium (Shaw, 2002; Zila & Kiselica, 2001). Increased media attention has raised awareness about this behaviour and its occurrence amongst adolescents; however, misconceptions regarding the correlates and function of SI persist in the general public. These misconceptions may affect the level of support provided to youth who engage in this behaviour. Our purpose is to reconceptualize self-injurious behaviour to be consistent with a resilience perspective. This will result in a more sensitive and comprehensive understanding of self-injurious behaviour among the global community of youth.

In this chapter, we provide knowledge about SI, including the definition, risk factors, prevalence, and function of the behaviour in a North American context. We then present an argument for understanding self-injurious behaviour within a resilience perspective, forming the foundation of a model for international interpretation. It is important that professionals working with youth invoke a more critical framework for the understanding of behaviours that often elicit strong negative reactions, such as SI. This chapter will therefore develop a framework for use in working with youth who self-injure that has the potential to be extrapolated to other negatively perceived behaviours. Through the development of a more complex understanding of SI one may gain a theoretically sound, culturally respectful approach to the evaluation and planning required for working with youth who self-injure.

## Resilience Theory

Resilience refers to a dynamic, developmental process involving positive adjustment in the face of significant adversity (Luthar, Cicchetti, & Becker, 2000). Two conditions are central to this definition: (1) exposure to considerable threat or adversity, and (2) the achievement of positive adaptation in spite of major assaults on one's development (Garmezy, 1990; Luthar & Zigler, 1991). 'Resilient' individuals are able to use internal and external resources to achieve age-appropriate developmental expectations (Cicchetti & Schneider-Rosen, 1986; Luthar et al., 2000; Masten & Coatsworth, 1998; Sroufe & Rutter, 1984; Waters & Sroufe, 1983). These resources are typically characterized as protective factors because they are consistently associated with positive functioning, despite significant adversity. Specifically, researchers have identified three primary factors implicated in the development of resilience in youth: the individual's interpersonal qualities, aspects of their families, and characteristics of their broader social environment (Masten & Garmezy, 1985; Werner & Smith, 1992).

Historically, researchers have relied on the absence of psychopathology or maladaptive behaviour as an indication of resilience in an individual exposed to extreme stress (Luthar & Zigler, 1991). Increasingly, though, researchers are looking at defining resilience in terms of competence demonstrated in multiple dimensions of life (Gerber, Ginsberg, & Reiff, 1992). The importance of utilizing multidimensional assessment measures is highlighted by studies of individuals who demonstrate competence in some domains but show difficulties in others. For example, in a study of inner-city ninth-grade students, Luthar (1991) determined that children identified as resilient were significantly more depressed and anxious than were competent children from less stressful environments. These findings suggest that resilience may be domain specific (Luthar, 1991, 1995) and emphasize the importance of distinguishing between adaptive behaviour and emotional health in studying positive adjustment (Luthar & Zigler, 1991).

Following on this, and as this chapter will demonstrate, SI is not necessarily a manifestation of severe psychopathology, but instead may signal otherwise resilient functioning. Indeed, to some, SI is considered the 'anti-suicide' because youth at high risk (e.g., those who are abused or homeless) report using SI to express overwhelmingly painful emotions (Favazza, 1987; Simpson, 1976). In this way, SI may be interpreted as a maladaptive coping mechanism in that it allows youth to express and, thereby, manage their pain. Walsh (2006) supports this notion in asserting that more concern is warranted when these youth cease to engage in self-injurious behaviours. If SI is used as a means of coping with overwhelming emotion, then prematurely eliminating these behaviours takes away the only known coping mechanism for these youth. This is an especially important point for those in the helping professions, who may perceive SI as a sign of serious psychological disturbance. For youth at high risk, however, SI may be a protective factor working to alleviate severe emotional distress.

## Definition of Self-Injury

SI is a low-lethality behaviour that involves the deliberate destruction of body tissue without suicidal intent (Favazza, 1989; Haines & Williams, 2003). Self-injurious acts include skin cutting (which is most common), skin burning, self-hitting, pinching, scratching, biting, and hair pulling (Gratz, 2003; Ross & Heath, 2002). SI does not include socially or group-sanctioned tissue damage such as tattooing, piercing, or ritual tissue mutilation. Self-injurious behaviour can be categorized along two dimensions. The first is severity based on degree of tissue destruction. Individuals may engage in major acts of SI (e.g., limb amputation and castration) or, more commonly, superficial forms of tissue damage (Favazza, 1998). A second dimension on which to evaluate self-injurious behaviour is frequency, ranging from occasional (or episodic) to repetitive SI. In recent years, researchers have found that some youth engage in self-injurious behaviour less frequently, and have termed this *occasional SI*. Skin cutting and burning are the most common forms of occasional SI (Favazza, 1998). An individual is considered a *repetitive self-injurer* when there is an overwhelming preoccupation with the behaviour. Favazza and Rosenthal (1993) define repetitive self-injurious behaviour as:

'(a) preoccupation with harming oneself, (b) recurrent failure to resist impulses to harm oneself physically, resulting in the destruction or alteration of body tissue, (c) increasing sense of tension immediately before the act of self-harm, (d) gratification or a sense of relief when committing the act of self-harm, and (e) the act of self-harm is not associated with conscious suicidal intent and is not in response to delusion or hallucination.' (p. 138)

The focus of our research includes the full range of frequency from occasional to repetitive, but is limited to superficial acts of self-injurious behaviour.

## Risk Factors and Correlates of Self-Injury

Much of the literature examining self-injurious behaviour in youth and young adults focuses on the potential risk factors or correlates. Two primary areas of risk have been documented: the first centres on clinical diagnoses that are associated with SI, and the second explores the role of childhood trauma or family dysfunction.

Historically, the discussion and understanding of SI has been the province of psychiatry. This behaviour was believed to occur almost exclusively in individuals with severe psychiatric pathology (Dulit, Fryer, Leon, Brodsky, & Frances, 1994; Griffin, Williams, & Stark, 1985) and was often associated with personality disorders (Zlotnick, Mattia, & Zimmerman, 1999). Nearly one-quarter of individuals who receive a diagnosis of a general personality disorder also report engaging in self-injurious behaviour (Favazza, 1987). For individuals with the specific diagnosis of borderline personality disorder (BPD), the percentage increases substantially (Gerson & Stanley, 2002; Paris, 2005; Zlotnick et al., 1999). However, this literature needs be interpreted with caution, as the presence of SI is frequently presumed to be indicative of BPD (Paris, 2005), which is not always the case. Additionally, self-injurious behaviour has been thought to co-occur with depression, post-traumatic stress disorders (Coons & Milstein, 1990; Greenspan & Samuel, 1989; Pitman, 1990), and eating disorders (Favaro & Santonastaso, 1998; Favazza, DeRosear, & Conterio, 1989; Garfinkel, Moldofsky, & Garner, 1980). Given a history of SI research focused on individuals who were already receiving psychiatric treatment, the occurrence of SI in these samples (which were largely composed of women) was interpreted as an indication that the self-injurious behaviour was pathological.

Recent research findings on SI in North American community samples indicate that the individuals engaging in self-injurious behaviour did not fit the traditional understanding of SI as symptomatic of underlying psychopathology. Instead, many of these individuals were using SI as a form of maladaptive coping (Favazza, 1998; Gratz, 2003; Ross & Heath, 2002, 2003). Youth who admitted to engaging in SI were functioning well in a high-school or university setting, and did not report clinical levels of depression, eating disorders, or anxiety. In fact, none of the sample had received a psychiatric diagnosis. Furthermore, they did not report child abuse or attachment issues (Heath, Toste, Nedecheva, & Charlebóis, 2008; Ross, 2004; Ross & Heath, 2002, 2003). Interestingly, in the absence of the traditional risk factors or correlates, participants from community samples who engaged in SI still reported difficulties with regulation of emotion (Heath et al., 2008). Such research findings support Favazza's (1987) conceptualization of SI as a 'morbid act of self-help,' indicating that SI serves to regulate over-whelming emotions. This suggests that self-injurious behaviour is not necessarily pathological, but represents a form of coping.

Although much of the literature on the correlates of, or risk factors for, SI has been drawn from clinical samples and thus must be interpreted carefully, there is a clear indication that individuals who self-injure typically have dysfunctional family histories. For example, Van der Kolk, Perry, and Herman (1991), in their study of young adults receiving treatment in a mental health clinic, found that individuals who cut themselves were much more likely to have had disruptions of attachment than their non-cutting peers. In addition, prolonged separation from caregivers was related to continued cutting and other forms of SI in this sample. Indeed, research findings indicate that self-injurious behaviour is significantly associated with physical and emotional neglect, as well as intrafamilial chaos (Boudewyn & Liem, 1995; Favazza & Conterio, 1989). Specifically, survivors of childhood sexual abuse frequently report engaging in SI (Favazza & Conterio, 1988). In their examination of 438 college students' experiences with childhood sexual abuse, Boudewyn and Liem (1995) found that men and women who had been sexually abused engaged in significantly more acts of SI than those who had not been abused. However, it is important to note that the higher rate of SI cannot simply be interpreted to indicate that those who engage in this behaviour have dysfunctional families and clinical diagnoses. In the media and some clinical circles, the literature demonstrating that individuals with family dysfunction are likely to self-injure has been interpreted as: 'If Mary engages in SI, she probably suffered childhood sexual abuse.' However, the literature does not support this statement. We would need to study all individuals who self-injure, including community samples, to determine if there is a higher incidence of family dysfunction in those who engage in SI, compared to a group who does not. Interestingly, the few studies that have done this provide a different picture.

## Self-Injury in Community Samples

In North American contexts, the field of SI research has expanded beyond psychiatric samples both concretely – by studying community samples – and abstractly – by suggesting that this behaviour is not exclusively pathological but a form of morbid self-help. Favazza, one of the first researchers to suggest that SI is not limited to psychiatric populations, has found that in community samples, 14% of young adults admitted to engaging in self-injurious behaviour (Favazza, 1989). More recent studies conducted in high schools have confirmed the prevalence rate of 14%. For example, in a study of a non-clinical sample of 440 adolescents in grades 7 to 11 (M = 14.5 years), approximately 20% indicated that they had hurt themselves on purpose at least once. Follow-up interviews indicated that 13.9% had self-injured at least once, with significantly more girls than boys reporting SI (Ross & Heath, 2002, 2003). Furthermore, Gratz (2001) found that 35% of university students reported engaging in self-injurious behaviour at least once in their lives, with 10% of this sample self-injuring habitually. It is important to note that Gratz recruited students 'interested in doing a study of SI' and thus probably had a selection bias. Nevertheless, researchers in the field suggest that these results are indicative of the increasing prevalence of SI within North America and Britain (Best, 2006; Lieberman, 2004; Walsh, 2006).

Unfortunately, there are very few investigations of SI within community samples outside of North America, although we know that self-injurious behaviour is not restricted to this continent (Yuri, 2005; Zoroglu et al., 2003). There is some limited research suggesting that SI is present in other cultures, but the paucity of literature makes it difficult to determine specific prevalence rates. In addition, methodological differences, including varying definitions of SI, further complicate the challenge of establishing prevalence estimates. Zoroglu et al. (2003) are among the few researchers who examined the prevalence of self-injurious behaviour within a community sample of adolescents outside of North America. Amongst a sample of Turkish high-school students, SI was reported at a rate of 21%.

Although self-injurious behaviour has been documented across cultures, the reasons for its occurrence within each culture are distinct. The meaning and interpretation of SI across cultures will be discussed in greater detail at a later point in this chapter. Future research is, however, certainly needed to explore aspects of SI in adolescents in the international community.

## Self-Injury as Coping

As previously suggested, emotional regulation appears to be the most consistently identified motivation for SI. Specifically, self-injurious behaviour serves to regulate overwhelming feelings of tension, anger, and sadness or to assist in terminating dissociative symptoms (Heath et al., 2008; Himber, 1994; Nixon, Cloutier, & Aggarwal, 2002; Pipher, 1994; Van der Kolk et al., 1991). Typically, individuals engaging in self-injurious behaviour are unable to identify the emotion they are feeling, but rather state that the emotion or tension is unbearable (Heath et al., 2008; Nock & Prinstein, 2004). Recently, Chapman, Gratz, and Brown (2006) proposed a model for conceptualizing SI as a behaviour 'that leads to the reduction or elimination of unwanted emotional responses, particularly the physiological aspects of the emotional response' (p. 379).

The use of SI as an affect regulator is supported by research in both at-risk, clinical samples and in more normative community samples. For example, samples of at-risk individuals such as those who have been victims of rape (Greenspan & Samuel, 1989), sexual or physical abuse (Briere & Gil, 1998; De Young, 1982; Shapiro, 1987; Van der Kolk et al., 1991; Wise, 1989), and homelessness (Tyler, Whitbeck, Hoyt, & Johnson, 2003) all report using SI to control overwhelming affect. Clinically, researchers examining SI in patients with BPD have found that SI is used to obtain relief from overwhelming negative moods and mental anguish, or to end a dissociative state. When used in response to a dissociative state, individuals report that SI serves to 'ground them,' to bring them psychologically back to their body, and terminate the dissociative state (Zlotnick et al., 1999; Zweig-Frank, Paris, & Guzder, 1994).

Researchers have reached similar conclusions with non-clinical samples. For example, Ross and Heath (2002) describe how, in a community-based sample of adolescents who self-injure, a stressful event is often followed by the use of SI to reduce the individual's depressed, anxious, or angry state. Similarly, in a recent study of university undergraduates, Heath et al. (2008) found no significant differences between students who self-injure and those who do not regarding risk factors such as childhood trauma, including abuse and insecure attachment. However, there was a significant difference on a measure assessing their ability to regulate emotions. Specifically, those who engaged in SI endorsed the following statements on the Difficulties in Emotion Regulation Scale (DERS [Gratz & Roemer, 2004]): 'I have difficulty making sense of my feelings'; 'When I'm upset, I feel out of control'; 'When I'm upset, it takes me a long time to feel better'; and 'When I'm upset, I have difficulty thinking about anything else.'

In light of the new perspective on SI as a form of coping, self-injurious behaviour is no longer considered a direct indication of severe underlying psychopathology. In fact, it has been suggested that there are two unique groups of adolescents who self-injure. The first, a small group of youth who likely suffer from other psychological difficulties, may have experienced severe childhood trauma and may engage in self-injurious behaviour more habitually over longer periods of time. The second, larger group, has only recently been discovered. These youth do not possess the traditional set of risk factors associated with SI in that they are functioning adaptively in other domains, and their reliance on self-injurious behaviour is transient rather than long standing (Heath et al., 2008; Paris, 2005). Currently, the existence of these two groups is largely a matter of conjecture; future research will serve to delineate more clearly these two groups for practitioners. In the interim, we may speculate that while SI is currently construed as a maladaptive coping mechanism to regulate emotion, the reliance on self-injurious behaviour does not necessarily signal a breakdown of resilience. On the contrary, SI may function to preserve adaptive functioning by helping youth control overwhelming negative emotions. By engaging in SI, youth may be using the strategies to which they have access to maintain functional mental health. This notion is further reflected by the term 'anti-suicide,' which has been used as an alternative to 'self-injury' (Simpson, 1976). The fact that a number of recent studies examining SI have been conducted with university undergraduate students attests to this notion; even within this 'high-achieving' sample, a high rate of self-injurious behaviour (11–35%) has been found (Gratz & Roemer, 2004; Heath et al., 2008).

**The Resilience Model**

The fact that North American youth in both clinical and community samples are engaging in SI shows clearly that such behaviour is not necessarily a predictor of poor overall adjustment. In order to work effectively with youth who self-injure, we need a more comprehensive understanding of this negatively perceived behaviour. To this end, we have developed a model that takes into consideration several key variables, with the goal of understanding self-injurious behaviour within a resilience framework. It is important to note that this model does not assume that all SI is a form of resilience but, rather, encourages consideration of this possibility for particular individuals within certain contexts.

*Factors in the Model*

Understanding adolescent SI within an international resilience perspective involves several critical considerations (see Figure 1). The first of these is the *meaning* of the behaviour for the individual, that is, the personal reasons for engaging in SI. The second consideration is the *interpretation* of the behaviour by the larger community, which refers to how the behaviour is understood by society. The third consideration is *time*. Time plays an instrumental role in bringing about societal, political, and economic changes that have the potential to affect both the meaning of the behaviour for individuals and the interpretation of the behaviour by the community. Neither meaning nor interpretation is static. Over time the meaning of behaviour may change for an individual, while the societal interpretation of the behaviour stays the same. Alternatively, the meaning of behaviour may remain consistent while the societal interpretation changes.

There are several unique features to this model, the first of which is that a clear distinction is drawn between meaning, or why an individual engages in self-injurious behaviour, and interpretation, or how this behaviour is understood by the larger community – although one clearly affects the other. The fact that meaning and interpretation are not synonymous concepts suggests a possibility for conflict, which has important implications for how professionals work with youth who engage in SI. Second, the model allows for an assessment of change in the meaning–interpretation dynamic as a function of the historical period (time). A third unique feature is the notion that SI may be perceived as a factor associated with resilient, as opposed to disturbed, functioning.

Figure 1:  Model for understanding of self-injurious behaviour

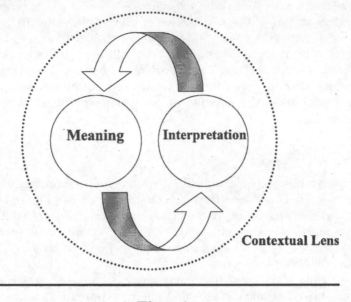

⇐ **Time** ⇒

## Implementation of the Resilience Model

*Contextual Lens*

The role of context is critical in gaining a more complete and accurate understanding of self-injurious behaviour. In this model, context represents the 'lens' through which we view the meaning and interpretation of SI across time. We will provide an overview of self-injurious behaviour in psychiatric, community, and prison settings, which will demonstrate the importance of the contextual lens in understanding the meaning and interpretation of SI. In each context, we will compare and contrast the meaning and interpretation of SI across different time frames.

*Psychiatric Samples*

In the context of psychiatric samples in North America, SI was historically (for at least thirty years) interpreted by the community as an indication of serious, underlying psychopathology. At that time, the meaning of SI for the individual appeared to be consistent with the interpretation, in that SI was almost exclusively found in association with severe psychopathology (Conterio & Lader, 1998; Favazza, 1987). Therefore, individuals engaged in SI as a manifestation of multiple psychiatric difficulties, and, as a result, research was primarily limited to inpatient psychiatric samples. To illustrate, Rosenthal, Rinzler, Walsh, and Edmund (1972) conducted a study of twenty-four individuals in an inpatient program who had a history of self-injurious behaviour. The researchers discovered that the majority of these individuals reported dissociative symptoms; half of the patients seemed to employ SI as a means of managing these symptoms. These patients described positive reactions in response to their cutting behaviour, and specifically at the sight of blood: 'They spoke of being "happy" at the blood, happy to see it, being fascinated by it' (p. 50). The majority of these patients no longer felt depersonalized or dissociated after the act of SI.

However, currently, the interpretation of SI in psychiatric samples appears to be in flux. Recent studies of adolescents in psychiatric inpatient samples have reported a general prevalence of SI ranging from 40% to 82.4% (Darche, 1990; DiClemente, Ponton, & Hartley, 1991; Nock & Prinstein, 2005). The rising prevalence of SI in inpatient settings is partly responsible for the changing attitudes towards SI in the psychiatric community. Specifically, self-injurious behaviour is not always being interpreted as severe psychopathology, but rather may be seen as a coping mechanism, a means of seeking assistance, or a corollary of BPD and other disorders (Nock & Prinstein, 2004, 2005; Paris, 2005). Currently, the meaning of self-injurious behaviour amongst psychiatric inpatient samples has broadened to encompass individuals who use SI to regulate emotions, as well as those who engage in SI as a manifestation of their psychological disturbance. For example, Nock and Prinstein found that 52.9% of their clinical sample of individuals who self-injure reported engaging in the behaviour to 'stop bad feelings' (2004, p. 888). Thus, a change in interpretation and meaning has occurred, but until the interpretation within this context solidifies, conflict will continue in our view of SI.

*Community Samples of Youth*

Within more normative community samples of North American youth, researchers are finding that the use of SI (i.e., meaning) has changed dramatically over the last twenty years (Gratz, 2003; Heath et al., 2008). Earlier community samples of youth who engaged in SI were thought to be doing so as a manifestation of severe underlying psychological disturbance. This interpretation was congruent with meaning, as SI was understood to be a reflection of mental health issues. In contrast, the meaning of self-injurious behaviour for current community samples of youth is no longer restricted to a manifestation of psychopathology, but has broadened to include emotion regulation. Despite this change in meaning, the present interpretation of SI in the community remains largely static. For example, many people in the general public, as well as some professionals, continue to perceive SI as a sign of emotional or mental disturbance (Best, 2004; Heath, Beettam, & DeStefano, 2005; Heath, Toste, & Beettam, 2006; Simeon & Hollander, 2001). To illustrate, Best (2004) examined the attitudes of teachers in regard to self-injurious behaviour, and found that SI was not seen as a maladaptive coping mechanism, but rather a pathological behaviour. Best reports teachers' expressions of shock, repulsion, 'alarm and panic' (p. 168), and that they were 'freaked out.' Additionally, he noted that teachers believe there is a definite link between self-harm, mental instability, and attempted suicide.

Clearly, the meaning of SI has changed over time while the interpretation has remained generally static, and thus conflict between the two perspectives has grown. The increasing conflict between the individual perspective (meaning) and the societal-community perspective (interpretation) may interfere with support received by youth who self-injure. The stigma associated with self-injurious behaviour is born out of the perception that it is a sign of psychiatric disturbance. This creates barriers to working with these youth by preventing them from seeking assistance (Conterio & Lader, 1998), increasing their alienation, interfering with the establishment of rapport between youth worker and client, and limiting the availability of appropriate referral services (Derouin & Bravender, 2004; Heath et al., 2005; White Kress, Gibson, & Reynolds, 2004).

*Prison Samples*

A third context in which the model may be utilized is within prison settings, where SI is very common (Conterio & Lader, 1998; Favazza, 1987). In one correctional institution for girls, 86% of inmates carved their skin (Ross & McKay, 1979, in Favazza, 1987). The majority of incidents involved carving initials of parents or close female friends in order to demonstrate affection or anger, seal a pact, or seek attention from staff. Researchers studying SI in male correctional facilities (Johnson & Britt, 1967) found that it was typically used to obtain transfers to other institutions or cell blocks or to receive narcotics (under the guise of injury). Of particular interest is that in this context SI has a completely different and unique meaning or purpose from that in any of the previously discussed contexts. For the prison staff, the interpretation of the use of SI in both female and male samples is largely consistent with the meaning. Specifically, prison staff usually understand this behaviour as an attempt to regain control and obtain a desired social outcome (e.g., transfer, affection, narcotics) rather than satisfy an internal need (e.g., emotion regulation). In regard to the time frame within this setting, little current research has been done, and therefore we can only surmise that both the interpretation and meaning have not altered substantially.

### South Asian Women in the United Kingdom

The model may also be used to illustrate the changing meaning and interpretation of SI in a different cultural context, namely amongst the population of South Asian women living in the United Kingdom. In this case, both the meaning and interpretation of self-injurious behaviour have changed. Recent research indicates that South Asian women are employing SI as a means of coping with cultural conflict (Thompson & Dinesh, 2000). Thompson and Dinesh argue that South Asian women, specifically adolescents, who have immigrated to the UK are using SI as a response to the pressure to function independently of family. This pressure is in direct conflict with their culture. In traditional South Asian cultures, these young women are expected to maintain a communal interdependence. However, in Western societies, young South Asian women experience pressure to separate from family, in combination with the pressures of adolescence. Therefore, similar to the North American community sample context, the meaning of self-injurious behaviour for this group of women has changed. Dealing with the cultural conflict inherent in emigrating to a new country represents a new reason for these women to engage in SI.

The interpretation of this behaviour by British society has also shifted. In 1994, the Department of Health in London recommended that the act of SI be interpreted as a possible response to cultural con-

flict. Although the psychiatric community argues that this understanding is overly simplistic (Loshak, 2003), SI has become widely
accepted as a response to cultural conflict.

## Implications for Intervention

The resilience model facilitates a more sensitive understanding of self-
injurious behaviour by emphasizing the role that contextual factors,
such as culture, play in shaping meaning and interpretation. In
working with youth who self-injure, professionals may want to consider why youth in their particular community have historically used
SI (i.e., what is the meaning of SI?) and whether it has changed for
youth within that context. What are the historical and societal interpretations of self-injurious behaviour in specific communities or cultural contexts? Is there presently a disconnect, or conflict, between the
meaning or use of SI by youth in this context and the societal interpretation of this behaviour?

There are a number of implications of the resilience model for intervention with youth who self-injure. These include the possible consequences of a conflict between the meaning and interpretation of SI, as
well as the strategies practitioners employ for treatment. As illustrated
earlier, a disconnect between meaning and interpretation may result in
any one (or more) of the following:

- Clients having more difficulty revealing their self-injurious behaviour (Conterio & Lader, 1998) and the practitioner finding it more
  difficult to establish and maintain a positive working alliance with
  the client (Derouin & Bravender, 2004; Heath et al., 2005; White
  Kress et al., 2004): If there is a greater disconnect and the youth is
  hesitant to reveal his or her behaviour, more time must be devoted
  to active listening without judgment; it is recommended that practitioners demonstrate a matter-of-fact demeanour when confronted
  with the details of SI. However, one should not dwell on the
  details, but rather focus on the underlying function of the behaviour for the youth. Similarly, in order to encourage youth to come
  forward for support around the issue of SI, the worker must be
  known in the community for their non-judgmental, supportive
  approach around this issue. This is particularly difficult for
  workers in contexts where there is a significant conflict between
  meaning and interpretation.

- Clients feeling increased stress, isolation, and alienation (www.selfinjury.org): With a greater disconnect, the youth's sense of isolation is heightened. Therefore, it is important to help the youth connect in a healthy way with others who share similar concerns. Given that this may frequently occur in contexts where there are no services that support the youth who engages in SI, we suggest encouraging the youth, wherever possible, to engage through healthy SI web sites. Alternatively, the youth's worker needs to provide the client with an understanding of the larger context of the behaviour. This may include sharing the prevalence of SI, and helping the youth de-pathologize the behaviour in his or her own mind.
- Greater difficulty in clients' accessing appropriate services (Lieberman, 2004): As the worker establishes a relationship with the youth, he/she will develop a better understanding of the purpose of the behaviour, and this will help determine what services would be most appropriate. In contexts where services are less available, it is suggested that the worker obtain resources through text, media, and the Internet that can be used to increase knowledge about this behaviour. Furthermore, the worker is encouraged to establish connections with other, like-minded professionals to create a network for sharing information and discussing issues that arise during work with youth who self-injure.
- A potential for clients to be more resistant to intervention (Nixon et al., 2002): Intervention should be conducted in a collaborative fashion with youth to establish goals. Wherever possible, families should be involved with the goal of helping them gain a better understanding of the meaning of SI for the youth. However, family involvement must be handled with caution, as frequently families are unaware of the youth's self-injuring and may have a strong negative response to this behaviour.

A cautionary note is warranted in regard to all intervention. There are certain markers that, independent of the degree of disconnect, may indicate the presence of more serious difficulties (e.g., suicide risk). These markers include, but are not limited to, previous suicide attempts, family history of suicide or depression, expressions of hopelessness by youth about their future, and finally, youth reporting that they do not feel better (i.e., a sense of release, calmness, or feeling more grounded) following self-injuring.

## Conclusion

Within the context of this volume, we have focused on understanding youth who engage in SI in a community setting. Indeed, the well-being of youth who self-injure cannot be addressed adequately without consideration of the community and societal interpretation of SI. Every youth who engages in SI will respond differently to intervention and will function differently in terms of his or her own well-being, depending on that youth's understanding and use of SI relative to context. In summary, we do not advocate working with youth who self-injure without consideration of this larger framework.

With reference to the relational aspects of resilience mentioned earlier, SI in youth appears to be strongly linked to a breakdown in relational strengths. Current research in North America suggests that the greatest difficulty these individuals have is in regulating emotion and relating to others around them on an emotional level. Working to build the relational resilience of these youth, and helping them learn to communicate effectively with others, holds the potential to eliminate this maladaptive coping mechanism. It may be that the increase in SI in the North American context is indicative of a lack of connectedness in our youth.

Furthermore, our model is closely linked to the notion of community responsiveness because its central tenet is the need for consistency between the individual's and the community's understanding of SI. Thus it is important to make communities responsive to youth. The issue of interpretation refers to the community's understanding and, on that basis, its response to youth engaging in SI. We would argue that communities need to constantly listen to youth, be critical of current interpretations of this behaviour, and be open to re-evaluating this interpretation over time.

Finally, government policy and service provision with respect to promoting resilience in youth are particularly relevant to the area of SI because the resources necessary to help youth are not available in many settings. Furthermore, our understanding of SI is changing so rapidly that service provision is not able to keep pace in some contexts. Service providers have difficulty accessing needed resources and training for managing self-injurious behaviour. One way of dealing with this is to use technology-based means of long-distance education to provide mental health professionals and youth workers with up-to-date information. Certain areas with many resources have cutting-edge information about SI, but some areas are completely lacking in this regard. Larger North American cities have treatment centres, but in more isolated areas youth are at greater risk of obtaining inappropriate or harmful responses to their behaviour due to a lack of information or awareness.

In conclusion, a more complete understanding of the meaning and interpretation of self-injurious behaviour is needed, one that is sensitive to the influence of the context and time in which SI takes place. Consideration of these two dimensions is necessary in obtaining an accurate understanding of the meaning of self-injurious behaviour for the individual and of the societal interpretation. An examination of different settings illustrates that the meaning and interpretation are context dependent. It is also evident that the meaning and interpretation of self-injurious behaviour change over time within the same context. The model presented in this chapter highlights the need to continually assess meaning for the individual as well as critically evaluate the contextual interpretation of SI, never assuming stasis.

## REFERENCES

American Self-Harm Clearing House (n.d.). *About self-harm*. Retrieved 6 October 2005 from http://www.selfinjury.org.

Best, R. (2004). *Deliberate self-harm in adolescents: An educational response*. Paper presented to the Annual Conference of the British Educational Research Association, Manchester, UK.

Boudewyn, A.C., & Liem, J.H. (1995). Childhood sexual abuse as a precursor to depression and self-destructive behavior in adulthood. *Journal of Traumatic Stress, 8*(3), 445–59.

Briere, J., & Gil, E. (1998). Self-mutilation in clinical and general population samples: Prevalence, correlates, and functions. *American Journal of Orthopsychiatry, 64*(4), 609–20.

Chapman, A.L., Gratz, K.L., & Brown, M. Z. (2006). Solving the puzzle of deliberate self-harm: The experiential avoidance model. *Behaviour Research and Therapy, 44*, 371–94.

Cicchetti, D., & Schneider-Rosen, K. (1986). An organizational approach to childhood depression. In M. Rutter, C. Izard, & P. Read (Eds.), *Depression in young people: Clinical and developmental perspectives* (pp. 71–134). New York: Guilford.

Conterio, K., & Lader, W. (1998). *Bodily harm: The breakthrough healing program for self-injurers*. New York: Hyperion.

Coons, P.M., & Milstein, V. (1990). Self-mutilation associated with dissociative disorders. *Dissociation, 3*, 81–7.

Darche, M.A. (1990). Psychological factors differentiating self-mutilating and non-self-mutilating adolescent inpatient females. *The Psychiatric Hospital, 21*, 31–5.

Derouin, A., & Bravender, T. (2004). Living on the edge: The current phenomenon of self-mutilation in adolescents. *American Journal of Maternal/Child Nursing, 29*(1), 12–18.

De Young, M. (1982). Self-injurious behaviour in incest victims: A research note. *Child Welfare, 61*, 577–84.

DiClemente, R.J., Ponton, L.E., & Hartley, D. (1991). Prevalence and correlates of cutting behavior: Risk for HIV transmission. *Journal of the American Academy of Child & Adolescent Psychiatry, 30*, 735–9.

Dulit, R.A., Fryer, M.R., Leon, A.C., Brodsky, B.S., & Frances, A.J. (1994). Clinical correlates of self-mutilation in borderline personality disorder. *American Journal of Psychiatry, 151*(9), 1305–12.

Favaro, A., & Santonastaso, P. (1998). Impulsive and compulsive self-injurious behavior in bulimia nervosa: Prevalence and psychological correlates. *Journal of Nervous & Mental Disease, 186*(3), 157–65.

Favazza, A.R. (1987). *Bodies under siege: Self-mutilation and body modification in culture and psychiatry*. London: Johns Hopkins University Press.

Favazza, A.R. (1989). Why patients mutilate themselves. *Hospital and Community Psychiatry, 40*(2), 137–45.

Favazza, A.R. (1998). The coming age of self-mutilation. *Journal of Nervous & Mental Disease, 186*(5), 259–68.

Favazza, A.R., & Conterio, K. (1988). The plight of chronic self-mutilators. *Community Mental Health Journal, 24*(1), 22–30.

Favazza, A.R., & Conterio, K. (1989). Female habitual self-mutilators. *Acta Psychiatrica Scandinavica, 79*, 283–9.

Favazza, A.R., DeRosear, I., & Conterio, K. (1989). Self-mutilation and eating disorders. *Suicide and Life Threatening Behaviors, 19*, 352–61.

Favazza, A.R., & Rosenthal, R.J. (1993). Diagnostic issues in self-mutilation. *Hospital and Community Psychiatry, 44*(2), 134–40.

Garfinkel, P., Moldofsky, H., & Garner, D. (1980). The heterogeneity of anorexia nervosa: Bulimia as a distinct subgroup. *Archives of General Psychiatry, 37*, 1036–40.

Garmezy, N. (1990). A closing note: Reflections on the future. In J. Rolf, A. Masten, D. Cicchetti, K. Nuechterlein, & S. Weintraub (Eds.), *Risk and pro-*

*tective factors in the development of psychopathology* (pp. 527–34). New York: Cambridge University Press.

Gerber, P.J., Ginsberg, R., & Reiff, H.B. (1992). Identifying alterable patterns in employment success for highly successful adults with learning disabilities. *Journal of Learning Disabilities, 25*, 475–87.

Gerson, J., & Stanley, B. (2002). Suicidal and self-injurious behavior in personality disorder: controversies and treatment directions. *Current Psychiatry Reports, 3*, 30–8.

Gratz, K. (2001). Measurement of deliberate self-harm: Preliminary data on the deliberate self-harm inventory. *Journal of Psychopathology and Behavioral Assessment, 23*(4), 253–63.

Gratz, K. (2003). Risk factors for and functions of deliberate self-harm: An empirical and conceptual review. *Clinical Psychology: Science and Practice, 10*(2), 192–205.

Gratz, K., & Roemer, L. (2004). Multidimensional assessment of emotional regulation and dysregulation: Development, factor structure, and initial validation of the Difficulties in Emotion Regulation Scale. *Journal of Psychopathology and Behavioral Assessment, 26*(1), 41–54.

Greenspan, G.S., & Samuel, S.E. (1989). Self-cutting after rape. *American Journal of Psychiatry, 146*, 789–90.

Griffin, J.C., Williams, D.E., & Stark, M.T. (1985). Self-injurious behavior: A statewide prevalence survey. *Applied Research Mental Retardation, 7*, 105–16.

Haines, J., & Williams, C.L. (2003). Coping and problem solving of self-mutilators. *Journal of Clinical Psychology, 59*(10), 1097–1106.

Heath, N.L., Beettam, E., & DeStefano, J. (2005, November). *Adolescent self-injury: What every high school teacher needs to know.* Paper presented at the annual convention of the Quebec Provincial Association of Teachers, Montreal.

Heath, N.L., Toste, J.R., & Beettam, E. (2006). 'I am not well-equipped': High school teachers' perceptions of self-injury. *Canadian Journal of School Psychology, 21*(1), 73–92.

Heath, N.L., Toste, J.R., Nedecheva, T., & Charlebois, A. (in press). An examination of non-suicidal self-injury among college students. *Journal of Mental Health Counseling.*

Himber, J. (1994). Blood rituals: Self-cutting in female psychiatric patients. *Psychotherapy, 31*, 620–31.

Johnson, E.H., & Britt, B. (1967). *Self-mutilation in prison: Interaction of stress and social structure.* Carbondale: Southern Illinois University Center for the Study of Crime, Delinquency, and Corrections.

Lieberman, R. (2004). Understanding and responding to students who self-mutilate. *Principal Leadership, 4*(7), 10–13.

Loshak, R. (2003). Working with Bangladeshi young women. *Psychoanalytic Psychotherapy, 17,* 52–67.

Luthar, S.S. (1991). Vulnerability and resilience: A study of high-risk adolescents. *Child Development, 62,* 600–16.

Luthar, S.S. (1995). Social competence in the school setting: Perspective cross-domain associations among inner-city teens. *Child Development, 66,* 416–29.

Luthar, S.S., Cicchetti, D., & Becker, B. (2000). The construct of resilience: A critical evaluation and guidelines for future work. *Child Development, 71,* 543–62.

Luthar, S.S., & Zigler, E. (1991). Vulnerability and competence: A review of research on resilience in childhood. *American Journal of Orthopsychiatry, 61,* 6–22.

Masten, A.S., & Coatsworth, J.D. (1998). The development of competence in favourable and unfavourable environments: Lessons from research on successful children. *American Psychologist, 53,* 205–20.

Masten, A.S., & Garmezy, N. (1985). Risk, vulnerability, and protective factors in developmental psychopathology. In B.B. Lahey & A.E. Kazdin (Eds.), *Advances in Clinical Child Psychology* (Vol. 8, pp. 1–52). New York: Plenum.

Nixon, M.K., Cloutier, P.F., & Aggarwal, S. (2002). Affect regulation and addictive aspects of repetitive self-injury in hospitalized adolescents. *Journal of the American Academy of Child & Adolescent Psychiatry, 41*(11), 1333–41.

Nock, M.K., & Prinstein, M.J. (2004). A functional approach to the assessment of self-mutilative behavior. *Journal of Consulting and Clinical Psychology, 72*(5), 885–90.

Nock, M.K., & Prinstein, M.J. (2005). Contextual features and behavioral functions of self-mutilation among adolescents. *Journal of Abnormal Psychology, 114*(1), 140–6.

Paris, J. (2005). Understanding self-mutilation in borderline personality disorder. *Harvard Review of Psychiatry, 13*(3), 179–85.

Pipher, M. (1994). *Reviving Ophelia: Saving the selves of adolescent girls.* New York: Ballantine.

Pitman, R.K. (1990). Self-mutilation in combat related post-traumatic stress disorder. *American Journal of Psychiatry, 147,* 123–4.

Rosenthal, R.J., Rinzler, C., Walsh, R., & Edmund, E. (1972). Wrist-cutting syndrome: The meaning of a gesture. *American Journal of Psychiatry, 128*(11), 47–52.

Ross, S. (2004). *Self-mutilation in a community sample of adolescents: A test of the anxiety model and the hostility model.* Unpublished doctoral dissertation, McGill University, Montreal.

Ross, S., & Heath, N.L. (2002). A study of the frequency of self-mutilation in a community sample of adolescents. *Journal of Youth and Adolescence, 31*(1), 67–77.

Ross, S., & Heath, N.L. (2003). Two models of adolescent self-mutilation. *Suicide and Life-Threatening Behavior, 33*(3), 277–87.

Shapiro, S. (1987). Self-mutilation and self-blame in incest victims. *American Journal of Psychotherapy, 41*, 46–54.

Shaw, S.N. (2002). Shifting conversations on girls' and women's self-injury: An analysis of the clinical literature in historical context. *Feminism & Psychology, 12*(2) 191–219.

Simeon, D., & Hollander, E. (2001). Self-injurious behaviours: Assessment and treatment. *Journal of the American Academy of Child & Adolescent Psychiatry, 41*(7), 210.

Simpson, M.A. (1976). Self-mutilation and suicide. In E.S. Schneidman (Ed.), *Suicidology: Contemporary developments* (pp. 286–315). New York: Grune and Stratton.

Sroufe, L.A., & Rutter, M. (1984). The domain of developmental psychopathology. *Child Development, 55*, 17–29.

Thompson, N., & Dinesh, B. (2000). Rates of deliberate self-harm in Asians: Findings and models. *International Review of Psychiatry, 12*(1), 37–43.

Tyler, K.A., Whitbeck, L.B., Hoyt, D.R., & Johnson, K.D. (2003). Self-mutilation and homeless youth: The role of family abuse, street experiences, and mental disorders. *Journal of Research on Adolescence, 13*(4), 457–74.

Van der Kolk, B.A., Perry, C., & Herman, J.L. (1991). Childhood origins of self-destructive behavior. *The American Journal of Psychiatry, 148*(12), 1665–71.

Walsh, B.W. (2006). *Treating self-injury: A practical guide.* New York: Guilford Press.

Waters, E., & Sroufe, L.A. (1983). Social competence as a developmental construct. *Developmental Review, 3*, 79–97.

Werner, E., & Smith, R. (Eds.). (1992). *Overcoming the odds: High risk children from birth to adulthood.* Ithaca, NY: Cornell University Press.

White Kress, V.E., Gibson, D.M., & Reynolds, C.A. (2004). Adolescents who self-injure: Implications and strategies for school counselors. *Professional School Counseling, 7*(3), 195–201.

Wise, M.L. (1989). Adult self-injury as a survival response in victim-survivors of childhood abuse. *Journal of Chemical Dependency Treatment, 3*, 185–201.

Yuri, D. (2005, June 19). *Pedidos de Socorro* (Calling out for help). *Folha de São Paulo* (newspaper), p. B4.

Zila, L.M., & Kiselica, M.S. (2001). Understanding and counseling self-mutilation in female adolescents and young adults. *Journal of Counseling & Development, 79*, 46–52.

Zlotnick, C., Mattia, J.I., & Zimmerman, M. (1999). Clinical correlates of self-mutilation in a sample of general psychiatric patients. *Journal of Nervous & Mental Disease, 187*(5), 296–301.

Zoroglu, S.S., Tuzun, U., Sar, V., Tutkun, H., Savas, H.A., Ozturk, M., et al. (2003). Suicide attempt and self-mutilation among Turkish high school students in relation with abuse, neglect and dissociation. *Psychiatry & Clinical Neurosciences, 57*(1), 119–26.

Zweig-Frank, H., Paris, J., & Guzder, J. (1994). Psychological risk factors for dissociation in female patients with borderline and non-borderline personality disorders. *Journal of Personality Disorders, 8*, 203–9.

# 3 Discovering How Resilient Capacities Develop in the Midst of Surviving Incest

KIM M. ANDERSON

Due to the intense psychosocial and physical stressors related to incest, child victims employ various coping methods in order to survive. The child who has experienced incest is under threat in the most intimate environment where ordinary systems of care that provide individuals with a sense of control, meaning, and connection are undermined (Herman, 1997). The essential ingredients for developing healthy relationships, such as trust, intimacy, security, and personal boundary setting, are taken from the child (Brierc & Runtz, 1993; Elliott, 1994). Childhood incest often continues for several years, leads to more severe sexual assaults, and is associated with greater negative long-term consequences (Courtois, 1988; Russell & Bolen, 2000; Valentine & Feinauer, 1993). As a result of experiencing childhood incest, individuals may exhibit significant impairment in their bio-psycho-social functioning (e.g., depression, anxiety, low self-esteem, and mistrust of others) if resulting issues are not addressed in treatment or in their natural environment.

Browne and Finkelhor (1986) identify the incest dynamics of traumatic sexualization (i.e., coerced sexual relations), betrayal, stigmatization, and powerlessness as being core experiences for psychological injury. Unless childhood coping methods are employed, an individual's sanity and will to live are seriously jeopardized because of the extreme consequences of incest (Himelein & McElrath, 1996). The child who has experienced incest is under a threat in the most intimate environment, which places her on constant guard because she does not know when the sexual abuse will occur again. To achieve feelings of safety, it is essential for the child to establish cognitive, behavioral, and emotional avenues of protection, escape, and resistance. These attempts to affect the abuse experience may start out as accidental, such as being sick. Recognizing that this prevents her from being sexually abused, however, the child may realize that this and other ways to influence the abuse situation, either directly or indirectly, exist (Ceresne, 1995). Focusing on child victims' resourcefulness draws on their resilience and helps mental health professionals gain a comprehensive view of the many possible dimensions of how a child not only survives incest, but thrives in spite of it. Child incest survivors may well prefer this focus on strengths and appreciate recognition for how they actively responded to adversity in the past. This can inspire them to channel their protective strategies into confronting present struggles.

This chapter presents a conceptual model of resilience that encompasses the resourcefulness of child victims as well as the damage inflicted upon them. Such a model nourishes and honours the potential in each individual who is coping or has coped with incest. A qualitative study of twenty-six female incest survivors provides the basis for this conceptual model. The study looks at protective strategies incest survivors develop to resist and overcome their victimization. At the time of their abuse and throughout their lives, even though they were seemingly powerless, their resistance to the domination of incest was significant to their survival and ultimately to their recovery. As Kelly (1988) explains, 'To resist is to oppose actively, to fight, to refuse to cooperate with or submit' (p. 161). Often in mental health treatment, resistance is viewed in a negative sense, as with the client who refuses treatment protocol or advice from the professional. In this study, resistance is a healthy indicator to surviving and persevering in life despite enduring childhood incest.

During childhood, participants in the study were not idle or silent regarding their victimization. They typically were resistant to their perpetrators' domination and used a variety of mental and behavioural strategies to prevent, withstand, stop, or oppose their subjugation and its consequences. Several of their childhood survival strategies were carried into adulthood and contributed to their ability to overcome childhood victimization. Examples drawn from interview transcripts (using pseudonyms) are presented to highlight incest survivors' perspectives regarding how traumatic events shaped their lives and how their own unique resilient capacities are related to these events. Mental health professionals may use this information to better understand how protective processes develop and contribute to hardiness in the case of female incest survivors. Information is provided on how helping professionals can mobilize the resilient capacities of child survivors. Since individuals often internalize shame and blame about their sexual abuse experiences (Draucker, 1995), providing a view of themselves as resourceful gives credit to their ability to persevere despite insurmountable odds. They may view themselves differently, particularly their strengths, by recognizing how they actively responded to adversity in the past, and may now channel their survival strategies into confronting present struggles.

## Resilience Research and Childhood Sexual Abuse

Resilience research primarily focuses on people whose constitutions or temperaments enable them to remain hardy despite enduring adverse circumstances (Fraser, 1997; Garmezy, 1987; Masten, 2001; Rutter, 1987; Werner & Smith, 1992). According to risk and protective studies, resilience describes people who escape harmful experiences with relatively few difficulties as measured at a particular point in time. Findings from studies of resilience show that some individuals develop healthy and stable personalities despite enduring trauma such as childhood sexual abuse (Byrd, 1994; Ceresne, 1995; Coffey, Leitenberg, Henning, Turner, & Bennett, 1996; Feinauer, Hilton, & Callahan, 2003; Himelein & McElrath, 1996; Liem, James, O'Toole, & Boudewyn, 1997; Scalzo, 1991). Resilience includes the protective factors that develop as one is faced with adversity. These factors range from attributes within individuals and their families to the external support systems of their community and culture that serve as protective mechanisms.

Current research on the effects of incest is directed at discovering what types of coping strategies minimize or exacerbate the after-effects of trauma (Draucker, 1995; Futa, Nash, Hansen, & Garben, 2003). As inquiry into the consequences of childhood incest has progressed, it is apparent that adaptation varies for each individual (Binder, McNiel, & Goldstone, 1996). Some individuals are debilitated by their childhood adversity, while others experience minimal symptoms. Research findings indicate that those who have endured intrusive and violent forms of incest are more prone to have difficulty functioning (Courtois, 1988; Trickett, Reiffman, Horowitz, & Putnam, 1997). Yet other studies show that characteristics of the abuse account for very little of the variance in psychosocial outcomes (Futa et al., 2003; Perrott, Morris, Martin, & Romans, 1998). Other mediating factors are therefore beginning to be explored with studies indicating that one's style of childhood coping is significant in determining long-term adjustment (Romans, Martin, Anderson, O'Shea & Mullen, 1995; Sigmon, Greene, Rohan, & Nichols, 1996).

Exploring how individuals grow and prevail in the aftermath of violence and traumatic events is a relatively new trend (Ai & Park, 2005). Resilience studies related to child sexual abuse suggest that there is a clear connection between childhood coping strategies and adult healing activities that promote positive functioning. Retrospective designs with adults are recognized as a potentially viable way to address gaps in knowledge about the long-term recovery process from childhood victimization (Feinauer & Stuart, 1996; Harvey, Mishler, Koenen, & Harney, 2000; Valentine & Feinauer, 1993). Although there is no theoretical framework that organizes the resilience literature into a coherent whole, the following four commonalities are found to be significant across studies regarding female survivors' childhood protective processes that help individuals to survive, heal, and thrive throughout their lives: (1) having an internal locus of control, (2) construing benefit from adverse experiences, (3) developing social networks, and (4) creating physical and mental escapes.

### Internal Locus of Control

Possessing an internal locus of control and having a sense of personal efficacy have received empirical support as important factors in overcoming child sexual abuse (Himelein & McElrath, 1996; Liem et al., 1997; Morrow & Smith, 1995; Valentine & Feinauer, 1993). During childhood, resilient survivors are able to recognize that they have personal power resulting in the development of an internal locus of control. These youth determine which parts of their adverse experiences they have control of, and let go of those aspects they cannot influence (Binder et al., 1996; Ceresne, 1995). These attempts to affect the abuse experience may start out as accidental, as mentioned above. Later, as in adulthood, resilient survivors remain determined to exert their autonomy. They may, for example, move away from their family of origin, further their education, and start a career (Valentine & Feinauer, 1993).

### Construing Benefit from Adverse Experiences

Research indicates that resilient sexual abuse survivors have a greater capacity to transform negative attributes into positive ones, including being grateful for what they have learned from overcoming adversity. Instead of living in despair and suffering, they are able to grow from their struggles. Resilient individuals reveal that they may have some difficulty making sense of what happened to them as children. Yet, even at a young age, they are able to understand that being sexually abused is not their fault. They are able to attribute the abuse to external circumstances, such as something being wrong with their abusers (Feinauer & Stuart, 1996; Valentine & Feinauer, 1993).

Adult survivors who find meaning in their struggle with adversity report better social adjustment, less psychological distress, and higher levels of self-esteem (Harvey et al., 2000; Silver, Boon, & Stones, 1983). Interpreting benefit from traumatic experiences is one way by which adult survivors find meaning (McMillen, Zuravin, & Rideout, 1995; Scalzo, 1991). For instance, Draucker's study (1992) of 142 incest survivors looked at the process of construing benefit from victimization and found that participants reported feeling an increased ability to relate to other victims and a greater appreciation of their own survival strengths. In adulthood, individuals channel these positive attributes into career choices that give them a sense of purpose and often involve helping others.

*Developing Social Networks*

Research on resilience also demonstrates the significant role of positive social relationships in overcoming childhood sexual abuse (Byrd, 1994; Feinauer et al., 2003; Liem et al., 1997; Romans et al., 1995; Scalzo, 1991). The significance of having *one* supportive adult in one's life is demonstrated in resilience studies highlighting the various functions such a relationship provides: being a role model for appropriate behaviour, offering affirmation, providing safety, and reinforcing the idea that the individual deserves to be loved. This adult may be a family member, friends' parent, teacher, clergy, coach, or other community member. During childhood, resilient individuals are also involved in extracurricular activities that provide opportunities not only to connect with supportive adults and peers, but also to get away from family problems. Activities such as being involved in church or athletics serve as opportunities to acquire safety and guidance (Hyman & Williams, 2001). Resilient individuals often extend their childhood activities or interests, such as sports, school, or an affiliation with a spiritual belief system, into their adult lives.

*Creating Physical and Mental Escapes*

During childhood, resilient individuals create distance from their sexual abuse by finding a protective place either psychologically, through fantasizing or dissociating, or behaviourally, through immersing themselves in satisfactory activities (Binder et al., 1996; Ceresne, 1995; Coffey et al., 1996). At the time of the abuse, they engage in fantasy and withdraw into their imaginations to combat the stress of their childhood adversity. Through fantasizing, these individuals create imaginary havens where they seek refuge from their brutal reality (Byrd, 1994). In addition to cognitive responses, other behavioural strategies in childhood provide distance from family problems, such as having a hiding place or engaging in distracting behaviours such as reading. Similarly, hiding and isolating themselves from their families provides a means for escape from the sexual abuse (Ceresne, 1995; Himelein & McElrath, 1996). This involves finding a safe place, such as fields, gardens, woods, closets, or under blankets, where they can momentarily escape what is happening to them. As adults, their desire to isolate themselves may remain important and they may continue to use their solitude as a means of finding a peaceful place for renewal.

## Studying Resilience through Listening to the Voices of Incest Survivors

Although research on resilience and sexual abuse survivors has identified key protective processes, there is little emphasis on *how* these processes develop (Feinauer et al., 2003; Himelein & McElrath, 1996; Liem et al., 1997). Consequently, understanding of the interplay between risk and protective factors remains underdeveloped. There is no explanation of how one's childhood adversity and trauma produce specific consequences that serve as a catalyst for resilient capacities to emerge. For instance, why do resilient persons connect with their personal power, particularly when sexual abuse often causes one to feel helpless (Browne & Finkelhor, 1986; Neumann, Houskamp, Pollock, & Briere, 1996)? And why do individuals cast their adversity in a positive light, when enduring sexual abuse often leaves one feeling devastated rather than 'grateful' (Herman, 1997; Romans, Martin, & Mullen, 1996)? Furthermore, how do survivors develop connections with others, when sexual abuse often causes one to feel distrustful of relationships (Briere & Runtz, 1993; Elliott, 1994)? Finally, how do they manage to create distance in families where secrecy and enmeshment prevail (Courtois, 1988; Russell & Bolen, 2000)? To truly understand coping, the context of adverse conditions from which protective processes emanate needs to be further explicated in resilience research and literature.

Little is known about how incest survivors regain a sense of order, coherence, and continuity after experiencing childhood trauma. Exploring incest survivors' perceptions of what happened to them both when the abuse was occurring and during their adult lives assists in understanding how resilience can emerge from adversity. Through research that asks participants to share their stories regarding adversity, the influences of context on experience and meaning can be explored. Consequently, the many ways in which incest survivors perceive, seek to make sense of, and respond to their traumatic experiences may be highlighted. The qualitative study presented in this chapter includes in-depth interviews with twenty-six women who are survivors of child-hood incest. The definition of resilience that shaped this study was: 'one's ability to survive traumatic and stressful events, and to persevere in life in spite of the trauma sustained' (Byrd, 1994, p. 12).

Since the intent of this study was to discover *how* one overcomes childhood incest, grounded theory was particularly suited, as its purpose is to identify complex and hidden psychosocial processes with the goal of developing theory (Glaser, 2001; Strauss & Corbin, 1998). In addition, developing theory from the perspectives of individuals experiencing the social problem directly helps to serve the population for which it is carried out. For the purpose of this study, incest was defined as sexual acts (i.e., non-genital and genital contact) between a female child and an adolescent or adult male family member.

The study focused on two research questions: (1) How do adult survivors perceive the impact of childhood incest on their lives? And (2) what are the protective processes that influenced the adult survivor's' ability to cope with childhood incest?

## Methodology

### Participants

The twenty-six women ranged in age from twenty-five to fifty-eight years old (M = 41). The majority were Caucasian (85%), two were African American, and two were biracial (i.e., Native American and

Caucasian). Seventeen of the participants were heterosexual, six were lesbian, and three were bisexual. The women were highly educated: twenty-two had completed junior college or higher (had a bachelor's, master's, or doctoral degree) and another four had at least some college education. All had received mental health services varying from a few outpatient sessions to several sessions over ten or more years. Three individuals had received mental health services during adolescence; however, in only one case was the topic of incest addressed. Thirteen (50%) of the participants had received *both* outpatient and inpatient services.

The majority of participants (61%) had experienced childhood incest for six or more years (M = 6.78). The age of onset ranged from two to twelve years old (M = 5.78). Sixty-five percent were sexually abused by more than one perpetrator. All participants were abused by male perpetrators, and in two cases additional perpetrators included females. Fifteen participants (58%) were sexually abused by their biological fathers or stepfathers. Other family members who sexually abused the participants were brothers, cousins, uncles, grandfathers, and a brother-in-law. One participant was sexually abused by her mother and another by her female cousin.

*Data Collection*

Participants were recruited by sending letters indicating the intent of the study, including a request for participants, to state-licensed clinical and master's level social work practitioners (who specialized in childhood sexual abuse) in a Midwestern metropolitan area. Based on theoretical sampling criteria, twenty-six individuals became research participants from among thirty-three respondents. Initial purposive sampling included the following criteria: women had to (1) be twenty-one years or older; (2) have experienced childhood incest; (3) be the victim of a male perpetrator who was perceived to be a family member; (4) have received mental health treatment services as an adult; and (5) have the ability to express thoughts, feelings, and opinions about their incest experiences in a manner that addressed *both* the effects of the trauma *and* their ability to survive and persevere. Subsequent theoretical sampling was based on the grounded theory criteria of saturation of conceptual information and code categories (Denzin & Lincoln, 1998; Oktay, 2004).

*Interview Procedure and Research Instrument*

Although a semi-structured interview guide (consisting of eleven open-ended questions) was used, the interview process remained open to the direction taken by participants. Each interview began by asking participants to share their perspectives regarding the impact of childhood incest on their lives. Participants were encouraged to disclose as much as possible of the background and context surrounding their experiences. As their stories unfolded, eight additional questions were asked regarding psychosocial protective factors pertaining to themselves, their families, and external support systems. The final two questions addressed recommendations for adult survivors and mental health service providers. Each in-depth interview took approximately an hour and a half. A follow-up thirty-minute telephone interview occurred after participants had received a summary of the findings to gain their insights regarding the final analysis.

*Data Analysis*

Data analysis was conducted using a constant comparative method, a qualitative procedure that identifies and extracts significant statements or 'meaningful units' from the transcripts to be conceptualized and reconstructed in new ways. This process included repeated sorting, codings, and comparisons that yielded increasingly complex and inclusive categories and continued until all of the data (i.e., interview transcripts) were accounted for in the core categories of the grounded theory paradigm model (Denzin & Lincoln, 1998; Glaser, 2001). Specifically, the process involved searching for units of data (e.g., risk and protective factors) that could stand on their own and were associated with the overall purpose of the study. Through coding, data were then grouped into final categories that represented key psychosocial issues and patterns (e.g., protective processes) related to adversity, which were analysed by comparing them with one another so that relevant themes (e.g., resistance to childhood victimization) addressing the research questions could emerge. Finally, a resilience conceptual model was generated around the core category (i.e., childhood victimization) that described the central phenomenon relating to participants' incest experiences.

## Findings

### Childhood Victimization

Figure 1 illustrates a set of conceptually meaningful categories for theory development. The core category of 'childhood victimization' provided a contextual thick description of the risk factors (i.e., abuse and violence) that participants had experienced and helped to explain *how* protective processes had developed. Because risk and protective factors are often studied separately in child sexual abuse research, the interplay between them is obscured with regard to how they prevent or promote resilience (Futa et al., 2003). In the present study, stories of childhood incest were explored in depth as a means of discovering how psychosocial protective factors developed in relationship to childhood victimization. As the data analysis progressed, it became clear that the roots of participants' resilience were actually forged in their resistance to abusive behaviour and domination by their perpetrators. Participants were not idle or silent in regard to their abuse. Their resistance included a variety of strategies to prevent, withstand, stop, or oppose their childhood victimization and its consequences.

All twenty-six individuals experienced traumatic sexualization, often committed forcefully, creating a childhood full of fear and terror. These women discussed how, in their intimate worlds, male relatives used their authority to control them. Sixteen participants reported being emotionally, physically, and sexually dominated by their perpetrators. The remaining ten individuals believed that they were taken advantage of due to their immaturity (i.e., preschool age) or emotional vulnerability, and at the time of the abuse were unaware that they were being dominated. The abusers were persistent and determined to undermine or thwart any avenues their victims used to protect themselves. The following quotation illustrates how a participant's life was confined and shaped by the actions of her stepfather:

> He started pawing me, and I didn't know what to do. Finally, he pinned me against the end of the divan. I scooted down, trying to get away and ended up on the floor, and he raped me. There was no one in the house to help and yelling didn't help. It seemed to make him enjoy it more. He slapped me around a little. He came to the bathroom while I was cleaning up and told me if I told anybody that they would blame me because I had tempted him and that it was my fault. I told him that he would

Figure 1: Conceptual model of adult incest survivors' resistance to childhood victimization

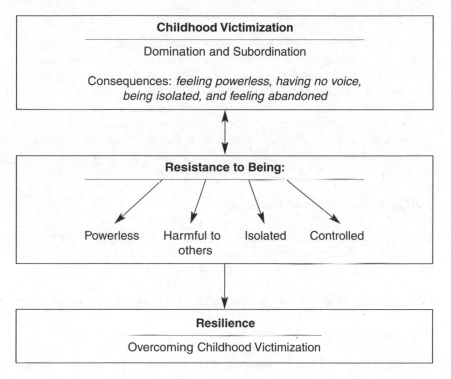

never do that to me again. He said, 'Oh, yes, I will. Anytime I want.' (Kelly, aged fifty-eight)

The consequences of participants' childhood victimization were enormous and yielded experiences of powerlessness, secrecy, isolation, and abandonment. Their trust in their familial support systems was undermined, as it was these same systems that often contributed to or ignored the incest rather than protecting the child from it. During childhood, participants discussed how their physical and mental health was negatively affected by the resulting stress they experienced. These effects included feeling lonely, suicidal, confused, and helpless. As demonstrated in the subsequent excerpt, participants' incest experiences contributed to a childhood during which they felt betrayed and disconnected from family members, that they had no control, and, finally, that they had to rely on themselves for protection:

> There are occasions that I was left with this step-grandfather [the perpetrator] and grandmother for weekends, and the abuse escalated about that time ... And I think it was the weekend that I was convinced he was going to rape me ... I blurted out at the dinner table, 'I don't wanna go. He's touching me. I don't wanna go.' I can remember my stepfather standing up and smashing his plate on the table. I just ran away from the table and went upstairs and nothing more was ever said about it. And when Friday came, we went. They [her parents] took me there and dropped me off. (Sarah, aged forty-four)

## Childhood Strategies of Resistance

Participants' strategies of resistance began as spontaneous protective reactions to their childhood victimization and, consequently, helped these women defend themselves against the destructive after-effects of their troubled childhoods. These childhood protective processes may be organized around four ontological themes. Participants expressed how their protective strategies helped them to resist being (a) powerless (e.g., 'I purposely did not do everything the abuser demanded of me'); (b) harmful to others (e.g., 'I promised myself that when I grew up I would not be like my abuser'); (c) isolated (e.g., 'I sought out connections with people who were safe and supportive'); and (d) controlled (e.g., 'I recognized cues in my abuser that alerted me to danger, so that I could then plan my escape').

*Resist Being Powerless*

Resilience research on sexual abuse survivors does not explain how individuals are able to develop a sense of power (i.e., one's ability to effect change) rather than powerlessness (i.e., being without options, doubts about one's efficacy) in the face of childhood incest (Himelein & McElrath, 1996; Morrow & Smith, 1995). As children, participants sometimes realized that their efforts did make a difference and began to slowly develop a sense of efficacy as a result. They may not have always been successful in stopping the abuse, but they were active in trying to resist, prevent, stop, or defy their perpetrators. In the following quotation, for example, Tracy shows how learning to confront her perpetrator helped prepare her to stand up for justice in general:

> I was trying, at least by the time I was sixteen, to get my mother to leave my dad [the perpetrator] ... I would contest what he would do ... I'd challenge him and, of course, then he'd get really abusive. He would consider that a threat to his power ... That's one thing I've continued to believe in, not necessarily the underdog, but to believe in what's right, and support what is right, and take a stand. I feel like standing up for what's right, even if it hurts me in some regard. (Tracy, aged forty-four)

Participants' strategies to resist powerlessness were adaptive given their abusive and violent family environments and evolved to become applicable to non-abusive environments as well. During childhood, they believed that their lives could get better and they were determined to make this happen in adulthood. Participants' brave acts of deviance provided the foundation for them to exert their autonomy in adulthood, including moving away from their families, finishing college, getting out of inpatient psychiatric treatment, and opposing mistreatment of themselves and others. The following passage highlights how a participant drew upon her survival strengths to make positive life changes during adulthood:

> When I started to get better and believe that I was worth something, then I started to correlate the strengths that I used to survive the incest to the strengths that I was able to use to move on in my life. (Erika, aged thirty-eight)

In the present study, childhood acts to gain power and exert autonomy were usually met with opposition from the perpetrators. Despite these insurmountable challenges, participants developed strategies to prevent, expose, or stop their childhood victimization that over time led to an internal sense of influence and control of one's life. Developing strategies that gave participants power helped them in other areas of their lives, including making a commitment to 'do no harm,' building supportive relationships, and getting 'on top' of traumatic after-effects.

*Resist Being Harmful to Others*

Previous resilience research gives no indication why adult survivors cast their negative experiences in a positive light (Feinauer & Stuart, 1996; Valentine & Feinauer, 1993). The current study's findings indicate that incest survivors' interpretation of benefits accruing from the abuse experience is connected to a commitment to 'do no harm.' They developed a resolve to be unlike their perpetrators, a resolve that served them well as they learned to live lives without hatred or destructiveness. They turned their struggles with adversity into a means of action to help, rather than hurt, others.

Participants' interpretation of benefit from their experience was also connected to their commitment to end the cycle of harm done to others. They were resolved to be different from their perpetrators. All twenty-six participants discussed how they chose to be caring and compassionate people rather than abusive and destructive. For example, their commitment to 'give back' to others was the central reason for their participation in the study. Because no one was there for them, they wanted to be there for others. Although some participants struggled with depression or suicide attempts, they did not pass on destructiveness to others. The next excerpt is an example of how during her childhood a participant chose to help others even though she was faced with her own victimization compounded by her family's poverty:

> When I was a little kid, when all this stuff [incest] was going on, I would go to a rummage sale and buy kids' clothes, wash them and iron them and find little dirty kids in the neighbourhood and go give them a bath and clean them up and feed them and send them home. I didn't bring home puppies. I brought home kids. (Jackie, aged forty-five)

Participants expressed such compassion in a variety of ways throughout their lives. The strengths they forged, such as courage and empathy, in regard to their adversity were thought to be of benefit to others who might be struggling to persevere. These women had a strong desire to give back to others and did so by entering into helping professions, doing volunteer work, contributing in group therapy, and/or advocating for others. As demonstrated in the next quotation, it was their hope that something good could come of the harm they had experienced, that often motivated them to reach out to others:

> I just felt like the abuse could affect me in some positive ways. I could go and help other people ... I think that the deep compassion I have for people has really helped, and I think that something good can come out of the abuse. (Shirley, aged thirty)

*Resist Being Isolated*

Resilience research details the types and benefits of social support for sexual abuse survivors. The effort put into acquiring and maintaining those relationships and the obstacles faced in doing so have not, however, been fully addressed (Byrd, 1994; Feinauer et al., 2003; Liem et al., 1997). In the present study, adult survivors developed meaningful connections with others in order to resist or counteract the isolation and alienation they felt within their own families. They lacked a close relationship with an adult, familial, caretaker; and no participant described her childhood as 'normal' or as one that provided an abundance of nurturing. Despite these challenges, as children they found creative ways to lessen their loneliness and have their needs met.

In resisting isolation, participants put tremendous energy into cultivating support systems and actively seeking out relationships. During childhood, this involved first searching for opportunities to connect with family members. Unfortunately, these attempts were often futile, leading them to seek relationships outside of the family, such as with teachers, coaches, and peers. Believing in God and being connected to a religious community also provided comfort and validation of their worthiness. The following two passages highlight participants' childhood strategies of accessing support:

> I used to stand and just stare at what my sister was doing, so I could get my mother's love. Never could figure that out ... My mother didn't want me touching her. But, my sister could touch her. What's the message there? I'm bad. I'm evil. (Holly, aged fifty-eight)

> The relationships I had from teachers I think were very important. I put a lot of energy into bonding with them on whatever they were in to. I wanted them to like me, so I tried to do real well at sports or music or English or whatever it was ... I was just always searching for that parent just everywhere. Probably still am. (Becci, aged thirty-four)

In adulthood, these women strove to have relationships that differed from the destructive ones they experienced in their own families of origin. Most found satisfaction and comfort in establishing close connections with others. They made a commitment to cultivate the social and spiritual dimensions in their lives. The subsequent quotation illustrates how a participant in her current role as a mother has recreated the childhood she wanted but never had:

> I raised myself, and I tell my parents sometimes I was cheated out of childhood, because ever since I was 8 or 9, it's like, 'Okay, you have to grow up pretty darn fast, girl.' I have been able to just relax and really fall into motherhood. I am able to relive my childhood again differently through my child in a positive way. (Vicky, aged thirty)

*Resist Being Controlled*

Resilience studies discuss how physical and mental escapes provide sexual abuse survivors with refuge because they are able to get away from the abuse both physically and emotionally (Binder et al., 1996; Ceresne, 1995). Yet research seldom focuses on the remarkable efforts children make to keep their perpetrators away and resist (e.g., prevent) further victimization. Participants in the present study were active in 'escaping' and in maintaining distance from their abusers, and did so in a determined manner. Findings demonstrate the courageous measures participants took to deny their perpetrators access to them. Throughout their lives they resisted having their incest experiences and the consequences of those experiences consume their identities. They took action to create and then sustain their own resilience.

Participants detailed the tremendous effort they used to gain control during childhood through 'cutting off' their perpetrators' access to them. They actively distanced themselves in order to circumvent further victimization. When they could not physically distance themselves, several participants discussed using dissociation to 'get away' from their traumatic experiences and overwhelming emotions. They reported that the abusers may have invaded their bodies, but they could not control their minds. The next passage illustrates a participant's exhaustive attempts to distance herself from her father in order to prevent further victimization:

> I always made sure that if my father was around that I was with my mother. I always arranged it so I would never be alone with my father. There was one point in time where I was supposed to ride the bus home, and my father worked out of the house, and rather than ride the bus home and get home early, I would sit in my mother's car, where she

worked at this clothing store, and I would sit in the car for three hours and wait for her to get off work, because I didn't want to be alone with my father. (Jennifer, aged thirty-five)

During their adult years, participants endured obstacles on their healing journeys, including problems accessing their memories, managing their emotions, and developing intimate relationships. Yet they strove to 'live well' to avenge their childhood victimization. They were persistent in pursuing help and determined to recover from their incest experiences. As one participant explained in relation to what made her resilient:

For me, it was to keep persevering and to keep going because I wanted to live differently. Perseverance is a good trait and an important trait. It's like you've got your bayonet and your war fatigues, and you just keep going through the terrain until you find a better life. (Becci, aged thirty-four)

*Summary*

To truly understand resilience, this study further explicates the context of adverse conditions (from which resilience emanates). A resilience theory was generated around the category of 'childhood victimization' to describe and explain the nature and workings of the psychosocial relations (i.e., strategies of resistance) within the conceptual model (see figure 1). Consequently, this study focused on *how* resistance to victimization can be a catalyst for strategies of survival and perseverance and serve as a foundation for resilience among survivors of childhood incest. The heightened focus on strategies of resistance encourages researchers and clinicians to get back in touch with the resourcefulness of survivors and provides a background for studying additional strengths. The study's findings help to expand previous discussions of strengths-based assessments and to inform strengths-based strategies by providing a conceptual framework for moving the assessment towards survival strengths by identifying experiences of and responses to childhood victimization.

**Helping Individuals Transcend Their Victimization**

Finding ways to provide effective treatment for child survivors remains a challenge for mental health professionals. Addressing the

Table 1: Questions for discovering acts of resistance

| | |
|---|---|
| I. *Resistance to Being Powerless*<br><br>What are the ways that you protected yourself from the abuser? | • Did you ever purposely not do everything your abuser* demanded of you<br>• Did you ever fight your abuser's violence in a way that surprised you?<br>• Did you ever fantasize or dream about having more power than your abuser?<br>• Did you ever challenge the name calling or stories your abuser said about you?<br>• Did you ever physically or verbally challenge the abuser?<br>• Did you ever tell someone about the abuse? |
| II. *Resistance to Harming Others*<br><br>What are the ways in which you tried to be different from your abuser? | • Did you ever promise yourself that when you grew up you would be different from the perpetrator?<br>• Did you ever try to fight and protect others from the abuse?<br>• Did you sense that something was not right about the abuse even though your abuser said it was?<br>• Did you ever stand up for someone who was in trouble?<br>• Is there anything you would like to do to help other kids who have been through what you have been through?<br>• When you grow up do you want to become someone who helps others (e.g., doctor, teacher, social worker)? |
| III. *Resistance to Being Isolated*<br><br>What are the ways that you defied being isolated? | • Did you seek out activities such as sports, art, music, or drama?<br>• Did you sense that there was a God or someone watching over you?<br>• Did you seek out friends?<br>• Did you seek out teachers, coaches, or other adults as role models or mentors?<br>• Did you volunteer or work?<br>• Did you connect with people because they felt safe and were supportive?<br>• Did you connect with pets? |

Table 1 (continued)

| IV. Resistance to Being Controlled | |
|---|---|
| What are the ways that you cut off your abuser's access to you? | • Did you recognize cues in your abuser that alerted you to danger? |
| | • Did you get involved in activities to get away from home? |
| | • Did you ever find ways to get away from what you were feeling through the use of art, music, or humour? |
| | • Did you escape into reading books or watching television? |
| | • Did you ever go away in your mind (e.g., daydream) when you were being abused? |
| | • Did you make plans of when you would leave home and imagine what life would be like? |
| | • Did you find a place or an activity that would provide an escape from the abuse? |

*As a means of familiarity and clarity for children, substitute 'dad,' 'brother,' etc., based on each individual's sexual abuse circumstances, instead of using the terms 'abuser' or 'perpetrator'.

effects of incest is an important therapeutic concern, such as with trauma-focused cognitive therapy (Cohen, Mannarino, & Knudsen, 2005). Incest survivors often underestimate their potential because their victimization has negatively affected their perceptions of self-worth. As a means of understanding or explaining why the sexual abuse occurred, they may blame themselves for not preventing or stopping it. Such internal causal attributions can lead to increased psychological difficulties, including depression and anxiety (Cohen et al., 2000). In addressing negative thoughts connected to trauma-related events, cognitive-behavioural therapy (CBT) has been shown to be a successful treatment intervention for children and adolescents (Deblinger, Steer, & Lippmann, 1999).

An important component of CBT is to reveal a client's cognitive distortions so that they can be corrected, decreasing psychological distress. For instance, a child survivor may state, 'I never did anything to stop the sexual abuse.' In exploring her reasoning for this negative thought she may indicate, 'I should have told my dad, "No".' Although these statements include several cognitive distortions, one in particular involves overgeneralization, as the child believes she did *absolutely nothing* to prevent or stop the sexual abuse because she did not say no. Because the child's coping methods are obscured by the trauma, the many ways she may in fact have tried to prevent the abuse and protect herself remain obscured to her. As a means of honouring and developing the survivor's resilience, a mental health professional could further explore her acts of resistance, replacing cognitive distortions of self-blame with ones of personal agency.

Table 1 provides a list of useful questions adapted from this study that may encourage the child to share his/her story and uncover experiences of and responses to victimization, including acts of protest involving resistance to being powerless, harming others, isolation, and being controlled. Developing one's story of personal agency may assist in facilitating individual awareness of one's inner strengths, worth, and resilience (Wood & Roche, 2001).

## Implications for Mental Health Professionals

In order to acknowledge, affirm, and extend the incest survivor's resilient capacities, helping professionals have to be knowledgeable about the protective strategies individuals used during childhood. These resilient capacities are often submerged beneath pain and discomfort and are difficult to access if sexual abuse survivors and practitioners do not view these protective strategies as strengths. A starting point to access these capacities may be the expression of compassion. Mental health professionals can express such compassion through actively listening to clients and validating their stories of victimization. Helping professionals need to be able to 'hear' their clients' incest stories in order to develop a contextual understanding of victimization and its consequences.

Practitioners who lack the ability to understand the full meaning of victimization and its consequences often interpret the pain and hurt expressed by incest survivors as evidence of psychopathology. A helping paradigm that operates from a pathogenic focus is less likely to tap into clients' resilience because 'we can only see and know that which our paradigms allow us to see and know' (Barnard, 1994, p. 137). This way of viewing individuals and their responses to trauma leaves many facets of their experiences unnoticed or distorted. A pathogenic focus does not take into account how incest survivors are actively engaged in 'health-inducing' (Wade, 1997) resistance to their childhood victimization and its consequences. Taking a resilience perspective does not deny the real trauma of sexual abuse. That perspective instead contests the belief that people who endure such hardships are incapacitated for life or are unable to achieve their potential. Viewing protective strategies as resistance to victimization is consistent with empowerment and strengths-oriented helping paradigms that emphasize individuals' strengths and resources (Gutierrez, Parsons, & Cox, 1998; Saleebey, 2006).

A rich source of understanding can be found in the personal stories of child incest victims (Mossige, Jensen, Gulbrandsen, Reichelt, & Tjersland, 2005). During exploration of these stories, the helping professional may ask questions similar to those used in this research in order to elucidate the means by which childhood victims redefine themselves as survivors and the strategies they use to cope. Identifying and building on the positive aspects of the self that have their origins in resistance to victimization then becomes the central focus in treatment.

McMillen et al. (1995) suggest that 'Clinicians cannot change the abusive experiences encountered by their clients; they can only hope to influence reactions to the abuse' (pp. 1042–1043). In keeping with this, findings from this study demonstrate that one of the foremost services a mental health professional can provide an incest survivor is to identify her resilient capacities. Doing so provides hope and opportunity for her to envision her life as successful (Wood & Roche, 2001).

## Conclusion

Previous research shows that survivors of childhood incest suffer adverse consequences that may leave them lacking in several areas of psychosocial functioning. Yet a list of symptoms tells us little about the worlds of violence through which survivors have travelled and about what they can teach us. Having individuals share their stories of childhood victimization validates their wisdom and experiences and, at the same time, helps to develop a deeper understanding of the many dimensions of healing from incest. The findings of this study uncover protective processes that help incest survivors resist the destructive experiences of their childhoods. Participants provided numerous examples of their resistance, such as defying their perpetrators, exercising their self-determination, accessing social support, giving back to others, and resolving to heal. Ultimately, sharing their experiences of trauma and recovery showed how survivors interact with stressors over time and are able to access resources within themselves and their environments that often go beyond initial coping efforts.

## REFERENCES

Ai, A.L., & Park, C.L. (2005). Possibilities of the positive following violence and trauma: Informing the coming decade of research. *Journal of Interpersonal Violence, 20*(2), 242–50.

Barnard, C. (1994). Resiliency: A shift in our perception? *American Journal of Family Therapy, 22*(2), 135–44.

Binder, R.L., McNiel, D.E., & Goldstone, R.L. (1996). Is adaptive coping possible for adult survivors of sexual abuse? *Psychiatric Services, 47*(2), 186–8.

Briere, J., & Runtz, M. (1993). Childhood sexual abuse: Long-term sequelae and implications for psychological assessment. *Journal of Interpersonal Violence, 8*(3), 312–30.

Browne, A., & Finkelhor, D. (1986). Impact of child sexual abuse: A review of the literature. *Psychological Bulletin, 99*(1), 66–77.

Byrd, R. (1994). Assessing resilience in victims of childhood maltreatment (Doctoral dissertation, Pepperdine University). *Dissertation Abstracts, 5503.*

Ceresne, L. (1995). Reflections on resilience: Narratives of sexually abused women's coping and healing strategies (Doctoral dissertation, Dalhousie University.) *Dissertation Abstracts, International, 35*(05), 2078A.

Coffey, P., Leitenberg, H., Henning, K., Turner, T., & Bennett, R. (1996). Mediators of the long-term impact of child sexual abuse: Perceived stigma, betrayal, powerlessness, and self-blame. *Child Abuse & Neglect, 20*(5), 447–55.

Cohen, J.A., Mannarino, A.P., Berliner, L., & Deblinger, E. (2000). Trauma-focused cognitive behavioural therapy for children and adolescents. *Journal of Interpersonal Violence, 15*(11), 1202–23.

Cohen, J.A., Mannarino, A.P., & Knudsen, K. (2005). Treating sexually abused children: One year follow-up of a randomized controlled trial. *Child Abuse & Neglect, 29*, 135–45.

Courtois, C.A. (1988). *Healing the incest wound: Adult survivors in therapy.* New York: W.W. Norton.

Deblinger, E., Steer, R.A., & Lippmann, J. (1999). Two-year follow-up study of cognitive behavioural therapy for sexually abused children suffering post-traumatic stress symptoms. *Child Abuse & Neglect, 23*(12), 1371–78.

Denzin, N.K., & Lincoln, Y.S. (Eds.) (1998). *The landscape of qualitative research.* Thousand Oaks, CA: Sage.

Draucker, C.B. (1992). Construing benefit from a negative experience of incest. *Western Journal of Nursing Research, 14*(3), 343–57.

Draucker, C.B. (1995). A coping model for adult survivors of childhood sexual abuse. *Journal of Interpersonal Violence, 10*, 159–75.

Elliott, D.M. (1994). Impaired object relations in professional women molested as children. *Psychotherapy, 31*, 79–86.

Feinauer, L., Hilton, H.G., & Callahan, E.H. (2003). Hardiness as a moderator of shame associated with childhood sexual abuse. *American Journal of Family Therapy, 31*, 65–78.

Feinauer, L.L., & Stuart, D.A. (1996). Blame and resilience in women sexually abused as children. *American Journal of Family Therapy, 24*(1), 31–40.

Fraser, M. (1997). *Risk and resilience in childhood: An ecological perspective.* Washington, DC: NASW Press.

Futa, K.T., Nash, C.L., Hansen, D.J., & Garben, C.P. (2003). Adult survivors of childhood abuse: An analysis of coping mechanisms used for stressful childhood memories and current stressors. *Journal of Family Violence, 18*(4), 227–39.

Garmezy, N. (1987). Stress, competence, and development: Continuities in the study of schizophrenic adults, children vulnerable to psychopathology, and the search for stress resistant children. *American Journal of Orthopsychiatry, 57*(2), 159–73.

Glaser, B.G. (2001). *The grounded theory perspective: Conceptualization contrasted with description.* Mill Valley, CA: Sociology Press.

Gutierrez, L.M., Parsons, R.J., & Cox, E.O. (Eds.). (1998). *Empowerment in social work practice: A sourcebook.* Pacific Grove, CA: Brooks/Cole.

Harvey, M.R., Mishler, E.G., Koenen, K., & Harney, P.A. (2000). In the aftermath of sexual abuse: Making and remaking meaning in narratives of trauma and recovery. *Narrative Inquiry, 10*(2), 291–311.

Herman, J. (1997). *Trauma and recovery.* New York: Basic.

Himelein, M.J., & McElrath, J.V. (1996). Resilient child sexual abuse survivors: Cognitive coping and illusion. *Child Abuse & Neglect, 20*(8), 747–58.

Hyman, B., & Williams, L. (2001). Resilience among women survivors of child sexual abuse. *Affilia, 16*(2), 198–219.

Kelly, L. (1988). *Surviving sexual violence.* Cambridge: Polity 161.

Liem, J.H., James, J.B., O'Toole, J.G., & Boudewyn, A.C. (1997). Assessing resilience in adults with histories of childhood sexual abuse. *American Journal of Orthopsychiatry, 67*(4), 594–606.

Masten, A.S. (2001). Ordinary magic: Resilience processes in development. *American Psychologist, 56*(3), 227–38.

McMillen, J.C., Zuravin, S., & Rideout, G.B. (1995). Perceptions of benefit from child sexual abuse. *Journal of Consulting and Clinical Psychology, 63*, 1037–43.

Morrow, S.L., & Smith, M.L. (1995). Constructions of survival and coping by women who have survived childhood sexual abuse. *Journal of Counseling Psychology, 42*(1), 24–33.

Mossige, S., Jensen, T.K., Gulbrandsen, W., Reichelt, S., & Tjersland, O.A. (2005). Children's narratives of sexual abuse: What characterizes them and how do they contribute to meaning? *Narrative Inquiry, 15*(2), 377–404.

Neumann, D. A., Houskamp, B. M., Pollock, V. E., & Briere, J. (1996). The long-term sequelae of childhood sexual abuse in women: A meta-analytic review. *Child Maltreatment, 1*(1), 6–16.

Oktay, J.S. (2004). Grounded theory. In D. Padgett (Ed.), *The qualitative research experience* (pp. 23–46). Belmont, CA: Wadsworth/Thomson Learning.

Perrott, K., Morris, E., Martin, J., & Romans, S. (1998). Cognitive coping styles of women sexually abused in childhood: A qualitative study. *Child Abuse & Neglect, 22,* 1135–49.

Romans, S.E., Martin, J.L., Anderson, J.C. , O'Shea, M.L., & Mullen, P.E. (1995). Factors that mediate between child sexual abuse and adult psychological outcome. *Psychological Medicine, 25,* 127–42.

Romans, S.E., Martin, J., & Mullen, P. (1996). Women's self-esteem: A community study of women who report and do not report childhood sexual abuse. *British Journal of Psychiatry, 169,* 696–704.

Russell, D., & Bolen, R.M. (2000). *The epidemic of rape and child sexual abuse in the United States.* Thousand Oaks, CA: Sage.

Rutter, M. (1987). Psychosocial resilience and protective mechanisms. *American Journal of Orthopsychiatry, 57*(3), 216–24.

Saleebey, D. (2006). *The strengths perspective in social work practice.* Boston: Allyn & Bacon.

Scalzo, J. (1991). Beyond survival: Keys to resilience among women who experienced childhood sexual abuse (Doctoral dissertation, Simon Fraser University). *Dissertation Abstracts International, 54*(04), 2222A.

Sigmon, S.T., Greene, M.P., Rohan, K.J., & Nichols, J.E. (1996). Coping and adjustment in male and female survivors of childhood sexual abuse. *Journal of Child Sexual Abuse, 5*(3), 57–76.

Silver, R.L., Boon, C., & Stones, M.H. (1983). Searching for meaning in misfortune: Making sense of incest. *Journal of Social Issues, 39*(2), 61–102.

Strauss, A., & Corbin, J. (1998). Grounded theory methodology: An overview. In N. Denzin & Y. Lincoln (Eds.), *Strategies of qualitative inquiry* (pp. 158–83). Thousand Oaks, CA: Sage.

Trickett, P.K., Reiffman, A., Horowitz, L.A., & Putnam, F.W. (1997). Characteristics of sexual abuse trauma and the prediction of developmental outcomes. In D. Cicchetti & S.L. Toth (Eds.), *Developmental perspectives on trauma: Theory, research, and intervention* (Vol. 8, pp. 289–314). New York: University of Rochester Press.

Valentine, L., & Feinauer, L.L. (1993). Resilience factors associated with female survivors of childhood sexual abuse. *American Journal of Family Therapy, 21*(3), 216–24.

Wade, A. (1997). Small acts of living: Everyday resistance to violence and other forms of oppression. *Contemporary Family Therapy: An International Journal, 19*(1), 23–39.

Werner, E., & Smith, R. (1992). *Overcoming the odds: High risk children from birth to adulthood*. Ithaca, NY: Cornell University Press.

Wood, G.G., & Roche, S.E. (2001). Representing selves, reconstructing lives: Feminist group work with women survivors of male violence. *Social Work with Groups, 23*(4), 5–23.

# 4 Fostering Post-traumatic Growth in Adolescent Immigrants

RONI BERGER

The model of *post-traumatic growth* (PTG) is one of the evolving theories of resilience (Calhoun & Tedeschi, 1999, 2006), focusing on the human potential to grow and achieve positive outcomes from encounters with highly stressful life events. Following previous conceptual frameworks that have been developed to explain the emergence of positive changes in the aftermath of trauma, PTG offers conceptualization and empirical credibility to the dimensions and process of gaining personal benefits from struggling with adversities in diverse, cross-cultural contexts. This chapter offers practice principles for applying the model of PTG to inform understanding and effective intervention for addressing the needs of individuals experiencing the dual stress of adolescence and immigration-related challenges.

It is estimated that 7% to 10% of the 191 million documented immigrants and refugees globally are adolescents, aged twelve to eighteen (Castles & Miller, 1998; Hernandez & Charney, 1998). Three different groups have been called immigrant adolescents: youth who are born in the culture of relocation to foreign-born parents, those who immigrate as children and become adolescents in the culture of relocation (named the '1.5 generation' [Portes & Rumbant, 1996]), and those who relocate during their adolescent years. The latter are the focus of this chapter.

Immigrant adolescents are positioned at the intersection of two challenging processes: the developmental coming of age and circumstantial relocation. Each of these processes in itself is stressful and involves multiple physical, emotional, and social losses. Transitions from one culture to another, and from childhood to adulthood, have been associated with challenging one's sense of self, tugging at the roots of one's identity, and raising fundamental issues of belonging (Berger, 1996; Blos, 1979; Erikson, 1968; Garza-Guerrero, 1974; Grinberg & Grinberg,

1989; Harper & Lantz, 1996; Ory, Simons, Verhulst, & Leenders, 1991). Crucial questions arise as to whether struggling with the adolescence-immigration intersection offers not only negative consequences, but also the potential for personal growth and for measures to enhance such growth. To date, these questions have not been addressed.

Traditionally, both empirical and clinical immigration literature have overemphasized pathology whilst minimizing the salutary effects of relocation during adolescence (Berger & Weiss, 2002; Witmer & Culver, 2001). Numerous studies have documented the negative effects of immigration and adolescence-related stress, but few have addressed post-traumatic growth relating to the achievement of positive changes either following immigration (Berger & Weiss, 2006) or during adolescence (Milam, Ritt-Olson, & Unger, 2004; Salter & Stallard, 2004). None, in fact, have addressed the question of what benefits and growth are shown by adolescent immigrants that derive from their unique experience. Given this dearth of data, this chapter is based on conceptual, anecdotal, and clinical knowledge of adolescent immigrants rather than empirical evidence.

The current work is informed by the PTG model, which addresses the human potential to grow and achieve positive outcomes following encounters with highly stressful events (Calhoun & Tedeschi, 2006). Specifically, the PTG model postulates personal growth as an outcome of cognitive-emotional processing of challenges triggered by a stressor event (Weiss & Berger, in press). Furthermore, trauma is understood as a subjective experience of a stressor event as shaking one's assumptions about the self and the world. In this regard PTG mirrors resilience theory, as both constructs highlight positive growth and development under adverse circumstances. The discussion of PTG in immigrant adolescents will have four parts. First, challenges of immigration, adolescence, and immigration during adolescence will be reviewed. Second, the construct of PTG and related concepts will be discussed. Third, a number of strategies for enhancing PTG in adolescent immigrants are suggested. Finally, the implications of this theoretical lens for future research and programming will be explored.

## Challenges

### Challenges of Immigration

Immigration has been described as an earthquake. It causes major disruption in a person's life, an uprooting which may lead to social, economic, and cultural insecurity, as well as creating an 'existential vacuum' and disconfirmation of one's core assumptions about the world (Berger, 1996; Garza-Guerrero, 1974; Grinberg & Grinberg, 1989; Harper & Lantz, 1996; Ory et al., 1991; Stewart, 1986). Immigration is an experience that involves multiple losses and major changes in one's life. *Objective changes,* conceptualized as *culture loss,* include loss of employment, financial security, social status, familiarity with one's physical environment, and relationships. Also potentially lost are an understanding of one's way of life and one's command of the language to frame ideas, communicate, and express oneself (Furnham & Bochner, 1986; Stewart, 1986). *Subjective changes,* called *culture shock,* include challenges to one's ability to adequately perceive reality and context, a diminished capacity to interpret reality as it is perceived, and the shaking up of emotions and one's self-definition.

These losses occur throughout the immigration process, in which three phases have been identified. The *departure* phase includes pre-immigration deliberation, planning, and preparations as well as separation from people, places, and possessions, sometimes irreversibly. The *transit* phase refers to the actual relocation from the country of origin to the new country, which may involve prolonged transition periods in refugee camps or detention centres as well as dangerous border crossings. The *resettlement* phase involves adjustment to the new culture, finding employment and housing, learning the language, rules, and norms of one's host community, and building a new life (Garza-Guerrero, 1974; Stewart, 1986).

Each of these phases carries its own stresses, which may create and intensify pre-immigration psycho-social issues, marital discord, and parent–child relationships. These stresses may also mutually exacerbate each other. For example, absence of command of the language can limit employment opportunities. Because of intensified stresses, immigration has been viewed as a potentially traumatic event, an experience that 'represents significant challenges to the adaptive resources of the individual' (Tedeschi & Calhoun, 2004, p. 1).

*Challenges of Adolescence*

Adolescence is a developmental period characterized by more biological, psychological, and social role changes than at any other stage of life except infancy (Feldman & Elliott, 1990; Holmbeck, 1994; Lerner, Villarruel, & Castellino, 1999). Making the transition from childhood to young adulthood involves coping with changes to one's body, cognitive ability, emotional development, and self-identity. At the same time society makes numerous demands on the individual, such as enhancing independence from one's family, establishing peer and inter-gender relationships, undertaking new roles and tasks, and making crucial educational and vocational decisions, some of which have long-term implications.

Given the magnitude of the aforementioned changes and their potential effects, it is not surprising that there are also significant changes in the types and frequency of health problems as well as psychological disorders during this particular period, as compared with childhood and adulthood. Major behavioural risks in adolescence include drug, alcohol, and substance use and abuse, unsafe sex, teenage pregnancy or fatherhood, school underachievement and abandonment, delinquency, crime, and violence (Williams, Holmbeck, & Greenley, 2002).

*Challenges for Immigrant Adolescents*

Adolescent immigrants face a double challenge. Coming of age in a foreign milieu requires making decisions under more stressful conditions – often with less help than is the case for non-immigrant adolescents. Immigrant youth cope with developmental and cultural transitional processes simultaneously, the effects of which are mutually exacerbated, often resulting in a 'pile-up' of stresses (Berger, 1996; Markowitz, 1997).

Adolescent immigrants experience immigration-related losses; social, economic, and cultural insecurity; and numerous changes in all aspects of their lives. At the same time they are struggling with age-related physical, cognitive, emotional, and social changes as well as new roles, responsibilities, and expectations, within an unfamiliar social and cultural context (Baptiste, 1993; Berger, 1996, 2005; Furnham & Bochner, 1986; Mirsky & Prawer, 1992; Stewart, 1986; Waters, 1996). Many of them also experience marginalization and discrimination because of their minority status. These combined challenges may be further intensified by the psychological burden of traumas related to war, natural disaster, torture, oppression, and persecution, experiences which many immigrant adolescents endure in their homelands prior to migration. In many cases the feeling of loss is further amplified by anger with parents who imposed the relocation.

These stressors contribute to unique vulnerabilities in adolescent immigrants and may manifest in mental health problems such as anxiety, confusion, identity crisis, decreased self-esteem, insecurity, frustration, anger, loneliness, and depression (Baider, Ever-Hadani, & Kaplan-DeNour, 1996; Berger, 1996; Drachman & Shen-Ryan, 1991; Garza-Guerrero, 1974; Harper & Lantz, 1996; Hernandez & Charney, 1998; Hulewat, 1996; Liebkind, 1992; Stewart, 1986).

Immigrant adolescents often have limited resources available to help them cope with these hardships. Immigration cuts them off from their natural support systems such as friends and extended family. The stability of their communities is shaken, the fabric of their culture unwoven. Their parents and other relatives are often unavailable to provide necessary help as a result of their own struggles with immigration-related challenges and lack of familiarity with the new culture.

Not surprisingly, because adolescents are immersed in their new culture at school and among their peers, they acculturate and acquire a new language more rapidly than their parents. Consequently, adolescent immigrants often serve as translators and cultural interpreters for their parents. This creates a reversal of roles, challenges the power structure in their families, and has the potential to spark intergenerational conflict. As a result, adolescents fail to see their parents as a resource to help them cope with the same environment that they are helping their parents to understand and manage (Gold, 1989; Landau-Stanton, 1985).

While they lack informal helping resources, immigrant adolescents are also often reluctant to use formal mental health services. Like many other adolescents, these youngsters tend to hold negative stereotypes of such services and are fearful that they will be stigmatized and considered 'crazy.' Furthermore, many immigrant adolescents come from cultures that disapprove of self-disclosure and the sharing of feelings and intimate information with extra-familial sources, especially representatives of the establishment. Talk therapy is therefore regarded as non-beneficial and use of traditional mental health services discouraged (Berger, 2005).

In spite of these difficulties and the identification of immigrant adolescents as high risk, studies show that in the United States 'the mental health and adjustment of children and youth in immigrant families appears to be similar to, if not better than, that of US-born children and youth in US-born families in most respects' (Hernandez & Charney, 1998, pp. 83–84). This indicates that in addition to considerable risk factors, adolescent immigrants can also be resilient in coping with the multitude of changes, stressors, and hardships of the immigration experience. They may even prosper and achieve personal growth through their experience.

## Maria: A Case Study

Maria was eleven when she moved to the United States with her mother and three older brothers to escape the political unrest and economic hardships of the Dominican Republic. They left behind Maria's primary caregiver, her grandmother, and a large extended family. The family crowded into a one bedroom apartment in a neighbourhood heavily populated by Dominicans in a northern section of New York City. Maria was enrolled in English as a second language (ESL) classes and soon gained sufficient mastery of the language. She spent most hours after school alone in the small apartment because her mother was working two jobs as a receptionist during the day and an elder caregiver during evenings and weekends while her brothers were busy with their own schooling, part-time jobs, and social lives.

As she entered middle school, Maria's teachers reported to the social worker that the girl was 'very quiet' and, though she seemed to be quite bright, she did not participate in class and appeared to be underachieving. The social worker initiated an appointment with Maria, who appeared depressed but denied any problems and declined counselling. Several months later, with her grades falling, a second interview with Maria was scheduled. This time she shared with the worker that she was being bullied by classmates and very much missed her grandmother who, in the Dominican way of 'doing things,' was her confidante and source of support. Furthermore, she refrained from sharing her difficulties with her strict and hard-working mother, whom she was afraid to disappoint and unwilling to overburden.

Maria agreed to meet with the worker during her lunch period to discuss how to address the bullying. The worker served primarily as a parental figure, listening to Maria's complaints, containing her pain, and 'lending her ego' by offering advice regarding helpful social strategies.

At one point of the relationship between Maria and the worker, Maria's mother came to the school furious, stating 'my daughter is not crazy; she does not need no shrink or psychologist.' The worker, recognizing the mother's frustration and exhaustion, was able to calm her and develop a 'parenting partnership' with her, with the worker's role defined as a helper to the mother in executing the latter's parental goals.

Gradually Maria developed a relationship with one classmate and her grades improved. Although she came to see the worker less often, Maria maintained some relationship with her until leaving for college, and continues to call for advice when encountering certain challenges.

## Post-traumatic Growth

Traditional trauma literature has been criticized for accentuating negative effects of highly stressful events on individuals and families, and minimizing salutogenic aspects of exposure to adversity. This is in spite of possibilities for growth following suffering and crisis presented in the literature and documented in cultures from ancient times. The traditional view has led us to overlook signs of resilience and the potential for post-traumatic growth (McMillen, 1999), both of which will be discussed here. During the last few decades, however, we have witnessed a growing recognition of the possibility for good outcomes following difficult experiences, accompanied by systematic empirical studies that lend credibility to this idea.

Four decades ago, Caplan (1964), for example, suggested that during marked psychological and physical disequilibrium, people make major cognitive and behavioural changes that could indicate psychological growth. One direction of such growth can be creating meaning. This is also suggested by Frankl (1984), who developed his *existential and humanistic psychology* following his experience in Nazi concentration camps. In *Man's Search for Meaning,* he described 'tragic optimism' as the human potential to turn suffering and encounters with traumatic events into achievement and accomplishment. A similar idea is echoed in Aldwin's (1994) *advanced system theory,* which suggests that adaptation to stress involves not only deviation countering, or maintaining homeostasis, but also a deviation amplification, or change-enhancing mechanism. It is this amplification that may create a positive feedback loop resulting in either long-term negative decline or, more optimistically, positive growth.

People are therefore capable of using traumatic experiences and adversities to gain wisdom for personal growth, to make positive personality changes, and to create more meaningful and productive lives. Such positive outcomes can and often do occur simultaneously with emotional distress, functional decline, and devastating outcomes created by atrocities and stressful events (Saakvitne, Tennen, & Affleck, 1998).

### Resilience

The human potential to cope and adapt successfully despite exposure to risk and adversity has been conceptualized as *resilience* (Rutter, 1987, 2001), *hardiness* (Kobasa, 1979), and *transformational coping* (Aldwin,

1994) and has been accompanied among professionals by practice models that include solution-focused, positive psychology and empowerment approaches to clinical work (DeJong & Miller, 1995; Fraser, 1997; Gutierrez, Parsons, & Cox, 1998; Saleeby, 1997; Werner & Smith, 1992). Some of these models emphasize the ability of individuals to 'rebound' (Kobasa, 1979; Rutter, 2001) while others emphasize the development of people's capacity to cope (Aldwin, 1994).

Conceptualizing, operationalizing, and measuring the construct of resilience has been controversial, and the debates regarding its meaning and nature, such as whether it is a trait, a process, or an outcome, have yielded numerous definitions, models, and methods of measurement (Fraser, Richman, & Galinsky, 1999; Glantz & Johnson, 1999; Lepore & Revenson, 2006). In spite of these controversies, a widely accepted definition of resilience is that it is the ability to bounce back after experiencing stress, trauma, and other negative life events (NASW, 2004) and to successfully adapt and recover despite challenging or threatening circumstances (Masten, Best, & Garmezy, 1990).

Resilience is viewed as a multidimensional and ever-changing product of individual and contextual factors (Ungar, 2001; Waller, 2001). Dimensions of resilience include *resistance, recovery*, and *reconfiguration*. Resistance refers to the ability to not be affected by the stressful event. Recovery is the ability to successfully overcome adversity, bounce back, and continue to develop in ways that are defined as normal by one's cultural group. Reconfiguration is the capacity to become stronger and more resourceful following adversity, so that one is better equipped to face and successfully cope with additional stressors that may present themselves in the future (Lepore & Revenson, 2006; Walsh, 1998).

*Individual factors* shaping resilience relate to recovery (as above). These factors include aspects of temperament, coping style, and personality traits such as assertiveness, self-efficacy, problem-solving skills, tolerance for uncertainty, hope and optimism, as well as gender and religiosity (Lepore & Revenson, 2006; O'Leary, Alday, & Ickovics, 1998; Ungar, 2001). Although there is ample evidence that the aforementioned personality traits are related to resilience, the mechanisms and pathways of this relationship remain unclear.

*Contextual factors* include relational, social, and cultural environments that bring with them social support from family, friends, and spiritual sources. The availability of effective parenting, mentors, and role models as well as access to community resources such as housing, education, employment, health, safety, spiritual, and recreational opportunities are also important contextual factors (Lepore & Revenson, 2006; Ungar, 2001). The interaction between individual and environmental factors as well as the degree of compatibility between them (that is, the degree to which the nature and availability of social resources fit the individual style) also determine and shape resilience (Lepore & Revenson, 2006).

*Post-traumatic Growth*

Concurrent with discussions of resilience, there has been growing interest in the concepts of post-traumatic growth (PTG) and *thriving* (O'Leary et al., 1998). These concepts suggest a 'value-added' model that posits not only ways of coping successfully with stressful and potentially traumatic events, but also achieving benefits from that struggle. Thus, events perceived as undermining one's basic assumption about self and the world, conceptualised as traumatic, may lead eventually to positive outcomes that may not have been achieved had the stressor event not occurred. Struggling with adversity therefore holds out the possibility of something more than survival or recovery to a previous state of equilibrium following exposure to a stressor. The stressful experience can also propel one towards achieving emotional and psychological development, functioning beyond one's previous level of adaptation and reaching states of well-being that would not have been reached without the occurrence of the stressful or traumatic event. These extra benefits have been conceptualized as PTG (Linley & Joseph, 2004; Tedeschi & Calhoun, 1995) and defined as an individual's perceptions of significant positive changes resulting from the struggle with a life crisis or trauma (O'Leary et al., 1998; Schaefer & Moos, 1992; Tedeschi & Calhoun, 1995, 2006; Weiss, 2004). Milam et al. (2004) explain that 'PTG is considered more than just adaptation or being resilient, it is thriving; moving beyond one's original levels of functioning' (p. 193).

Various approaches to understanding the mechanism that enables growth following suffering have been suggested. Kelly (1955) has identified two distinct processes in which personal benefits from trauma transpire: *gradual growth*, which involves an ongoing process in which a new system is elaborated upon, and *sudden restructuring*, referring to instantaneous insight that leads to significant change. Similarly, Lazarus and Folkman (1984), who studied stress and coping, introduced in their *transactional model* the idea of cognitive appraisal of events. When people are exposed to stressful events, they can appraise the situation as *harmful* (that is, damage or injury that has already occurred), a *threat* (potential damage or injury), or a *challenge* (an opportunity for growth and mastery). Importantly, recognition of the potential for post-traumatic growth does not imply that the stressor event is traumatic in the sense that it represents a threat to one's assumptions about self and the world as well as one's well-being, causing emotional distress. Rather, the potential for post-traumatic growth postulates personal growth as an outcome of cognitive-emotional processing of the challenges triggered by the stressor event.

Furthermore, according to the related *social-cognitive transition (SCT)* model, people have an *assumptive world*, a complex mental representation of the world shaped by sociocultural context and revised according to personal circumstances, that informs reactions to events and circumstances in one's life. When faced with an extreme event or life crisis, one's assumptive world alters to fit the experience. This change may be both positive and negative (Brennan, 2001). In this regard, Calhoun and Tedeschi (2006) emphasize the cognitive process of *rumination*, i.e., repeatedly thinking, reminiscing, and reflecting upon elements of the stressor event in an effort to make sense of the event can lead to growth.

The phenomenon of positive psychological consequences arising specifically as a result of persons coping well with stress is an emerging area of study, yielding strong support for the concept of PTG. Perceived benefits from coping with varied forms of adversity have been reported in 45% to 90% of the respondents in studies across different cultures (O'Leary et al., 1998; Tedeschi & Calhoun, 2004). Reports of post-traumatic growth have been documented following events such as severe, chronic, and life-threatening diseases (such as HIV/AIDS, arthritis, cancer, heart attacks, bone marrow transplants), infertility, birth of a seriously ill or disabled child, caring for sick relatives, natural and technological disasters, accidents, rape and sexual assault, child sexual abuse, death of a loved one, parental grief, being children of Holocaust and genocide survivors, military combat exposure, shootings, injury, and recovery from substance addiction (Affleck, Tennen, Croog, & Levine, 1987; Berger & Weiss, 2006; Calhoun & Tedeschi, 1999; Cordova, Cunningham, Carlson, & Andrykowski, 2001; Dunbar, Mueller, Medina, & Wolf, 1998; Fromm, Andrykowski, & Hunt, 1996; Lev-Weisel & Amir, 2003; Linley & Joseph, 2004; Milam et al., 2004; Weiss, 2004; Znoj & Keller, 2002).

Furthermore, the existence of PTG has been affirmed in contexts as varied as Bosnia (Powell, Rosner, Butollo, Tedeschi, & Calhoun, 2003), China (Ho, Chan, & Ho, 2004), Turkey (Kilic, personal communication, 11 June 2006), Germany (Maercker & Herrle, 2003), Israel (Berger & Weiss, 2006; Ho et al., 2004; Lev-Wiesel & Amir, 2003; Powel et al., 2003; Tedeschi & Calhoun, 2004), and, more recently, Latina immigrant communities (Berger & Weiss, 2006). However, the dimensional structure of PTG appears to be culture specific and its nature coloured by the cultural background of the individual and specific environment (Cohen, Cimbolic, Armeli, & Hettler, 1998; Weiss & Berger, 2005).

As with resilience theories, the PTG model regards the specifics of the traumatic event, the individual's personality, and his or her social context all as crucial to determining the degree of perceived PTG. It is, however, difficult to know what effects PTG has in children, adolescents, and adult immigrants given that, with very few exceptions (Berger & Weiss, 2006; Milam et al., 2004; Yaskowich, 2003), the concept has hardly been explored (Berger & Weiss, 2002).

## Fostering PTG in Immigrant Adolescents

Given the stress immigration causes adolescents and the potential for personal growth and benefits from coping with such stressful experiences, the question arises as to the role of practitioners when working with immigrant adolescents. How can we facilitate this potential for growth, and what types of intervention strategies are effective in bringing about such growth? Clinical experience offering several principles (Berger & Weiss, 2002) will be discussed and illustrated here. Within this intervention framework, principles of effective strategies for fostering PTG in adolescent immigrants include: creating a space for mourning immigration-related losses; recognizing the possibility of growth; refraining from imposing expectation for growth; creating an environment receptive of growth; creating conditions to enhance reflective rumination; exercising patience; providing role models and mentoring; using creative means of expression such as theatre and non-verbal intervention strategies (e.g., music, drawing, sculpture); and working in collaboration with adolescents' families and communities.

It is worth stating that PTG focuses on *integrating* the growth perspective into common therapeutic strategies rather than proposing an additional, specialized intervention model or method (Tedeschi & Calhoun, 2006; Weiss & Berger, in press). This is in contrast to traditional therapeutic approaches to trauma work such as EMDR (Eye Movement Desensitization Reprocessing) and cognitive-behaviour therapy approaches, which use specific intervention techniques designed to aid clients struggling with the aftermath of trauma in processing the experience and its effects.

*Creating a Space for Mourning Immigration-Related Losses*

Immigrants, when they dare to talk about their immigration-related losses, frequently report encountering comments such as, 'Your conditions here are much better so why do you complain?'; 'What did you have there that you don't have here?'; 'If things were so good there, why did you chose to come here?'; 'Why don't you go back to all those "wonderful" things that you miss?' As a result, a major challenge for the practitioner in PTG is creating conditions favourable to recognizing the losses created by immigration, losses that are often overlooked or rejected by broader society.

While for many, immigration improves economic and political conditions as well as educational opportunities, a large percentage of immigrants face a worsening of their housing conditions, fewer opportunities for employment, and a drop in social status. All immigrants encounter, at least temporarily, loss of familiarity with their physical, social and cultural environments as well as loss of language, social support systems, and identity (Berger, 2004). Furthermore, even for those whose situation improves objectively in regard to personal safety, living conditions, and medical, financial, educational, and social resources, the loss of their past is real and needs to be acknowledged before they can move forwards. Just like abused children who long for their abusive parents from whose 'care' they were removed, people relocating from the direst of circumstances in their 'motherland' may still feel a sense of loss.

For immigrant adolescents, these feelings of loss may be even more intense as a result of their often being sheltered by their parents from negative experiences that propelled the immigration decision. These adolescents may be angry with their parents for what they see as the 'arbitrary, inconsiderate, and unfair decision to relocate' (personal communication with Ana, aged fifteen, relocated with her parents and grandparents from the former Soviet Union, 15 March 2006).

Acknowledging immigration-related losses, helping adolescents to think of themselves as having experienced immense losses, giving them permission to mourn these losses, and encouraging them to find ways of processing these losses are crucial in therapeutic interventions designed to promote post-traumatic growth. Because the possibility of achieving PTG depends on attaining a certain degree of emotional regulation (Tedeschi & Calhoun, 2006), it is important to help clients normalize emotional post-traumatic reactions, allowing PTG to occur later. For example, Vilma, fifteen, and her family escaped their war-stricken homeland of Colombia and relocated to a neighbourhood heavily populated by Spanish-speaking immigrants in the Bronx, New York City. Vilma, who had aspired to a career in journalism, felt that her parents' decision to move to the United States deprived her of her language proficiency and thus of her hopes for a future as a writer. However, when she tried to express these feelings, she was often scolded by others in her community: 'You should be grateful that they took you out of the dangerous zone of political unrest and brought you to a place where you can live safely.' Such reactions have blocked Vilma's ability to openly mourn her loss.

## Recognizing the Possibility of Growth

Once these losses have been recognized, clinical interventions should focus on recognizing the possibility of growth in addition to the feelings of pain. The worker's role at this stage is to listen carefully and to identify and highlight client statements that indicate potential for positive change. As such, the worker does not instil hope in the client but cultivates the hope that the client expresses, thus enhancing recognition of potential growth as part of the client's repertoire of reactions in the aftermath of immigration. This can be done by supporting cognitive-emotional processing of the immigration experience. By fostering family rituals such as storytelling about the immigration experience, for example, professionals can help adolescents and their families identify and remove potential obstacles to the process of PTG.

## Refraining from Imposing Expectation for Growth

Whilst it is important that the professional recognize positive potential for growth following immigration, all efforts should be made to refrain from creating more stress by imposing expectations for such growth. The role of the worker is not directly to elicit PTG, but rather to help the client rebuild her damaged or shattered world view, developing a new life narrative that incorporates loss in a meaningful way (Tedeschi & Calhoun, 2006). The following dialogue with Vilma, conducted during an interview with the author, illustrates the fine line practitioners are walking between enabling and not pushing:

VILMA: There is no point in making the effort. I am never going to make it. It is a lost cause. I do not have the words; there are all these Americans who are better at that than me. I ... [shrugs her shoulders]

WORKER: This sounds really difficult. Can you describe to me an example when you felt like you needed words that you did not have?

VILMA: That other day in class the teacher wanted us to talk about a situation that changes our life. I wanted to explain how difficult it is to leave your country and home and friends and pet and family, but they would not understand and I did not even know how to begin to say it, and in English too.

WORKER: You have all these experiences and you could not find at that moment a way to let others know about them.

VILMA: I am not sure if I ever will be able to.

WORKER: You really make me understand clearly your doubt if you will be ever able to share your feeling here in the U.S.

VILMA: Right. It is so difficult.

WORKER: Yes, you make me see clearly how difficult it is for you.

VILMA: How can you understand if you never had to deal with it?

WORKER: Well, I am not sure if I do understand as well as you would like me to, but I really think that you make me see how it is for you. At least a little bit.

VILMA: Well, I do not know. I will have to think if I can try to make the teacher and students in my class understand too. Maybe ...

*Creating an Environment Receptive of Growth*

In addition to recognizing potential for PTG, the worker can offer legitimization and validation of this by creating an environment that is receptive of growth. This is particularly important when social expectations for continuing grief discourage relating positive changes to the specific trauma, and is especially true for refugees who have escaped war, natural disaster, and political strife. They often hesitate and feel guilty when experiencing positive changes following their adversity. The worker can alleviate such emotions by establishing an environment that is receptive and sympathetic to such changes.

*Creating Conditions to Enhance Reflective Rumination*

Cognition is central in the transformation of trauma into triumph: cognitive appraisal of stressor events and rumination are key to PTG. Because effective rumination, focusing on one reaction to and coping with the difficulty, is more likely to produce PTG than brooding rumination, or constantly revisiting the traumatic events in detail (Tedeschi & Calhoun, 2006), it is advisable to create conditions that enhance the former. This means helping the client to redefine basic concepts, such as strengths (Calhoun & Tedeschi, 1999), as well as exploring successful coping with previous traumatic events. The practitioner should also keep in mind that PTG may be more a phenomenological than behavioural change, where the person reports feeling transformed for the better rather than manifesting observable and measurable change. Attending to existential, spiritual, and religious themes or dilemmas of the immigrant is therefore important.

*Exercising Patience*

PTG requires going through a painful process of trauma-related rumination (Berger & Weiss, 2002; Calhoun & Tedeschi, 1999). Furthermore, recognizing and achieving growth after struggling with a stressor event can be a lengthy process (Lepore & Revenson, 2006), with PTG manifesting later in intervention rather than sooner. Short-circuiting this process should therefore be avoided, making the timing of this processing critical in the therapeutic process. The worker needs to be patient, teaching her client to be patient with the pace of the progress. Particularly following immigration, reaching PTG may be delayed because of the unique nature of the event as a stressor process. The extensive logistical and practical activities in the post-migration phase, such as learning a new language and adjusting to a new school system and social norms, often require immigrants to be immersed in these activities (Drachman & Paulino, 2005) and to delay addressing the stress of immigration, including potential PTG.

*Providing Role Models*

One means of facilitating PTG is by exposing adolescents to role models who have experienced similar traumatic stressors and achieved personal growth. This can be done by involving the immigrant adolescent in a group with other immigrant adolescents, some of whom may be closer to realizing PTG and are now ready to help others. The effectiveness of group work with immigrants in general and with immigrant adolescents in particular has been documented elsewhere (Berger, 1996; Glassman & Skolnik, 1984). Using the group modality to enhance PTG among adolescent immigrants can help achieve two goals concurrently. First, the group may serve as a source of social support and compensate for the loss of the natural peer group caused by immigration. Second, the group may offer models for PTG. A group composed of participants who have differing amounts of distance from traumatic stressors will increase the likelihood that some members have already reached PTG and can serve as role models to others.

### Providing Mentoring

An additional way to support PTG in immigrant adolescents is through personal mentoring. According to this model, a volunteer builds a professionally supported one-on-one relationship to help guide at-risk children and youth. The use of self by a practitioner or mentor who has himself experienced PTG following immigration or other stressor-related growth may serve to make youth aware of opportunities for positive changes by offering them insights into their own experience as well as advice and encouragement. Although there is little empirically based consensus on the effectiveness of mentoring programs or on the core principles and components that define effective mentoring (Bellamy, Springer, Sale, & Espiritu, 2004; Royse, 1998), a small number of studies suggest that mentoring enhances academic achievement and employment success. It also contributes to decreasing substance abuse by teens (De Anda, 2001; Rhodes, Reddy, & Grossman, 2005). This model and the preferred characteristics of the mentor (for example, the relative benefits of a volunteer who is an immigrant) should be adjusted to address the specific needs of immigrant adolescents.

### Using Creative Means

An additional way to develop PTG is by means of creative writing, non-verbal techniques, community theatre, and additional expressive strategies that enable adolescents to process their experience and explore paths for growth from a safe emotional distance (Berger, 1994).

*Working in Collaboration with Adolescents' Families and Communities*

Practitioners should be willing and able to work in collaboration with the adolescent family and community. Collaborating with teachers, informal mentors, sport group leaders, and other adults involved in the adolescent's life can be beneficial. Extra-therapeutic factors such as soliciting empathy, validation, and acceptance from family, colleagues, and other significant figures in the adolescent's life play a major role in enhancing PTG (Woodward & Joseph, 2003).

Finally, to create conditions conducive to PTG in immigrant youth, communities of compatriots and other immigrants and non-immigrants need to be informed about PTG. Social support has been suggested as of importance in enhancing PTG, although research findings regarding the association of PTG and the availability of social support have been inconsistent. For example, a recent study of PTG in Latina immigrants to the United States failed to find such a relationship (Berger & Weiss, 2006). Nevertheless, community education programs can increase awareness of the issues of immigrants and help reduce prejudice, xenophobia, and racism. The lessening of the marginalization of immigrants and the opening of venues for better integration are also potential benefits (Berger, 2004).

## Conclusion

Relocating from one's culture of origin is difficult under the best of circumstances, as is coping with the transition from childhood to adulthood. The combined challenge of these processes creates a stressor event that situates adolescent immigrants as a population at risk (Berger, 2005). However, adolescent immigrants also possess the capacity to cope with and prosper amid the multitude of changes and hardships presented by the immigration experience, whilst simultaneously struggling with age-related development. A critical role of youth workers serving this population group is, therefore, to facilitate this process of prospering.

To effectively achieve the goal of facilitating PTG in immigrant adolescents, it is of utmost importance to maintain a double lens: while the practitioner needs to recognize, understand, and acknowledge the multiple losses, challenges, and pain of coming of age in a new, unfamiliar, and often hostile and xenophobic environment, she needs to simultaneously educate herself regarding the potential for growth following the struggle with traumatic events. She must remain open to this possibility and attentive to cues from the client that indicate these benefits from the experience. Thus, the practitioner needs to develop the ability to concurrently accompany adolescents in the process of mourning while facilitating their growth. This can be achieved by validating and normalizing adolescents' feelings, cultivating their expressed hopes, supporting their struggle to process the immigration experience, and patiently providing a holding environment that is receptive of the adolescent's effort to engage in the rumination process.

Focusing on the individual level in serving adolescent immigrants is not enough. Working with the adolescent's immediate and extended family and peer group can help promote relational aspects of resilience. Given that adolescent immigrants tend to socialize with youth who share their situation (Eisikovits, 2000), and because other family members also face immigration-related challenges, it is important to work with adolescents in the context of their familial and sociocultural environments.

In addition, using media, continuing education programs, theatre, art exhibitions, publicity campaigns, and similar public venues to inform the public at large on the topics of immigration-related stressors and PTG may help to create a supportive environment. These can enhance positive growth in immigrant youth as well as appropriate meaningful policies. For example, encouraging productions in community theatres or initiating murals in public locations (schools, churches, parks, and municipal buildings) that present challenges and growth potential following immigration are some of the ways in which awareness of and support for immigrant communities can be promoted.

While practice-based experience allows the suggestion of guidelines for enhancing PTG among immigrant adolescents, many questions remain open for empirical inquiry. Such questions include: What is the differential potential for PTG in various groups of youth, and what personal and environmental factors correlate with this potential? Which of the specific intervention strategies are most effective in enhancing PTG in immigrant adolescents? What is the differential effectiveness of diverse strategies with specific population groups (relative to age, culture of origin, immigration status, family configuration) of immigrant adolescents? What processes and mechanisms associated with each intervention strategy best enhance PTG in immigrant adolescents? Answers to these and related questions would advance professional understanding of PTG and development of training programs to equip practitioners in the helping professions with the knowledge and skills necessary to enable and support PTG in immigrant adolescents.

## REFERENCES

Affleck, G., Tennen, H., Croog, S., & Levine, S. (1987). Causal attribution, perceived benefits, and morbidity after a heart attack: An 8–year study. *Journal of Consulting and Clinical Psychology, 55*, 29–35.

Aldwin, C.M. (1994). *Stress, coping and development: An integrative perspective.* New York: Guilford Press.

Baider, L., Ever-Hadani, P., & Kaplan-DeNour, A. (1996). Crossing new bridges: The process of adaptation and psychological distress of Russian immigrants in Israel. *Psychiatry: Interpersonal and Biological Processes, 59*, 175–83.

Baptiste, D. (1993). Immigrant families, adolescents, and acculturation: Insights for therapists. *Marriage and Family Review, 19*, 341–63.

Bellamy, N.D., Springer, U.F., Sale, E.W., & Espiritu, R. (2004). Structuring a multi-site evaluation for youth mentoring programs to prevent teen alcohol and drug use. *Journal of Drug Education, 34*, 197–212.

Berger, R. (1994). *Using community theater in group work with adolescent immigrants: The Russian experience.* Paper presented at the 16th Annual Symposium, Association for the Advancement of Social Work with Groups, New York.

Berger, R. (1996). Group work with immigrant adolescents. *Journal of Child and Adolescent Group Therapy, 6*, 169–79.

Berger, R. (2004). *Immigrant women tell their stories.* New York, NY: Haworth Press.

Berger, R. (2005). It takes a community to raise an adolescent: Community based clinical services for immigrant adolescents. In A. Lightborn & P. Sessions (Eds.), *Community based clinical practice* (pp. 441–58). New York: Oxford University Press.

Berger, R., & Weiss, T. (2002). Immigration and posttraumatic growth: A missing link. *Journal of Immigrant & Refugee Services, 1*(2), 21–39.

Berger, R., & Weiss, T. (2006). Posttraumatic growth in Latina immigrant women. *Journal of Immigrant and Refugee Studies, 4*, 55–72.

Blos, P. (1979). *The adolescent passage.* New York: International University Press.

Brennan, J. (2001). Adjustment to cancer: Coping or personal transition? *Psycho-Oncology, 10*, 1–18.

Calhoun, L.G., & Tedeschi, R.G. (1999). *Facilitating posttraumatic growth: A clinician's guide*. Mahwah, NJ: Lawrence Erlbaum.

Calhoun, L.G., & Tedeschi, R.G. (Eds.). (2006). *Handbook of posttraumatic growth*. Mahwah, NJ: Lawrence Erlbaum.

Caplan, G. (ed.). (1964). *Principles of preventive psychiatry*. New York: Basic Books.

Caplan, G. (1981). Mastery of stress: Psychosocial aspects. *American Journal of Psychiatry, 138*, 413–420.

Castles, S., & Miller, M.J. (1998). *The age of migration: International population movements in the modern world*. New York: Guilford Press.

Cohen, L.H., Cimbolic K., Armeli S.R., & Hettler, T.R. (1998). Quantitative assessment of thriving. *Journal of Social Issues, 54*, 323–35.

Cordova, M.J., Cunningham, L.C., Carlson, C.R., & Andrykowski, M. (2001). Posttraumatic growth following breast cancer: A controlled comparison study. *Health Psychology, 20*, 176–85.

De Anda, D. (2001). A qualitative evaluation of a mentor program for at risk youth: The participants' perspective. *Child and Adolescent Social Work Journal, 18*, 97–117.

DeJong, P., & Miller, S.D. (1995). How to interview for client strengths. *Social Work, 40*, 729–36.

Drachman, D., & Paulino, A. (Eds.) (2005). *Immigrants and social work*. New York: Haworth Press.

Drachman, D., & Shen-Ryan, A. (1991). Immigrants and refugees. In A. Gitterman (Ed.), *Social work practice with vulnerable populations* (pp. 618–46). New York: Columbia University Press.

Dunbar, H.T., Mueller, C.W., Medina, C., & Wolf, T. (1998). Psychological and spiritual growth in women living with HIV. *Social Work, 43*, 144–54.

Eisikovits, R.A. (2000). Gender differences in cross-cultural adaptation styles of immigrant youth from the former Soviet Union. *Youth & Society, 31*, 310–31.

Erikson, E. (1968). *Identity: Youth and crisis*. New York: W.W. Norton.

Feldman, S.S., & Elliott, G.R. (Eds.). (1990). *At the threshold: The developing adolescent*. Cambridge, MA: Harvard University Press.

Frankl, V.E. (1984). *Man's Search for Meaning*. New York: Washington Square Press.

Fraser, M.W. (Ed.). (1997). *Risk and resilience in childhood: An ecological perspective*. Washington, DC: NASW Press.

Fraser, M.W., Richman, J.M., & Galinsky, M.J. (1999). Risk, protection and resilience: Toward a conceptual framework for social work practice. *Social Work Research, 23,* 131–43.

Fromm, K., Andrykowski, M.A., & Hunt, J. (1996). Positive and negative psychosocial sequelae of bone marrow transplantation: Implications for quality of life assessment. *Journal of Behavioral Medicine, 19,* 221–40.

Furnham, A., & Bochner, S. (1986). *Culture shock: Psychological reactions to unfamiliar environments.* New York: Methuen.

Garza-Guerrero, A.C. (1974). Culture shock: Its mourning and the vicissitudes of identity. *Journal of the American Psychoanalytic Association, 22,* 408–29.

Glantz, M.D., & Johnson, J.L. (1999). *Resilience and development: Positive life adaptations.* New York: Kluwer Academic/Plenum.

Glassman, U., & Skolnik, L. (1984). The role of social group work in refugee resettlement. *Social Work with Groups, 7,* 45–62.

Gold, S.J. (1989). Differential adjustment among a new immigrant family members. *Journal of Contemporary Ethnography, 17,* 408–34.

Grinberg L., & Grinberg, I. (1989). *Psychoanalytic perspectives on migration and exile.* New Haven, CT: Yale University Press.

Gutierrez, L.M., Parsons, R.J., & Cox, E.O. (Eds.). (1998). *Empowerment in social work practice: A sourcebook.* Pacific Grove, CA: Brooks/Cole.

Harper, K.V., & Lantz, J. (1996). *Cross-cultural practice: Social work with diverse populations.* Chicago: Lyceum.

Hernandez, D.J., & Charney, E. (Eds.). (1998). *From generation to generation: The health and well-being of children in immigrant families.* Washington, DC: National Research Council and Institute of Medicine.

Ho, S.M.Y., Chan, C.L.W., & Ho, R.T.H. (2004). Posttraumatic growth in Chinese cancer survivors. *Psycho-Oncology, 13,* 377–89.

Holmbeck, G.N. (1994). Adolescence. In V.S. Ramachandran (Ed.), *Encyclopedia of human behavior* (Vol. 1, pp. 17–28). Orlando, FL: Academic Press.

Hulewat, P. (1996). Resettlement: A cultural and psychological crisis. *Social Work, 41*(2), 129–35.

Kelly, G.A. (1955). *The psychology of personal constructs.* New York: Norton.

Kobasa, S.C. (1979). Stressful life events, personality and health: An inquiry into hardiness. *Journal of Personality and Social Psychology, 37,* 1–11.

Landau-Stanton, J. (1985). Adolescents, families and cultural transition: A treatment model. In A. Mirkin & S. Koman (Eds.), *Handbook of adolescents and family therapy* (pp. 360–369). New York: Gardner Press.

Lazarus, R.S., & Folkman, S. (1984). *Stress, appraisal and coping.* New York: Springer.

Lepore, S.J., & Revenson, T.A. (2006). Resilience and posttraumatic growth:

Recovery, resistance and reconfiguration. In L. Calhoun & R. Tedeschi (Eds.), *Handbook of posttraumatic growth: Research and practice* (pp. 24–46). Mahwah, NJ: Lawrence Erlbaum.

Lerner, R.M., Villarruel, F.A., & Castellino, D.R. (1999). Adolescence. In W. Silverman & T. Ollendick (Eds.), *Developmental issues in the clinical treatment of children* (pp. 125–36). Boston, MA: Allyn & Bacon.

Lev-Wiesel, R., & Amir, M. (2003). Posttraumatic growth among holocaust child survivors. *Journal of Loss and Trauma, 8*, 229–37.

Liebkind, K. (1992). Ethnic identity: Challenging the boundaries of social psychology. In G. Breakwell (Ed.), *Social psychology of identity and the self concept* (pp. 147–85). London: Surrey University Press.

Linley, P.A., & Joseph, S. (2004). Positive changes following trauma and adversity: A review. *Journal of Traumatic Stress, 17*, 11–21.

Maercker, A., & Herrle, J. (2003). Long-term effects of the Dresden bombing: Relationships to control beliefs, religious belief, and personal growth. *Journal of Traumatic Stress, 16*, 579–87.

Markowitz, F. (1997). Diasporas with a difference: Jewish and Georgian teenagers' ethnic identity in the Russian Federation. *Diaspora, 6*, 331–53.

Masten, A.S., Best, K.M., & Garmezy, N. (1990). Resilience and development: Contributions from the study of children who overcome adversity. *Development and Psychopathology, 2*, 425–44.

McMillen, J.C. (1999). Better for it: How people benefit from adversity. *Social Work, 44*, 455–68.

Milam, J.E., Ritt-Olson, A., & Unger, J.B. (2004). Posttraumatic growth among adolescents. *Journal of Adolescent Research, 19*, 192–204.

Mirsky, Y., & Prawer, L. (1992). *Immigrating as an adolescent, being an adolescent as an immigrant.* Jerusalem: Elka & Van Leer Institute. (in Hebrew)

NASW (National Association of Social Workers). (2004). *Resiliency: NASW research website.* Retrieved 16 October 2004, from http://www.socialworkers.org/research/naswResearch/0804Resiliency.

O'Leary, V.E., Alday, C.S., & Ickovics, J.R. (1998). Models of life change and posttraumatic growth. In R. Tedeschi, C. Park, & L. Calhoun (Eds.), *Posttraumatic growth: Positive changes in the aftermath of crisis* (pp. 127–51). Mahwah, NJ: Lawrence Erlbaum.

Ory, F.G., Simons, M., Verhulst, F.C., & Leenders, F.R. (1991). Children who cross cultures. *Social Science and Medicine, 32*, 29–34.

Portes, A., & Rumbant, R. (1996). *Immigrant America.* Berkley, CA: University of California Press.

Powell, S., Rosner, R., Butollo, W., Tedeschi, R.G., & Calhoun, L.G. (2003).

Posttraumatic growth after war: A study with former refugees and dis-
placed people in Sarajevo. *Journal of Clinical Psychology, 59,* 71–83.
Rhodes, J.E., Reddy, R., & Grossman, J.B. (2005). The protective influence of
mentoring on adolescents' substance use: Direct and indirect pathways.
*Applied Developmental Science, 9,* 31–47.
Royse, D. (1998). Mentoring high-risk minority youth: Evaluation of the
Brothers project. *Adolescence, 33,* 145–58.
Rutter, M. (1987). Psychosocial resilience and protective mechanism. *Ameri-
can Journal of Orthopsychiatry, 57,* 316–31.
Rutter, M. (2001). Psychosocial adversity: Risk, resilience and recovery. In J.
Richman & M. Fraser (Eds.), *The context of youth violence: Resilience, risk and
protection* (pp. 13–41). Westport, CT: Praeger.
Saakvitne, K., Tennen, H., & Affleck, G. (1998). Exploring thriving in the
context of clinical trauma theory: Constructivist self development theory.
*Journal of Social Issues, 54,* 279–300.
Saleeby, D. (Ed.). (1997). *The strengths perspective in social work practice.* New
York: Longman.
Salter, E., & Stallard, P. (2004). Posttraumatic growth in child survivors of a
road traffic accident. *Journal of Traumatic Stress, 17,* 335–40.
Schaefer, J.A., & Moos, R.H. (1992). Life crises and personal growth. In B.
Carpenter (Ed.), *Personal coping: Theory, research, and application* (pp.
149–70). Westport, CT: Praeger.
Stewart, E.C.P. (1986). The survival stage of intercultural communication.
*Tokyo: International Christian University Bulletin, 1*(1), 109–21.
Tedeschi, R.G., & Calhoun, L.G. (1995). *Trauma and transformation: Growing in
the aftermath of suffering.* Thousand Oaks, CA: Sage.
Tedeschi, R.G., & Calhoun, L.G. (2004). Posttraumatic growth: Conceptual
foundations and empirical evidence. *Psychological Inquiry, 15,* 1–18.
Tedeschi, R.G., & Calhoun, L.G. (2006). Expert companions: Posttraumatic
growth in clinical practice. In L. Calhoun & R. Tedeschi (Eds.), *Handbook of
posttraumatic growth: Research and practice* (pp. 291–310). Mahwah, NJ:
Lawrence Erlbaum.
Ungar, M. (2001). Constructing narratives of resilience with high-risk youth.
*Journal of Systemic Therapies, 20,* 58–73.
Waller, M.A. (2001). Resilience in ecosystemic context: Evolution of the
concept. *American Journal of Orthopsychiatry, 71,* 290–7.
Walsh, F. (1998). *Strengthening family resilience.* New York: Guilford.
Waters, M. (1996). The intersection of gender, race and ethnicity in identity
development of Caribbean American teens. In B.J. Leadbetter & N. Way

(Eds.), *Urban girls: Resisting stereotypes, creating identities* (pp. 65–81). New York: New York University Press.

Weiss, T. (2004). Correlates of posttraumatic growth in husbands of women with breast cancer. *Psycho-Oncology, 12*, 1–9.

Weiss, T., & Berger, R. (2005). Reliability and validity of a Spanish version of the Posttraumatic Growth Inventory. *Journal of Social Work Research, 16*, 191–9.

Weiss, T., & Berger, R. (in press). Posttraumatic growth and immigration: Theory, research and practice implications. In S. Joseph & P. A. Linley (Eds.), *Trauma, recovery, and growth: Positive psychological perspectives on posttraumatic stress*. Hoboken, NJ: John Wiley and Sons.

Werner, E., & Smith, R.S. (1992). *Overcoming the odds*. Ithaca, NY: Cornell University Press.

Williams, P.G., Holmbeck, G.N., & Greenley, R.N. (2002). *Adolescent health psychology, 70*, 828–42.

Witmer, T.A., & Culver, S.M. (2001). Trauma and resilience among Bosnian refugee families: A critical review of the literature. *Journal of Social Work Research, 2*, 173–87.

Woodward, C., & Joseph, S. (2003). Positive change processes and posttraumatic growth in people who have experienced childhood abuse: Understanding vehicles of change. *Psychology and Psychotherapy: Theory, Research and Practice, 76*, 267–83.

Yaskowich, K.M. (2003). Posttraumatic growth in children and adolescents with cancer. *Dissertation Abstracts International, 63*(8–B), 3948.

Znoj, H.J., & Keller, D. (2002). Mourning parents: Considering safeguards and their relation to health. *Death Studies, 26*, 545–65.

# 5 Building a Better Mousetrap: Risk and Resilience Processes, the DSM, and the Child Psychiatrist

NORMAND CARREY

> Learning is not compulsory ... neither is survival.
>
> W. Edwards Deming

Child psychiatry and allied child mental health disciplines have seen an explosion of theory, models, and new treatments for children, adolescents, and families in the last two to three decades. To emerge as a field in its own right, child psychiatry has had to shake off its former influences of psychoanalytic theory and adult descriptive nosology, as applied to child and family problems. Still today, child psychiatry occupies an uncertain middle ground between adult psychiatry on the one hand and paediatrics on the other. As such, the field remains heavily medicalized in its approach. At the same time it has benefited from advances in attachment theory, behavioural genetics, developmental psychopathology, and psychopharmacology.

The field, from a research and practice perspective, has not, however, integrated new findings into a resilience or strengths-based perspective. This chapter explores the integration of the traditional DSM (Diagnostic and Statistical Manual of Mental Disorders) approach with emerging findings in developmental psychopathology and attachment theory, and how they can be reframed into a resilience or strengths-based perspective. I will then demonstrate through case studies how child mental health practitioners can enhance resilience processes at several levels. This chapter seeks to integrate new theories of resilience and positive youth development with more traditional areas of child psychiatry where the emphasis has been on diagnosis and treatment. It is my belief that resilience research and practice can significantly enhance traditional child psychiatric theory and practise. Although most comments in this chapter are addressed as if speaking to child psychiatrists, the comments assume a multi-disciplinary setting with child psychiatrists as team members or collaborative consultants.

## The DSM and Resilience Theory

Criticizing the DSM has become common, especially among non-medical professionals who accuse it being reductionistic and decontextualized and of pathologizing otherwise normal aspects of everyday life. Together with this, psychiatrists have been accused of being obsessed with 'labelling' (i.e., lumpers or splitters). For those not familiar with the DSM, the manual either inspires uncritical awe or is summarily dismissed as totally irrelevant. Yet the popularity and influence of this 'psychiatric bible' have been undeniable for the success of psychiatry in particular and have struck a cord that resonates with Western cultural values.

I will make two arguments to put the DSM in a context where it can be integrated within a resilience framework. The first argument is that there was a need for a DSM type of classification system in psychiatry. The DSM-III in particular, with its research diagnostic criteria, was responding to a need for a 'universal' classification system that could be agreed upon by practitioners and researchers across different countries. For example, with the same operational diagnostic criteria, a person could be diagnosed with bipolar disorder whether his psychiatrist was from New York, London, or Beirut. The appeal of universal categories in medicine was precisely what made this model so powerful and successful. As such, the pathology or organic deficit model of pathophysiology in psychiatry was borrowed from medicine. The second argument I will make is that, while the DSM has succeeded to a certain extent as a classification system, especially for traditional adult psychiatric disorders such as bipolar disorder and schizophrenia, its so-called atheoretical stance has led to its inability to incorporate more complex models of health and well-being such as developmental psychopathology and attachment theory. Such theories can inform practitioners and researchers about how positive adaptation takes place. It therefore becomes important to know how the two processes interact to complement or modify each other.

The original impetus for a DSM classification of mental disorder came from a need to obtain statistics on mental disorders as well as categorize disorders in the same manner as other branches of medicine and science. While this 'modernistic' project of psychiatry and medical power can be decried, the tradition of separating phenomenon into categories is traditionally the first step in the development of a science. Once the concept of an organic mental disorder (derangement of the brain as opposed to demonic possession) was established at the end of the eighteenth century, classification of psychiatric disorders became intricately part and parcel of treatment (Goldstein, 1987). For example, French psychiatrist Phillip Pinel's (1800) classification system distinguishing between mental retardation and functional psychoses had implications not only for diagnosis but for treatment, affecting the social and legal status of these patients. Subsequently, nosology evolved according to national traditions or schools of thought. Confusion between practitioners then ensued due to the absence of a common language and the resulting variety of interpretations given to the same phenomenon. While an oversimplification, two contemporary schools of psychiatry developed: organic/directive and psychodynamic/non-directive (Schowalter, 1989).

Early establishment of the DSM occurred simultaneously with an administrative need to categorize Second World War veterans, filling up veteran's hospitals as a result of stress-related combat disorders. DSM-I and DSM-II were conceived with this need in mind. Categorization was heavily psychoanalytic in nature, with most disorders conceptualized as 'reactions.' Subsequent incarnations of the DSM were influenced by Feighner et al.'s (1972) research criteria that operationalized specific symptoms for specific disorders (RDC or research diagnostic criteria). DSM committees were established to reach consensus for each category of diagnoses based on the RDCs. These committees were progressively composed of psychiatrists more organically oriented (the so-called neo-kraepelineans), spearheaded by the chairman of the DSM-III and III-R editorial committee, Robert Spitzer. Spitzer had a major influence on reshaping the new direction of the DSM and American psychiatry (for an interesting account of Spitzer's life, see Spiegel [2005]). This corresponded in turn with a waning influence of psychoanalysts in major teaching and research centres. New drugs for the treatment of the major psychiatric disorders, such as CPZ for psychosis, lithium for manic-depressive illness, and imipramine for the treatment of severe depression, were being increasingly utilized by psychiatrists as they abandoned the couch. At the same time, this meant a broad-base reintegration of psychiatry with the medical sciences of epidemiology, neurosciences, and genetics.

In addition to the Feighner research criteria introduced in DSM-III, a multi-axial system of classification was proposed as a comprehensive way to enhance diagnosis. Axis 1 was for major psychiatric disorders, Axis 2 was for intellectual impairments in children or personality disorders in adults, Axis 3 for medical conditions impacting on Axis 1 presentation, Axis 4 for psychosocial adversity, and Axis 5 for a rating of the highest level of functioning in the past year. This multi-axial system was introduced by Spitzer in DSM-III and was seen as significant innovation to capture other relevant variables. While there are specific DSM criteria for guiding the clinician or researcher on Axis 1 and 2, it is often left up to individual discretion as to how to conceptualize risk and resilience factors from Axis 4 in the case formulation. Most of the time clinicians, depending on their backgrounds, simply list the stressors and ignore protective factors, including psychosocial, religious, cultural and political cultural factors. This is confusing for psychiatry students and novice practitioners, who must reconcile the complex genetic and environmental interactions (including both risk and resilience factors) between the different axes. This has led to a 'hierarchical' emphasis of axis 1 type of diagnoses over other, just as important risk and resilience factors listed on the other axes.

Although the DSM claims to be 'atheoretical' by choosing to keep its descriptions at the behavioural level, any system of classification becomes the lens through which the world is apprehended. The lens that the DSM has chosen, consistent with the axial system, is the categorical as opposed to the dimensional approach. Aberrant, maladaptive behaviours or symptoms are counted until they reach a threshold for determining 'caseness' or severity. The diagnosis of a 'case' of, for example, attention deficit hyperactivity disorder (ADHD) or conduct disorder (CD) is then made. The convention of thinking of individuals as 'cases' of course rings true with the accepted nomenclature of medicine (for example, a 'case' of tuberculosis or pneumonia). Thinking about cases leads to categorical, yes/no answers with the accompanying sense of certainty: you either have a case of TB or not. These conventions are also useful in epidemiology, where cases can be counted at the population level and determine broad indices of disease such as prevalence. However, an alternative and not necessarily contradictory approach is to think of behaviour or traits as varying along a continuum or a dimension. Traits such as aggression, hyperactivity, extra-version, shyness, and intelligence, for example, can all vary along a dimension or continuum. Examples of medical parameters varying along a continuum include blood pressure, blood sugar level, and cho-lesterol levels, with the extreme end of a continuum, such as elevated blood pressure or blood sugar, defined as a maladaptive or disease state.

As it applies to child psychiatry, the DSM categorical approach has been helpful in raising awareness of the onset of various serious psy-chiatric disorders in young children. It is now known that in the major-ity of patients with anxiety disorders such as obsessive compulsive disorder (OCD), there was either a partial or a full onset of symptoms in childhood (Swedo & Pine, 2005). Mood disorders can have their onset in childhood, although it appears that in a considerable number of cases a child or a young person's mood is more reactive to environ-mental stressors and is certainly influenced by attachment status and developmental period. While the DSM has also raised awareness of first-episode mood disorders and psychosis, the hunt for precursors (early signs of psychosis) or variants (paediatric bipolar disorder) has had mixed results, generating controversy about subjecting children and youth to the effects of labelling and long-term psycho-pharmaco-logical treatment.

The emphasis by DSM researchers on family history, in an attempt to ferret out possible genetic contributions of psychiatric disorders across generations (susceptibility genes), has produced increased awareness of psychiatric disorder transmission in families. In a family therapy context this can have the effect of relieving a parent of guilt and self-blame and, if warranted, lead to them seeking treatment for themselves. There has, however, been a tendency for non-medical practitioners to consider genetic explanations in psychiatry as deter-ministic. Genes may operate at several levels (individual characteris-tics affecting parenting, family life, etc.) and recent explanatory models advocate both risk and resilience factors operating through genetic–environmental interactions.

There are advantages and disadvantages to both approaches, but the choice of the DSM to adopt a strictly categorical approach prevents an understanding of underlying significant risk and resilience factors that may vary along different dimensions. The categorical approach may be somewhat suitable for certain psychiatric disorders, such as schizo-phrenia, bipolar disorder, or autism, although other mediating features, such as severity of the disorder, response to treatment, psychosocial support, and modes of inheritance, may vary along a dimension. The dimensional approach suggests a much more nuanced view of development across the lifespan but does not lend itself well to the sense of certainty associated with the categorical disease approach. Risk and resilience factors may interact in ways that modify each other, so that an individual may be in a developmental trajectory at one time and at another point at another time. In the next four sections, I explore how the DSM categorical approach could be incorporated into a dimensional developmental trajectory of risk and resilience framework while taking into account cultural factors, before ending with three case studies.

## Developmental Psychopathology and Resilience

Developmental psychopathology from its very inception included assessing the impact of risk and adversity on developmental adaptation. Standard developmental research designs measure multiple domains of functioning across time, incorporating how contextual processes modify risk and resilience factors (Cicchetti, 1993). This is different from a DSM categorical approach where counts of symptoms (which may vary along a dimension) reach a threshold to 'lock in' a diagnosis as invariant. In the DSM's effort to achieve diagnostic uniformity across the lifespan, it simply concedes that certain disorders have their onset in childhood (disorders usually first diagnosed in infancy, childhood, or adolescence [DSM-IV-TR, p. 39]). As a classification system, the DSM does not take into account the effect of risk and resilience variables on developmental outcome.

A more nuanced view of development needed to start by understanding the operation of what has been termed 'cumulative' risk factors. Rutter et al. (1975) and, subsequently, Sameroff, Morrison Gutman, & Peck, 2003 have documented the adverse effect of cumulative risk on developmental psychopathology. The six significant predictors of child psychopathology in the Rutter study were severe marital discord, low SES, large family size, parental criminality, maternal mental health and out-of-home placement. Children with one risk were not affected, whereas children with four or more risks had a tenfold risk for maladjustment. Appleyard, Egeland, van Dulmen, & Sroufe (2005), analyzing longitudinal data from the Minnesota at-risk urban children study, were able to demonstrate that cumulative risk was additive but that there was no evidence of a 'threshold effect' for psychopathology. That is, cumulative risk did not lock in a categorical diagnosis at one point in time. From these longitudinal studies on risk and psychopathology there was an emerging understanding that one risk does not cause one outcome, but rather multiple risks are necessary and, in addition, the same risk factors lead to multiple outcomes (e.g., maternal rejection leading to depression or conduct disorder in the child) or different risk factors interact to produce the same outcome (Burt et al., 2005; Formoso, Gonzales, & Aiken, 2000). The implication for the clinician is that cumulative and interactive risk is best conceptualized as a dimensional construct rather that a categorical construct with cut-offs and thresholds.

Recently, the field has evolved towards looking at interactions between multiple risk and resilience factors in longitudinal studies sensitive to developmental variations (Brame, Nagin, & Tremblay, 2001; Broidy et al., 2003; Moffitt, Caspi, Harrington, & Milne, 2002; Romano, Tremblay, Boulerice, & Swisher, 2005; Shaw, Gilliom, Ongoldsby, & Nagin, 2003). Statistical modelling has been utilized to separate out different developmental trajectories using person-centred analyses (Nagin & Tremblay, 1999) as opposed to variable-centred analyses. Developmental trajectories have not only allowed a more nuanced understanding of the interplay between risk and resilience, but have also provided information on how risk and resilience modify each other across developmental periods (Carrey & Ungar, 2007; Phelps et al., 2007)

This modelling work has significant implications for how we view developmental trajectories, placing the practitioner in a stronger position to understand processual factors and assisting the clinician to achieve a more comprehensive formulation and treatment plan. For example, Romano et al. (2005) studied longitudinally 'externalizing disorders' or 'disruptive behavior disorders' and found that a small but significant number (4–6%) of young children persist in their aggressive behaviour throughout childhood through adolescence and into adulthood, whereas one large group desists quickly and another large group desists later on. Shaw and colleagues (2003) were able to demonstrate the impact of maternal variables (maternal depression and maternal rejection) on the persistence of aggressive behaviour. In addition to the challenge this developmental research has for a reconceptualization of the static categories of 'externalizing disorders,' it tells us something important about intervention; some trajectories of aggressive behaviour can be prevented by early intervention targeting maternal factors, which in turn strengthen long-term attachment behavior (Shaw et al., 2003).

These longitudinal studies, by emphasizing pathways to competence through individual, familial, and community factors, have illustrated the second key point in understanding the development of resilience. Competent individuals are involved in interactional transactions with supportive or empowering persons or environments. Resilience research sensitive to ecological variables has sought to understand how individuals gain access to available resources in their environment. Although there are several examples of excellent longitudinal studies illustrating risk and resilience across time, a few in particular lend themselves well to informing a strengths-based clinical practice.

One of the oldest longitudinal studies is Project Competence, based at the University of Minnesota. Masten and O'Connor (1989) investigated the development and the role of competence in positive adaptation in children. They found that intelligence and parenting could significantly moderate the effects of adversity on psychopathology. In other words, children who had experienced adversity and had low cognitive ability (as measured by IQ, attentional difficulties, or executive functions) or inadequate parenting were more susceptible to developing conduct problems than were children facing similar risk but who had higher intelligence and better parenting. It appeared that the competent and resilient children had more resources at hand, including access to effective adults. Conversely, maladapted children seemed to have fewer internal and external resources. Accordingly, Masten and O'Connor strongly urge that we change the way we conceptualize our theories to incorporate a resilience framework into policy and intervention.

Ferguson and Horwood (2001) have published follow-up results from the twenty-one-year Christchurch Health and Development Study. The most significant findings include: (1) early conduct problems in the absence of attentional problems are associated with increased risks of later delinquency and substance abuse but are not associated with later educational failure; (2) early attentional problems in the absence of conduct problems are associated with increased risks for school failure but not increased risk of delinquency and substance use; and (3) children with both conduct problems and early attentional problems are at increased risk of later delinquency, substance abuse, and school failure. In addition the study found that children with the most severe problems (conduct, substance abuse, police contact, and mental health problems) had the highest number of adversities. In fact, the 5% of children exposed to the greatest adversity had risks of multiple problems that were one hundred times those of children in the most advantaged 50% of the cohort. This study reemphasized the adverse effect of cumulative risk and the importance of early intervention to prevent what the authors termed the 'cascade effect'.

Wyman and colleagues (1992), who conducted the Rochester Child Resilience Project, followed two cohorts of children (seven to nine and ten to twelve) longitudinally over two to six years. All children came from highly adverse environments, but were labelled as stress resistant or stress affected depending on how they rated on scales of competent adjustment in multiple spheres. Stress-resistant children demonstrated realistic control attributions about family stressors, feelings of self-efficacy to master challenges, positive future expectations, and empathy. Protective effects for children were also found in parents' competencies. However, the positive adaptation to adversity depended on the context. For example, whereas interpersonal and affective distancing and low expectations for parent involvement are generally associated with poorer child adaptation, those qualities were adaptive for children in families that functioned poorly.

Finally, the work of McGloin and Widom (2001) illustrates how developmental research incorporating both the DSM and a resilience framework complement each other. They studied abuse victims and a socio-economically matched control group of children and followed them to adulthood, measuring multiple domains of functioning with DSM diagnoses and resilience indices as outcome measures of adaptation. Using a quite stringent definition of 'resilience' or successful adaptation across multiple domains across time, they found that 22% of the abuse sample met their criteria for resilience at adulthood, compared to 41% of the control group, with important gender differences emerging (with females adapting better than males). In their discussion they sounded a cautionary note that the field of child maltreatment has traditionally assumed an overall negative effect of abuse on development and a subsequent inevitable negative outcome. While acknowledging child abuse as a risk, the authors suggested that this focus on the negative has overshadowed understanding of how some abused individuals adapt and thrive. The study also illustrates that a comparison to a 'normal sample' indicated a continuum rather than a sharp cut-off demarcating 'normal' from 'abnormal.' In a developmental perspective where risk and resilience modify each other, DSM diagnoses need to be contextualized as either a process variable (that is, one of many risk variables operating together) or an outcome variable (several stressors or risk factors leading to a final pathway that then in itself becomes another risk factor).

As such, these models subsumed under the interactional-developmental label offer a richer view of context, interactions, and development than the simple categorical models of psychopathology of the DSM. Child psychiatric labels as offered through the DSM can produce a bewildering array of co-morbidities that may have as much to do with context as with individual diagnoses. For example, young children with aggression problems will tend to see those problems persist if they are exposed to a classroom where there are other aggressive children (Kellam, Ling, Merisca, Brown, & Lalongo, 1998). Similarly, studies of youths' conduct problems have shown that the social context (deviant peer group or pro-social norms) are influential in determining whether the conduct problems remain stable, increase, or decrease (Loeber & Stouthamer-Loeber, 1998).

Very rarely do families present with a single diagnosis or risk factor. Families struggle against a host of both genetic and environmental risk factors exposing them to the effects of cumulative risk and adversity. For example, in our clinic a family presented with an angry acting-out pre-teen. The family had multiple risks, including maternal depression, a biological father with conduct disorder, spousal violence, poor attachment to the child, parental separation, multiple partners and, not surprisingly, the child's poor school adjustment and peer relations. It is likely the boy also inherited susceptibility genes for CD or depression. Furthermore, the mother lacked support and had been cut off from her biological family. For families with such multiple risks and overwhelming adversity, a DSM framework may be somewhat inadequate to capture the complexity of intergenerational risk and resilience patterns.

The results of the above studies have added immensely to our knowledge of how development is affected by adversity and what it takes to move towards competence and positive development. There are many implications for the resilience-informed practitioner who intervenes at the individual, family, or community level. Since theory informs what we look for, assessments and interviews need to change from an exclusive focus on individual problems to include context and interactions. An overemphasis on diagnosis and medication can contribute to a de-emphasis on contextual factors that in turn affect the choice of intervention. To illustrate, a model school program to combat high rates of absenteeism and delinquency in a socially deprived area of Montreal in Quebec, Canada, separated boys from girls in classrooms and provided hands-on learning that emphasized doing rather than listening. The program was a phenomenal success; not only did absenteeism all but vanish, but students were re-engaged in learning. However, the program's future was uncertain as it was more costly to administer than regular school programs. In the absence of such a program many of these children and teens may be referred individually for acting-out behavior to a clinic and diagnosed and treated for individualistically based disorders.

However, for the resilience-based practitioner it can be a disservice to a youth and family to over- or under-utilize the DSM as a diagnostic tool and/or therapeutic approach. To deny that a young individual may have a serious psychiatric disorder (e.g., severe depression with suicidal ideation or severe conduct disorder) and only focus on positive aspects when other interventions are needed (e.g., hospitalization, containment, psychopharmacology, respite care) is to deny valuable help and guidance to the child and family. There has been a tendency in the strengths-based approaches and certain family therapies (solution focused or narrative) to look only at strengths and to overcompensate for the previous tendency in the biomedical approaches to pathologize all behaviour. In addition, serious psychiatric pathologies in and of themselves can diminish factors that make the person or environment resilient. Depression and schizophrenia, for example, diminish the person's self-esteem and impair competence, while ADHD and CD affect impulse control, familial bonds, and peer relationships

Revisiting the notion that the glass is half-full from the developmental psychopathology point of view has meant that, in addition to assessing psychopathology and risks, we must also consider the development of competencies that promote resilience in the child and family. A focus on promoting competence, however, is not incompatible with assessing psychopathology, but rather redresses the previous imbalance of focusing on deficits. Within the context of a child mental health service, a resilience approach means taking the time necessary to conduct a comprehensive assessment of individual, family, and community risks and assets in a multidisciplinary team.

Mental health workers by their training and in response to what is expected of them professionally, as well as a consequence of the power delegated to them by our culture as 'specialists,' are expected to make individual diagnoses that detail deficits and weaknesses rather than strengths. Psychiatrists, along with psychologists and social workers, need to rethink whether their traditional roles as expected by society (diagnosing and treating), within the broader context, are helpful in enhancing resilience or not (Carrey, 2007).

## Attachment Theory and Resilience

Attachment theory has become the pre-eminent theory in child psychiatry (as well as other child mental health disciplines), serving as the impetus for new areas of research and generating new therapeutic approaches. While susceptible to some of the same criticisms as psychoanalytic theory in that it blurs the lines between normal and abnormal, the theory, because it is operationalizable, makes it theoretically possible to gather data on attachment. Attachment theory is compatible with developmental psychopathology and with the DSM in the sense that it is an innate biological property of primates to bond with their primary caretakers in environmentally mediated ways. The infant needs to attach in order to survive. A healthy attachment is necessary for normal development, including emotional, endocrinological, and neurological development (Carrey, Butter, Bialek, & Persinger, 1995; Perry, 2002; Sapolsky, 2004; Zhang, Chretien, Meaney, & Gratton, 2005). The inability to satisfy this basic security need through the mother-child or caretaker-child dyad (as compromised through child abuse, family violence, repeated placements) results in serious psychopathology. A child's resilience can be enhanced by safeguarding primary attachments (promoting secure attachments) and preventing unnecessary disruptions.

While the DSM has specific diagnostic criteria for children who have disrupted attachments, the incorporation of attachment status and how it affects development in both the child and caregiver (through intergenerational attachment) has not been standard practice in child and family assessments. It would seem logical to codify this in some way on axis 2, currently reserved in the DSM for long-term behaviour patterns such as personality disorders in adults. In this section I selectively review some of the research findings on attachment and DSM diagnoses, as well as a new hypothesis about intergenerational transmission of attachment quality. I conclude by discussing how child protective service interventions need to be more sensitive to attachment disruptions in both child and adult clients. Clearly the potential exists for either diminishing or enhancing resilience through the quality of attachment, one of the most powerful proximal factors affecting child development and psychopathology.

Relational trauma, ranging from neglect to physical, sexual, or emotional abuse to exposure to domestic violence in the early attachment years, plays a role in various DSM-designated disorders later in childhood, adolescence, and adulthood. While much work needs to be done on what risks as a result of the attachment disruptions lead to what outcomes, practically any psychopathology can in some way be linked either causally or as a mediating factor to disrupted attachment.

For example, as a sequelae of childhood sexual abuse, the empirical literature demonstrates that depression, anxiety, post-traumatic stress, dissociation, low self-esteem, somatization, behaviour problems, delinquency, substance abuse, sexual promiscuity, prostitution, aggressivity, and relational problems are all possible outcomes (Briere & Elliott, 1994; Green, Russo, Navratil, & Loeber, 1999; Grilo, Sanislow, Fehon, Martino, & McGlashan, 1999; Mennen & Meadow, 1993; Silverman, Reinherz, & Giaconia, 1996; Wolfe & Birt, 1995; Wright, Friedrich, Cinq-Mars, Cyr, & McDuff, 2004). Van der Kolk and colleagues (1991) as well as Herman (1992) have argued convincingly that even severe personality disorders such as the so-called borderline personality have a higher (up to 75%) incidence of childhood sexual abuse and may in fact represent emotional dysregulation and failure to self-soothe as secondary to relational trauma.

Multiple longitudinal studies have examined the relationship between maternal depression and/or maternal rejection of preschool toddlers and later development of child conduct problems. Raine, Brennan, and Mednick (1994) in a Danish sample of 4,269 live male births found that birth complications and maternal rejection at age one interacted to predict later violent offending at age eighteen. Toddlers who experienced maternal hostility as a result of maternal depression and punitive parenting were more physically aggressive as school-aged children (Romano et al., 2005) or had more conduct disorder behaviours as adolescents (Foley et al., 2004). Presumably the developmental pathway here involves the interaction between maternal factors via the quality of attachment, other environmental adversity risks (low birth weight), or an underlying genetic susceptibility (i.e., susceptibility to develop an externalizing disorder).

Disrupted attachment leading to maladaptive development and later to psychopathology is multiply determined by factors such as gender, perinatal complications, cognitive skills, and of course protective factors such as the availability of alternative, secure attachment figures (Egeland, Jacobvitz, & Sroufe, 1988). The question remains, however, why some abused children are not as susceptible to psychopathology. Some researchers have argued that all abused children show signs of maladaptation if the children are followed long enough, since one of the strongest proximal factors affecting positive or negative developmental outcomes is the quality of the child–parent relationship (Bolger & Patterson, 2001a, 2001b). Other contextually sensitive research has shown that maltreated children remain resilient by maintaining affective and interpersonal distance, hence decreasing their distress (Wyman et al., 1992). Sroufe (2005), reviewing findings from the thirty-year Minnesota study, observed that secure attachment predicted the quality of resilience capacities such as self-reliance, emotional regulation, and the emergence and course of social competence in adulthood.

It is a well-known clinical observation that some parents who have difficulty bonding with their newborns had poor attachments to their own parents; this has been termed the 'intergenerational transmission of poor attachment.' Over twenty years ago, Main, Kaplan, and Cassidy (1985) documented that a mother's state of mind about her own attachment was strongly correlated to the quality of her own child's attachment to her at year one. This finding has been replicated by other researchers, confirming that the mother's capacity to regulate her own thoughts and feelings about relationships with her primary caregivers is linked to her capacity to respond in a sensitive manner to her child (referred to as 'affective attunement').

Main asked the care-giving adults of children she was researching to describe their own early attachment experiences, including separation, loss, trauma, and rejection. While at first she thought that it would be the events in the parent's lives that would affect attachment quality, results had more to do with how much the parents had integrated and made sense of their own early childhood experience (termed 'secure internal working models of attachment,' [Main et al., 1985]). Fonagy and colleagues (2002, 2005) refined this notion further, labelling it as the parent's or the mother's 'reflective function,' or how the mother gives meaning to the child's affective experience and re-presents this experience to him or her in a regulated fashion. In so doing, the mother sets the stage for the development of a sense of security, authenticity, and safety. From this perspective, reflective capacity is the caretaker's ability to access his or her own store of emotions and memories relevant to early attachment experiences and provide this as a secure base for his or her child.

These concepts are important for the resilience-informed clinician, since they broaden the therapeutic scope to include the context of the parent's own attachment history. Other parents may have unresolved losses (mothers with difficult, painful pregnancies, stillborns, death of a child in the family, medical illness or disability in an infant) or have been the victims of spousal or family violence, which in turn affects the quality of attachments to their own children. As a result, many of these caregivers may have internalized distorted views of the child or themselves as these relate to the attachment relationship ('I'll never be a good enough mother for him' or 'that child was put on earth to punish me'). Clearly the therapist must not only be attuned to strengths but open to exploration of sensitive emotions and their impact on relationships. Specific forms of child-parent dyadic therapies that seek to strengthen the quality of attachment have recently been developed (Chambers, Amos, Allison, & Roeger, 2006). In work with children and families it is important to think of enhancing resilience in relationships rather than individualistically.

Conversely, children and young adults with serious psychopathology (serious conduct disorder, depression, schizophrenia, manic-depressive illness, panic disorder, obsessive compulsive disorder, anorexia nervosa) may tax the resources of the family and test the bonds between parent and child. In these instances, it is very important for the therapist to determine the direction of causality in order not to confuse cause and effect. For example, a child with a serious conduct problem (assuming it is not the result of a family problem) may have taxed parents' resources and 'deskilled' the parents to such an extent that they feel demoralized and ineffective in their parenting. In these instances a DSM diagnosis may help identify a serious impairment in the young person. While it is always important to bring out strengths and coping skills and maintain optimism and hope, parents might perceive that the therapist is minimizing parental concerns if the seriousness of a problem is not acknowledged. A resilience or strengths-based approach should not be unrealistically optimistic and naive, but recognize limitations and challenges as well.

Finally, it is important to consider particularly difficult circumstances that exist for children who have been removed from their homes and subject to multiple placement breakdowns and hence disrupted attachments under mandates with child protective services. Social services seem to be in a Catch-22 situation about what is in the child's best interest: keep them in the home and subject to possible ongoing neglect and abuse or remove them and expose them to the multiple perils of the foster care, group home, residential care, and psychiatric inpatient system. Koslowska and Foley (2006) have specifically outlined the risks associated with alternate care that may place children at further risk: (1) physical or sexual abuse is still a possibility; (2) foster families, if not properly screened, may have their own challenges, seeing fostering as a second chance to resolve personal or intergenerational problems; (3) poor funding and support of foster families faced with difficult children leads to burnout and a cycle of frequent placement breakdown and further disrupted attachment for the child; (4) biological parents lose motivation to invest in the relationship; (5) biological parents can become alienated from the system; and (6) the child's attachment with other biological extended family members is disrupted.

Research about intervening more aggressively and preventatively to preserve the mother-infant bond is emerging and is cautiously optimistic. Cicchetti, Rogosch, and Toth (2006) report encouraging results when biological parents who had maltreated their infants are provided with in-home, preventative support. The result of this intervention showed increased maternal sensitivity and increased secure attachment when compared with a control group.

Arguably, breaking intergenerational cycles of multiple adversities, violence, and maltreatment ultimately makes sense on economic as well as humanitarian grounds. Resilience-informed clinical work must hold a broad mandate that includes consultation, support, and education of other colleagues and allied agencies in attempts to secure and preserve long-term relationships between children and their biological families or long-term caregivers.

## Culture, Resilience, and the DSM

Major criticisms directed at the DSM, in addition to those mentioned above, have been that it does not take into account social, cultural and political factors, reflecting only American culture, and values. One striking example of this is that people with schizophrenia seem to have better outcomes in non-Western, majority-world countries than in Western, minority-world countries (Sartorius Gulbiwat, Harrison, Laska, & Siegel, 1996). Possible explanations include closely knit families in non-Western settings who ensure the client takes medication and is compliant with treatment, reducing the risk of relapse. Therefore, while there is agreement on a cross-cultural diagnosis of schizophrenia, the prognosis or severity of the disorder can be influenced by sociocultural factors. A strengths-based approach here would not deny the existence of a serious psychiatric disorder in the individual, but would seek to increase capacity in the family and community to prevent relapse, hospitalization, and institutionalization.

Ultimately, the DSM is a cultural document, and it would be foolish to say that any classification system is value free. As a nod to acknowledging the impact of culture on diagnosis, the latest version of the DSM (DSM-IV-TR) has an appendix devoted to a cultural formulation and a glossary of culture-bound syndromes. The description of syndromes with unfamiliar names like *amok, ataque de nervios, boufee delirante,* and *koro,* to name just a few, masks the inability of dominant culture to step outside of itself and recognize how all descriptions must pass through a cultural filter particular to that historical time frame. Many syndromes that are very common in North America or other Western industrialized countries, such as anorexia nervosa and borderline personality disorder, are rare or unheard of in other countries. This has implications for enhancing resilience at a cultural level as well as at a policy level, since many of our well-intended therapies (or industries) may in fact be maintaining patterns of ill health rather than promoting well-being.

## Case Studies

### Case 1: Mitigating Family Adversity

Two individuals from the same family, a girl aged fourteen and a boy aged twelve, were referred for serious suicide attempts. While there had been chronic stressors in the family, the precipitant appears to have been an unexpected suicide by an aunt a year ago. The family members accompanying the teenagers to treatment included their mother and maternal grandmother. After the second session it was evident that the mother and grandmother had been severely traumatized by the aunt's suicide and were barely functioning. The mother in particular was depressed (stating that her sister had been 'my best friend'). She would come home from work and withdraw from her children. Additional stressors included the children's witnessing the mother being sexually assaulted when they were younger. Both youth had dropped out of school.

Strengths for the family included a younger brother who appeared quite resilient. The family had an ethic of sticking together and standing up for each other. In addition, the mother was determined to keep the family together despite a perceived threat that Child Protection Services might remove her children from her home.

Three experienced therapists from the child and family outpatient mental health service immediately made themselves available for the family. Each young person saw their own individual therapist while the third therapist addressed the unresolved grief issues for the mother and grandmother.

*Comment*: Our team of service providers recognized the tremendous adversity this family and each member had had to face. To create conducive conditions for resilience in this family it was necessary to recognize not only their strengths, but also the tremendous pain and grief they were dealing with. Under such circumstances it was necessary for the clinic to invest more resources before the family could start to function again. The mother also had to be reassured that it was the clinic's philosophy that the children's best place was  with their family at home.

*Case 2: Bureaucracies That Defeat Resilience*

Mrs T had consulted social services for her ten-year-old son who had become aggressive, staying out late at night and starting to break the law. He was admitted to a residential program for assessment and treatment. While the boy was in the program, evidence came to light of the mother's physically abusive treatment of him. Mrs T herself had been raised in a series of foster homes. Child Protective Services decided to terminate her rights, which seriously traumatized the young man, who despite the mother's harsh treatment of him was still quite attached to her. Mrs T's visits with her son became erratic and unpredictable. The degree of animosity between the mother and staff was quite evident, as Mrs T felt betrayed given that she had voluntarily sought help.

The client was told that a foster home would be found for him. Due to his needs and behaviour, however, it was evident that a specialized foster home was necessary. Unfortunately, finding him a permanent foster home was not at the top of the Department of Community Service's (DCS) priorities.

This was in part because the number of available families in the jurisdiction had drastically dwindled from 600 to 250 in preceding years (fostering in this jurisdiction is seen as voluntary, with minimal per diem payment and foster parent support). Ironically, children were being placed instead in costly specialized group homes.

In spite of improvements in the boy's behaviour during the first year at the residential centre, together with a clear indication of his intelligence and passion for animals, after two years his behaviour began to deteriorate. This was due in part to the fact that he had lost hope of an alternative placement being found. Furthermore, he seemed to be the only child who had no one visiting him, and would spend holidays and vacations in the institution. As well, the relationship between the staff and the boy's mother continued to deteriorate. The boy was sometimes told about special family events by his mother but was rarely allowed to attend. His behaviour continued to deteriorate (e.g., hitting staff), and a relationship of mutual distrust characterized interactions between him and centre staff. His misbehaviour was interpreted as a sign of calculated malice rather than an expression of his lack of hope or desperate attempts to save attachments.

His mother became pregnant and gave birth to a baby brother. The child was automatically removed by DCS and placed in another foster home. Although the boy had been allowed to be present at the birth, he was now banned from seeing his brother. His placement issue was still unresolved after two and a half years. The local legal aid service was contacted so that a lawyer could advocate on his behalf. A young couple finally responded to an ad DCS placed in the newspaper to recruit foster parents. However, the couple was deemed to be too inexperienced to handle the boy. The boy continued his placement in the institution, now completing his third year.

*Comment*: This case is presented to highlight how some institutions are actually harmful and create more damage by exposing vulnerable children to risks associated with alternate care. All principles to build resilience were ignored here. This boy's attachments have been greatly disrupted and damaged, presenting an example of how institutions set up individuals for the next generation of problems. Part of a resilience-based practice is to advocate politically against such institutional neglect, especially when multiple agencies are involved. Additionally, when children must be placed, some jurisdictions are shifting resources to specialized foster care rather than dehumanizing imper-sonal group homes.

## Case 3: Resilience through the Community

J was eight years old when he and his younger brother were appre-hended by DCS. His mother had a substance abuse problem and was physically abusive to the two children, and the father had not been on the scene for several years. For the ensuing three years J went through a series of twenty-two foster homes. Foster home breakdown was pre-sumed to be due to J's aggressive behaviour. He was referred to a res-idential program for behaviour stabilization. After nearly two years he was discharged to a group home with the diagnoses of ADHD and ODD. He was taking Risperidone and Dexedrine. His behaviour sta-bilized at the group home although there were rare incidents of self-harm that J rationalized as being adaptive. Better to hurt himself, he said, than others.

J had asked his social worker several times to contact his younger brother (it had been seven years since their last contact), but appar-ently the adopted family refused. He had also asked his social worker for a foster family but was told this was highly unlikely since 'teenagers don't get placed in foster families.' J was intelligent, sensi-tive, and expressed the opinion that 'group homes are no places for people to grow up in' after being there for three years. Through a network of friends an ad was placed in a local community bulletin to see if any family was interested in fostering a teen. Two families responded. He chose one family and he has been with this family for seventeen months now.

*Comment*: The family that agreed to foster this teen had stated that they had raised their family and were thinking of how they could make a further contribution to the community. This teen valued the placement. To J, the importance of belonging was part of his resilience.

## Conclusion

Never say you know the last word about any human heart.

Henry James

Diagnoses as defined by the DSM are only starting points in the context of challenges and adversities facing children and youth at risk. Understanding a child and his family must involve understanding the myriad of influences affecting the child's development, including genetic factors, attachment, and family and community environments. The study of developmental psychopathology and attachment provides a context for understanding the interplay of risk and resilience factors. As reviewed above, one risk does not cause one outcome; rather, multiple risks are necessary and cumulative. In addition, the same risk factors can produce multiple outcomes and different risk factors may interact to produce the same outcome. The implication for the clinician is that risk and resilience are best conceptualized as developmental dimensional constructs rather that a static categorical construct.

The implications of the above-mentioned studies for developing resilience in children, youth, and families across the life span force child mental health professionals to view their interventions at multiple levels and across generations. Our role must be to break cycles of intergenerational despair and nurture resilience over time. As illustrated in the case examples, both resilience and adversity can be transmitted across generations. Multiple adversities or risks are cumulative within certain individuals or families. At the same time, institutions charged with the mandate to 'build resilience,' such as health, education, child protection, community services, and youth correction agencies, may inadvertently do exactly the opposite. Part of a resilience and strengths-based practice may necessarily involve advocacy at higher levels for what we know is deliberately diminishing resilience and human dignity.

There needs to be a lot more 'cross-talk' between resilience practitioners and researchers and more traditionally oriented clinicians and practitioners involved in child development. Resilience concepts are principles that can be applied across disciplines or theoretical orientation. Nothing that has been said in this chapter is meant to trivialize the importance of acknowledging serious psychiatric psychopathology. Resilience and strengths-based approaches must be realistic in not minimizing impairments caused by crippling psychiatric symptoms. While maintaining hope, our clients and their parents expect realistic help with whatever practical and conceptual tools are available.

## REFERENCES

Appleyard, K., Egeland, B., van Dulmen, M., & Sroufe, L.A. (2005). When more is not better: The role of cumulative risk in child behavior outcomes. *Journal of Child Psychology and Psychiatry, 46*, 235–45.

Bolger, K., & Patterson, C. (2001a). Developmental pathways from child maltreatment to peer rejection. *Child Development, 72*(2), 549–68.

Bolger, K., & Patterson, C. (2001b). Pathways from child maltreatment to internalizing problems: Perceptions of control as mediators and moderators. *Development and Psychopathology, 13*, 913–40.

Brame, B., Nagin, D.S., & Tremblay, R.E. (2001). Developmental trajectories of physical aggression from school age. *Journal of Child Psychology & Psychiatry and Allied Disciplines, 42*, 503–12.

Briere, J.N., & Elliott, D.M. (1994). Immediate and long-term impacts of child sexual abuse. *Future of Children, 4*(2), 54–69.

Broidy, L.M., Nagin, D.S., Tremblay, R.E., Bates, J.E., Brame, B., Dodge, K.A., et al. (2003). Developmental trajectories of childhood disruptive behaviours and adolescent delinquency: A six-site cross-national study. *Developmental Psychology, 39*(2), 222–45.

Burt, K., Carlivati, J., Sroufe, L.A., Appleyard, K., van Dulmen, M., Egeland, B., et al. (2005). Mediating links between maternal depression and offspring psychopathology: The importance of independent data. *Journal of Child Psychology and Psychiatry, 46*(5), 409–99.

Carrey, N. (2007). Practising psychiatry through a narrative lens: Working with children, youth and families. In C. Brown & T. Augusta-Scott (Eds.), *Narrative therapy: Making meaning, making lives* (pp. 77–103). Thousand Oaks, CA: Sage.

Carrey, N., Butter, H., Bialek, R., & Persinger, M. (1995). Physiological and cognitive correlates of child abuse. *Journal of the American Academy of Child and Adolescent Psychiatry, 34*(8), 1067–75.

Carrey, N., & Ungar, M. (2007). The Diagnostic Statistical Manual and resilience theory: Incompatible bed fellows? In N. Carrey & M. Ungar (Eds.), *Resilience: Child and Adolescent Psychiatric Clinics of North America* (monograph), *16*(2), 497–514.

Chambers, H., Amos, J., Allison, S., & Roeger, L. (2006). Parent and child therapy: An attachment based intervention for children with challenging problems. *Australian New Zealand Journal of Family Therapy, 27*(2), 68–74.

Cicchetti, D. (1993). Developmental psychopathology: Reactions, reflections, projections. *Developmental Review, 13*, 471–502.

Cicchetti, D., Rogosch, F., & Toth, S. (2006). Fostering secure attachment in infants in maltreating families through preventative interventions. *Development and Psychopathology, 18*, 623–49.

Egeland, B., Jacobvitz, D., & Sroufe, L. (1988). Breaking the cycle of abuse. *Child Development, 59*, 1080–88.

Feighner, J.P., Robins, E., Guze, S.B., Woodruff, R.A., Winokur, G., & Munoz, R. (1972). Diagnostic criteria for use in psychiatric research. *Archives of General Psychiatry, 26*, 57–63.

Ferguson, D., & Horwood, L. (2001). The Christchurch Health and Development Study: Review of findings on child and adolescent mental health. *Australian and New Zealand Journal of Psychiatry, 35*(3), 287–96.

Foley, D.L., Eaves, L.J., Wormly, B., Silberg, J.L., Maes, H.H., Kuhn, J., & Riley, B. (2004). Childhood adversity, monoamine oxidase A genotype, and risk for conduct disorder. *Archives of General Psychiatry, 61*, 738–44.

Fonagy, P., Gergely, G., Jurist, E., & Target, M. (2002). *Affect regulation, mentalization, and the development of the self.* New York: Other Books.

Fonagy, P., & Target, M. (2005). Bridging the transmission gap: An end to an important mystery of attachment research? *Attachment and Human Development, 7*(3), 333–43.

Formoso, D., Gonzales, N.A., & Aiken, L.S. (2000). Family conflict and children's internalizing and externalizing behavior: Protective factors. *American Journal of Community Psychology, 28*, 175–99.

Goldstein, J. (1987). *Console and classify: The French psychiatric profession in the 19th century.* Cambridge: Cambridge University Press.

Green, S.M., Russo, M.F., Navratil, J.L., & Loeber, R. (1999). Sexual and physical abuse among adolescent girls with disruptive behavior problems. *Journal of Child & Family Studies, 8*(2), 151–68.

Grilo, C.M., Sanislow, C., Fehon, D.C., Martino, S., & McGlashan, T.H. (1999). Psychological and behavioral functioning in adolescent psychiatric inpatients who report histories of childhood abuse. *American Journal of Psychiatry, 156*, 538–43.

Herman, J.L. (1992). Complex PTSD: A syndrome in survivors of prolonged and repeated trauma. *Journal of Traumatic Stress, 5*(3), 377–91.

Kellam, S., Ling, X., Merisca, R., Brown, C., & Lalongo, N. (1998). The effect of the level of aggression in the first grade classroom on the course and malleability of aggressive behavior in middle school. *Development and psychopathology, 10,* 165–85.

Koslowska, K., & Foley, S. (2006). Attachment and risk of future harm: A case of non-accidental brain injury. *Australian and New Zealand Journal of Family Therapy, 27*(2), 75–82.

Loeber, R., & Stouthamer-Loeber, M. (1998). Development of juvenile aggression and violence: Some common misconceptions and controversies. *American Psychologist, 53*(2), 242–59.

Main, M., Kaplan, N., & Cassidy, J. (1985). Security in infancy, childhood and adulthood: A move to the level of representation. In I. Bretherton & E. Waters (Eds.), *Growing points of attachment theory and research* (Monographs of the Society for Research in Child Development) 50(1–2, serial no. 203), (pp. 66–107).

Masten, A., & O'Connor, M.J. (1989). Vulnerability, stress and resilience in the early development of a high risk child. *Journal of the American Academy of Child and Adolescent Psychiatry, 28,* 274–8.

McGloin, J.M., & Widom, C. (2001). Resilience among abused and neglected children grown up. *Development and Psychopathology, 13*(4), 1021–38.

Mennen, F.E, & Meadow, D. (1993). The relationship of sexual abuse to symptom levels in emotionally disturbed girls. *Child & Adolescent Social Work Journal, 10*(4), 319–28.

Moffit, T. E. (2005). Genetic and Environmental Influences on Antisocial Behaviours: Evidence from Behavioural – Genetic Research. *Advances in Genetics, 55,* 41–104.

Moffit, T., Caspi, A., Harrington, H., & Milne, B. (2002). Males on the life course persistent and adolescence limited antisocial pathways: Follow-up at age 26. *Development and Psychopathology, 14,* 179–206.

Nagin, D.S., & Tremblay, R. (1999). Trajectories of boys' physical aggression, opposition, and hyperactivity on physically violent and non-violent juvenile delinquency. *Child Development, 70,* 1181–96.

Perry, B. (2002). Childhood experience and the expression of genetic potential: What childhood neglect tells us about nature and nurture. *Brain and Mind, 3,* 79–100.

Phelps, E., Balsano, A., Fay, K., Peltz, J., Zimmerman, S., Lerner, R., & Lerner, J. (2007). Nuances in early adolescent developmental trajectories of positive and of problematic/risk behaviours: Findings from the 4–H study of positive youth development. In N. Carrey & M. Ungar (Eds.), *Resilience: Child and Adolescent Psychiatric Clinics of North America* (monograph) *16(2),* 473–96.

Pinel, P. (1800). *Analectes sur le traite medico-philosophique sur l'alienation mentale ou la manie.* Paris: Richard, Caille et Ravier Librairies, no. 11, an. IX.

Raine, A., Brennan, P., & Mednick, S.A. (1994). Birth complications combined with early maternal rejection at age 1 year predispose to violent crime at age 18 years. *Archives of General Psychiatry, 51,* 984–8.

Romano, E., Tremblay, R.E., Boulerice, B., & Swisher, R. (2005). Mulitlevel correlates of childhood physical aggression and prosocial behavior. *Journal of Abnormal Child Psychology, 33*(5), 565–78.

Rutter, M., Yule., B., Quinton, D., Rowlands, O., Yule, W., & Berger, M. (1975). Attainment and adjustment in tow geographical areas, III: Some factors accounting for area differences. *British Journal of Psychiatry, 126,* 520–33.

Sameroff, A., Morrison Gutman, L., & Peck, S. (2003). Adaptation among youth facing multiple risks. In S. Luthar (Ed.), *Resilience and vulnerability: Adaptation in the context of childhood adversity* (pp. 364–91). Cambridge: Cambridge University Press.

Sapolsky, R. (2004). Mothering style and methylation. *Nature Neuroscience, 7,* 791–2.

Sartorius, N., Gulbiwat, R., Harrison, G., Laska, E., & Siegel, C. (1996). Long term follow-up of schizophrenia in 16 countries: A description of the International Study of Schizophrenia conducted by the World Health Organisation. *Social Psychiatry and Psychiatric Epidemiology, 31*(5), 249–58.

Schowalter, J. (1989). Psychodynamics and medication. *Journal of the American Academy of Child and Adolescent Psychiatry, 28*(5), 681–4.

Shaw, D.S., Gilliom, M., Ongoldsby, E.M., & Nagin, D.S. (2003). Trajectories leading to school age conduct problems. *Developmental Psychology, 39*(2), 189–200.

Silverman, A.B., Reinherz, H.Z., & Giaconia, R.M. (1996). The long-term sequelae of child and adolescent abuse: A longitudinal community study. *Child Abuse & Neglect, 20*(8), 709–723.

Spiegel, A. (2005, January 3). The dictionary of disorder: How one man revolutionized psychiatry. *New Yorker*, pp.1–18.

Sroufe, L.A. (2005). Attachment and development: A prospective, longitudinal study from birth to adulthood. *Attachment and Human Development,* 7(4), 349–67.

Swedo, S., & Pine, D. (2005). *Anxiety disoders.* In S. Swedo & D. Pine (guest editors), *Child and Adolescent Clinics of North America,* 14(4).

Van der Kolk, B.A., Perry, J.C., & Herman, J.L. (1991). Childhood origins of self-destructive behavior. *American Journal of Psychiatry, 148*(12), 1665–71.

Wolfe, V.V., & Birt, J.-A. (1995). The psychological sequelae of child sexual abuse. *Advances in Clinical Child Psychology, 17*, 233–63.

Wright, J., Friedrich, W., Cinq-Mars, C., Cyr, M., & McDuff, P. (2004). Self-destructive and delinquent behaviors of adolescent female victims of child sexual abuse: Rates and covariates in clinical and nonclinical samples. *Violence and Victims, 19*(6), 627–43.

Wyman, P., Cowen, E., Work, W., Raoof, A., Gribble, P., Parker, G., & Wannon, M. (1992). Interviews with children who experienced major life stress: Family and child attributes that predict resilient outcomes. *Journal of the American Academy of Child & Adolescent Psychiatry, 31*, 904–10.

Zhang, T., Chretien, P., Meaney, M., & Gratton, A. (2005). Influences of naturally occurring variations in maternal care on prepulse inhibition of acoustic startle response and the medial prefrontal cortex dopamine response to stress in adult rats. *Journal of Neuroscience, 25*(6), 1493–1502.

# 6 Promoting Resilience and Coping in Social Workers: Learning from Perceptions about Resilience and Coping among South African Social Work Students

LINDA SMITH AND SANDRA J. DROWER

The South African context provides a rich and unique opportunity to examine issues of resilience and coping among its people generally and among young people in particular. Apartheid, with its policies of violent oppression, has left a legacy of inequality and social disadvantage. However, in the face of this extreme inequality and hardship, South African society is characterized by immense strength and resilience.

Within this context, South African social workers face particular challenges where poverty and inequality is compounded by the current HIV/AIDS epidemic. According to the United Nations Regional Information Network (IRIN, 2004), with an increasing number of children orphaned by HIV/AIDS seeking foster care, the HIV/AIDS epidemic is placing enormous pressure on an already over-burdened child welfare system. Social workers are grappling with heavy caseloads of up to four hundred children each. In this regard, perceived declines in the productivity of social workers are ascribed to 'high case loads, emotional and other trauma experienced by social workers in service delivery, high stress levels due to management and societal demands, and lack of resources to deliver their mandate' (Department of Social Development, 2006, p. 20). It is important, therefore, that social service professionals pay particular attention to their own levels of coping, resilience, and protective and risk factors if they are to be able to render effective and appropriate services.

This chapter explores understandings of resilience amongst social work students at the University of the Witwatersrand, Johannesburg, South Africa. Findings shed light on how social work professionals in training ascribe meaning to resilience in individuals, groups, and communities, as well as their own resilience as they prepare for a demanding practice context.

We believe that the unique South African context produces unique resiliencies. Reflecting on insights about resilience and coping amongst South African students studying social work provides an opportunity to understand these issues away from dominant minority-world constructs. In social work training, students are often required to reflect on and evaluate strengths and resilience in individuals and communities. Their unique perspectives, born of their own experiences of living and working in South Africa, offer rich opportunities for personal and professional reflection and growth. Many of these students themselves have to navigate the full range of challenges of the past and present, which include the violent and oppressive legacy of apartheid, the country's endemic poverty, and the HIV/AIDS epidemic. Thus, students' own strengths and resilience come into play in their practice with individuals, families, and communities. These reflections provide an opportunity for resilience researchers to better understand the dynamics of strengths within frontline workers themselves. However, we need to keep in mind that a critical stance in relation to structural issues should still be adopted when using the concept of resilience, as it is open to ideological and political manipulation at the macro level through the shifting of responsibility for structural reform onto individuals (Garmezy & Rutter, 1988).

**The South African Context**

The census of 2001 showed that South Africa had a population of 44.8 million, of which 9.9 million were children (*South Africa at a Glance*, 2005). Based on the racial groupings and definitions of the previous apartheid government, the population is currently 79% black, 9.6% white, 8.9% coloured, and 2.5% Asian. According to the then Population Registration Act, a 'coloured person' was defined in negative terms as someone who was neither black nor white, and today is understood as someone of mixed-racial heritage (black and white). Although these categories are obsolete today, figures such as these are useful for the information they offer about racial stratification and inequality and disadvantage. Eleven official languages are spoken, with Zulu, Xhosa, Afrikaans, Pedi, Tswana, English, and Sotho being listed most frequently as home languages (listed in declining order).

Before 1994, only English and Afrikaans (a language derived from seventeenth- and eighteenth-century Dutch combined with the dialects of black and coloured slaves) were official languages. The 1976 uprisings amongst youth were spurred by dissatisfaction with Afrikaans being the enforced language of instruction in black schools at the time.

When the first democratic government was elected in 1994, the euphoria of a people filled with hope and anticipation for the future was an expression of the struggle and hardship of the preceding era. Apartheid legislation and policies had institutionalized racism, poverty, and disadvantage stemming from colonial rule for half a century; human rights abuses were the order of the day.

The extreme context of racism and oppression in South Africa was reliant on extreme forms of social control. Bulhan (1985) describes how, during oppressive regimes, all areas of life are subjected to curtailment and infiltration. These areas of curtailment include the freedoms of movement, expression of opinion, and assembly. They affect ideas, the ecology, social networks, and family and community life. Finally, they involve the obliteration of the past and the falsification of history. Specifically, Bulhan (1985) argues that 'such methods of social control, best exemplified in slavery and apartheid, make the psyche and social relations of the oppressed the locus of control and domination' (p. 122). In this context of oppression and struggle, resilience grew among South Africans. Aziz observes, 'this hope and resilience is a spirit that pervades the politics of liberation ... that expresses the power of the powerless ... that spontaneously unifies and raises the voices above the sorrows and wounds – that vivifies and energizes' (as cited in Schmukler, 1993, p. 15).

Today, institutionalized racism in the form of apartheid has ended. The overt, external 'enemy' of the people has ceased to exist. However, structural oppression, racism, and internalized oppression continue to be a challenge. Sewpaul and Holscher (2004), for example, point out that 'the impact of oppression is such that oppressed people eventually turn societal oppression into self-oppression' (p. 100). It is therefore necessary to focus on efforts to promote strengths and healthy outcomes among individuals, groups, and communities. It should come as no surprise, then, that South Africa has been described as one of the most unequal societies globally, with poverty and inequality still skewed along racial lines. The *South African Human Development Report* of 2003 states that poverty and inequality continue to exhibit strong spatial and racial biases, and that income distribution remains highly unequal and has deteriorated in recent years as reflected in the high Gini-coefficient, which rose from 0.596 in 1995 to 0.635 in 2001 (United Nations Development Programme, 2003). According to a report of the Human Sciences Research Council (2004), 57% of individuals in South Africa were living below the poverty line in 2001, a proportion unchanged from 1996 (p. 2). However, according to the report, the poverty gap, which measures the annual income that a poor household would require to bring them out of poverty, has grown, indicating that poor households have sunk deeper into poverty. Furthermore, 'in a society in which existing levels of social inequality and poverty are already very stark as a result of previous apartheid economic policies, the interaction between local inequalities and emerging forms of inequality due to globalization may lead to unsustainable levels of marginalization, vulnerability, and poverty' (Department of Social Development, 2000, p. 8).

The position of children within this context of marginalization and inequality is precarious at best. Despite South Africa's ratifying the United Nations Convention on the Rights of the Child in 1995 and committing to 'put children first' in policies and budgetary considerations, childhood is for many in the country fraught with difficulties. Such difficulties include orphanhood and poverty.

Children seem to be the worst victims of poverty. October household survey results of 1999 indicate that 75% of children in the country live in poverty (cited in Meintjies, Budlender, Giese, & Johnson, 2003). According to the Human Sciences Research Council (2004), the local context is such that nearly a third of children across the country live in households with self-reported hunger or food insecurity and that this 'deprivation of resources associated with unemployment and reduced livelihood options affects children's growth, health, well-being and education; ... and the care of dependant and vulnerable family members' (p. 38). The spread of HIV/AIDS further exacerbates this situation.

The HIV/AIDS pandemic is, together with poverty and malnutrition, one of Africa's greatest threats. According to Carter (2004), an estimated 25.4 million people live with HIV in southern Africa, and 3.1 million adults and children were newly infected with HIV in the region in 2004 alone. The situation regarding HIV/AIDS in South Africa is particularly alarming. A recent Treatment Action Campaign report (2006) indicated that there are approximately 1,400 new HIV infections and 800 AIDS-related deaths in South Africa daily. The consequences of such a pandemic are far reaching and require urgent intervention.

Many children in South Africa have lost one or both parents as a result of the illness, posing an extremely serious risk factor to coping and survival. The United Nations states that, globally, the number of children under the age of fifteen years that have lost one or both parents due to AIDS is estimated at 13.2 million, and 90% of these children live in sub-Saharan Africa (IRIN, 2004). These statistics reflect an enormous shift in traditional family and household composition, as well as the need for a change in childcare arrangements. Child-headed households have become commonplace as an alternative family form. A protective factor in this regard is evident in the flexibility of family forms such as extended family arrangements like *babamkulu* and *babamcane* (literally, 'father-great' and 'father-uncle') and *mamamkulu* and *mamamcane* ('mother-great' and 'mother-aunt').

The problem of violence is a further exacerbating factor in the South African context. According to Duncan and Rock (1997), South Africa has been described as one of the most violent countries in the world. Of particular concern to these writers is the 'disturbing consequence of the high levels of violence in this country is that violence has come to be expected and has, to a degree, been normalized' (p. 146) – violence is commonly perceived to be the only means to resolve difficulties and conflict. In a Human Sciences Research Council report, Dawes (2003) describes a survey of children aged eleven and fourteen in low-income areas that showed that 90% of these children had witnessed some form of assault and 47% had been victims of assault.

It is clear, therefore, that the South African context is fraught with challenges and difficulties for individuals, families, and communities in terms of survival and coping. At the same time, government and policy makers must find ways to develop policies, facilitate structural arrangements, and create resources to promote healthy development of all South Africans. As part of government policy and community efforts, South Africa celebrates an annual 'Child Protection Week' event, which strives to create public awareness of the need for special measures for the protection of children. In his address on the occasion of the launch of the 2005 Child Protection Week to the National Assembly (Department of Social Development, 2005), Dr Zola Skweyiya, Minister for Social Development, encouraged the ethic of *Umntwana wakho ngumntwana wam* (every child is my child), which emphasizes the (currently neglected) traditional view that there exists a communal, collective obligation to take care of all children. Such attention to societal responses to children seems to be important if a commitment to children's well-being is to be prioritized by policy makers.

Social workers and other frontline workers do not merely find themselves in a responsive role to these challenges. They find themselves in the same subjective space and context in which they seek to make a difference. It is therefore vital that social workers, especially at the level of training and preparation for practice, have the opportunity to develop knowledge and reflective skills about their own resilience and coping.

## Social Work in South Africa

Historically, social work in South Africa has undergone many changes. The definition of social work as described by the International Association of Schools of Social Work (IASSW) states that social work

> promotes social change, problem solving in human relationships, and the empowerment and liberation of people to enhance well-being. Utilizing theories of human behaviour and social systems, social work intervenes at the points where people interact with their environments. Principles of human rights and social justice are fundamental to social work. (Sewpaul & Jones, 2004, p. 2)

Social work in South Africa has, however, been shaped by the social welfare policy of any given time. According to MacPherson and Midgely (1987, as cited in Patel, 2005, p. 66), both colonialism and apartheid shaped the evolution of the nature, form, and content of social welfare policy in South Africa. They argue that colonialism disrupted and denigrated most traditional forms of social welfare. As forms of social relations changed in accordance with colonial societies and economies, traditional modes of social provision were eroded. As such, social work in South Africa has itself been indicted with having supported and upheld the oppressive apartheid status quo. McKendrick (2001) describes how under the previous government, social work's major beneficiaries were the group that needed these services the least. The field did not prioritize black poverty and overwhelmingly emphasized social casework.

In spite of government departments' collusion with the oppressive regime, various non-governmental and community-based organizations remained committed to the ideals of liberation from oppression. Social workers operating in these groups were often victimized, detained, and banned from participation in public activities. This history of engagement and participation in the struggle for liberation found expression through community development work (Smith, 2004). Resistance to the regime within sections of the informal welfare sector became especially evident during the Truth and Reconciliation process, when social workers and representatives from NGOs voiced their experiences during the apartheid era (Patel, 2005).

Social work services in South Africa have undergone a major transformation during the past ten years, guided primarily by the 1997 *White Paper for Social Welfare*. This policy document for welfare in the 'new' South Africa, drawn up with full and broad participation of stakeholders, states in its preamble:

> South Africans are called upon to participate in the development of an equitable, people centred, democratic, and appropriate social welfare system. The goal of developmental social welfare is a humane, peaceful, just, and caring society which will uphold welfare rights, facilitate the meeting of basic human needs, release people's creative energies, help them achieve their aspirations, build human capacity and self-reliance, and participate fully in all spheres of social, economic, and political life. (Department of Social Development, 1997, p. 2)

The profession has embraced the vision of developmental social welfare where development is linked to empowerment. The *White Paper for Social Welfare* defines development as the 'process of increasing personal, interpersonal, and political power to enable individuals or collectives to improve their life situation' (Department of Social Development, 1997, p. 80). The *White Paper* further states that the vision is to achieve a system that facilitates the development of human capacity and self-reliance within a caring and enabling environment. In line with this, greater emphasis is placed on developmental, empowerment, and strengths based perspectives in social work practice itself.

A change in the training of social workers has followed these shifts in paradigm, moving beyond the 'casework-community work' dichotomy towards that of contextualization within social development, as called for by Lombard at a 1998 conference on the transformation of social work education. According to Noyoo (1998), this shift towards social development was initiated successfully following the change of government. Training of social workers has become more focused on the empowerment of people, and non-remedial forms of intervention have been implemented. Concern with participation and people's networks has been established, as well as concern with economic development and independence (Gray & Simpson, 1998, as cited by Noyoo, 1998, p. 46). This shift reflects arguments about promoting resilience and coping.

## Social Work Perspectives and Resilience

In South Africa, the current reformation of social work services calls for a *social development, strengths-based*, and *ecological* approach that is coherent and has a focus on resilience. According to Peirson (2005), these approaches redirect attention from a deficit orientation towards a focus on strengths of families living in adverse conditions. However, it is also crucial to maintain a *critical* and *anti-oppressive* perspective in order to avoid the possibility of a narrow focus on resilience, coping, and strengths, and inattention to structural inequalities and oppression. In this regard, a *constructionist* approach is beneficial. This section examines these perspectives and approaches in social work practice for understanding resilience and coping.

Social development is, by definition, an approach that focuses on the strengths of people and communities. According to Patel, 'developmental welfare services emphasize the empowerment of individuals, families, groups, and communities to manage human relations, social problems, and needs optimally whilst building on the strengths of client systems' (Patel, 2005, p. 160). This developmental model of welfare services has relevance for resilience discourse, as it emphasizes the need for both micro and macro approaches to intervention (Patel, 2005), emphasizing the examination of strength and resilience at levels beyond that of the individual to include family, community, and the wider society.

In the study of resilience, incorporation of the individual's broader context or system in which he is found is reflective of the ecological perspective. For example, the importance of a nurturing environment during early childhood development is widely recognized, as is the role of secure attachments with significant others in identity formation, development of relationship competence, and low levels of anti-social behaviour (Bowlby, 1979; Helton & Smith, 2004). Attachment theory considers early experiences of attachment to secure and responsible adults (usually parents) as being a foundation for later social competence. Similarly, it is argued that warmth, mutuality, support, and security are qualities of early relationships that tend to produce coherent, well-organized later selves (Payne, 2005).

A 'system-based' view aligns well with understanding human resilience from an ecological perspective because it shifts from an intra-psychic focus on the individual to the relationships and processes of which the individual is a part. It is the context within which individuals find themselves that resilience may be produced. Walsh (1998), for example, maintains that families can be successful despite diversity of forms and functionalities – that it is family processes rather than family forms that affect healthy functioning. The ecological view supports the argument that resilience is based in the larger system of community or culture, directing attention to the role that processes and quality of interrelationships play in determining healthy outcomes 'despite adversity.'

According to Ungar (2004), within this perspective resilience factors would include compensatory characteristics in the individual or the environment that neutralize risk; challenging factors that 'inoculate' individuals against future stress; and multidimensional protective factors that reduce the potential for negative outcomes. Similarly, Newman and Blackburn (2002) maintain that according to the *saluto-genic model* in health care research, resilience is composed of a person's emotional and material defences together with an ability to render the world understandable and, hence, manageable. They maintain that 'resilience develops through the positive use of stress to improve competencies ... The key quality needed to trigger resilience and recovery is the ability to see childhood adversities in a new way, and to recognize that one is not a powerless actor in a drama written by others' (p. 8), suggesting incorporation of a *strengths perspective* in approaches to resilience.

In his description of empowerment in the strengths perspective, Saleebey (2002) argues that 'to discover the power within people we must ... provide opportunities for connections to family, institutional, and community resources' (p. 9). He goes on to describe resilience as being, not the disregarding of difficulties and traumatic life experiences, but rather the ability to 'bear up' in spite of these ordeals. It is a process of continuing growth and articulation of various virtues derived through meeting demands and challenges. A strengths perspective, then, adopts the view that the client has untapped reserves and capacities within both herself and her broader context that, if recognized, elevate motivation and potential. The worker is, therefore, called upon to develop an understanding of how the client has managed to cope and survive in an oppressive, chaotic environment (Sheafor, Horesji, & Horesji, 1994).

Following on such holistic views of resilience processes, a *constructionist interpretation* would describe resilience as successful negotiation with the environment for resources that define the self as healthy even during adversity. Resilience factors are, thus, viewed as multidimensional and unique to each context, where individuals and their reference group define health outcomes. Given an interpretivist approach to resilience, the relationship between risk and protective factors is complex, socially constructed, and relative to the views of successful outcomes of a particular group (Ungar, 2004). Similarly, resilience is considered to be socially constructed and formed between and among people, and constructed in and through shared meanings (Ratele, 2006).

Links may also be made between resilience and an *empowerment approach*. In the narrowest sense, 'empowerment' connotes only a psychological and personal sense of well-being; it is depoliticized and not useful for institutional change. However, when including the concept of liberation in describing those processes and objectives that challenge oppression, empowerment is restored to its intended meaning. Lee (2001) describes this meaning as the development of a more positive and potent sense of self, the construction of knowledge and capacity for critical comprehension of the web of social and political realities of one's environment, and the cultivation of resources and strategies for a more functional competence in the attainment of personal and collective goals. Empowerment approaches, however, often focus exclusively on the functioning and competence of the individual, failing to embrace fully the imperative of promoting the challenging of oppressive social structures. Regarding political empowerment, Lee (2001) states, 'All empowerment work is political' (p. 285). This is especially true of community work. We have demonstrated that the actions of empowered community members can achieve desired change and tip the power balance in their favour. In a shift from the individual to the collective focus of empowerment work, Thompson (2005) maintains that empowerment is 'geared towards helping to equip people for the challenges of tackling social disadvantages and inequalities they face ... it involves playing a part in connecting the personal to the political' (p. 125).

In addition to the above, a *critical, anti-oppressive approach* to social work practice is necessary in achieving resilience. According to Thompson (1998) practices can either 'condone, reinforce, or exacerbate existing inequalities or they can challenge, undermine or attenuate such oppressive forces' (p. 38). Accordingly, all practice should take into account oppression and domination. A critical, anti-oppressive approach ensures commitment to practice itself being self-critical and aware of oppressive power relations during intervention. It ensures the working against oppression of individuals and society. Practice without a political dimension, even in the promotion of resilience work, would be inadequate. In this regard, Dominelli (2002) maintains that social work is in danger of exhibiting oppressive capacities, which have been generated largely through the reproduction of everyday relations of domination, through the support of more overtly fascist policies, or even through cultural genocide of aboriginal peoples. She maintains that 'further oppressive relations are produced when, for example, practitioners hold people individually responsible for their position and urge them to change their behaviour without protesting the inequities in the social system in which they reside' (p. 68).

## Research Study

### Aims of the Study

The broad aim of this study was to explore students' thoughts and understanding of the concepts of 'resilience,' 'strength,' and 'coping' with respect to both their client systems and their personal worlds. Specifically, the study sought to explore students' perceptions of:

- factors that they thought enhanced resilience in childhood, families, communities, and society;
- cultural contributions to the development of resilience in individuals, families, and communities; and
- 'protective' and 'risk' factors present in people's lives in the South African context that may facilitate or impede human capacity for resilience.

*Research Design and Methodology*

In order to explore social work students' perceptions of resilience and coping, a qualitative approach was adopted using an exploratory, descriptive design. The fourth-year social work class of 2005 (eighteen students) at the University of the Witwatersrand, Johannesburg, South Africa, were invited to write an assignment on resilience and coping as part of their Social Work Theory and Practice IV course, Direct Methods of Social Work Practice.

Letters were distributed that described the rationale, aims, and procedures to be followed in the study. In these letters, students were invited to return on the following morning for a two-hour seminar if they were interested in participating. Confidentiality and voluntary participation were assured. No names or personal details were required on the worksheets, and it was explained that responses would not be for examination purposes. Sixteen students volunteered.

The assignment consisted of seventeen questions with subsections. The questions related to students' views of how resilience and coping are demonstrated; what contributes to the development of resilience in individuals, families, and communities; and the link between resilience and culture. The assignments were to be written on an answer sheet seven pages in length and did not require reference to literature.

Thematic content analysis was used to analyze data. This form of analysis is described as the classification of text into categories and drawing of inferences from textual material (Rosenthal & Rosnow, 1991, p. 158).

*Social Work Training at the University of the Witwatersrand*

Currently, approximately 170 undergraduate students and 40 postgraduate students are registered in the Department of Social Work. These students are predominantly black, representing all South African language groups. For 95% of students, English is their second or third language. One-fifth are male, and approximately half of the students are from rural areas. Most are from financially disadvantaged backgrounds. Students' ages range from twenty to forty years (M = 25). All students have roots in the context of apartheid, its racial oppression and violence, as well as in the HIV/AIDS epidemic.

In order to register with the Council for Social Service Professions, social workers are required to graduate with a four-year professional degree. Social work is a major course, and an elective second major is chosen in psychology or sociology to the third-year level. Emphasis is placed on both theoretical and practical content (which comprises a minimum of one thousand hours), including skills training, experiential learning, student participation, self-awareness, and reflection. The focus is on general training with the possibility of postgraduate specialization. To graduate, students are required to complete theory and practice as well as field instruction courses and to complete a research study.

Training incorporates the theoretical perspectives discussed earlier in this chapter, with a focus on ecosystemic perspectives, strengths perspectives, developmental social work, the empowerment approach, and anti-oppressive practice. Training also reflects a commitment to a shift away from a linear, causal, pathologizing paradigm. It is, therefore, important to examine and understand resilience and coping in relation to the professional self as well as in relation to the client system (individuals, families, groups, and communities) during training and preparation for practice.

## Social Work Students' Descriptions of Resilience and Coping

This section examines and discusses how social work students define and describe resilience and protective and risk factors and how growing up in the South African context may have affected these. Themes discussed are outlined in Table 1, along with extracts of student narratives illustrating each theme. This section also examines students' views about individual, family, and community factors as well as religious, cultural, societal, and structural factors that affect resilience and outcomes. The section concludes with an exploration of students' views of resilience in social workers and how this knowledge may be helpful for preparation for practice as social workers.

### Defining and Describing Resilience, Coping, and Strengths

Students regard resilience as the ability to 'bounce back,' 'overcome,' or 'deal with' difficult experiences and trauma and as 'surviving' or 'moving forward' in spite of strain and hardship. They describe resilience as comprising inner qualities such as 'hope,' 'help seeking,' and 'learning from hardship.' These descriptions concur with existing

Table 1: Student perceptions of resilience and coping

| | |
|---|---|
| Defining and describing resilience, coping, and strengths | 'to overcome suffering and still bounce back to life after a traumatic experience in life'<br>'one's ability to rise above any challenges or problems'<br>'ability to deal with injury, problem/constraint in positive way by bouncing back – "*kgotlelela*" – resilience in *seTswana*'<br>'to overcome feeling of hurt and discouragement, and to persevere'<br>'to be able to survive during or in a poverty-stricken family' |
| Describing protective factors | 'support from people, community, society, human rights'<br>'family, love, society supports, spiritual beliefs'<br>'safe community environment'<br>'living in a safe environment free from violence, poverty, crime and having a source of income and other supporting systems' |
| Risk factors and vulnerability | 'things that make people weak, e.g., domestic violence; neglect; crime and pollution can affect people from coping with their difficulties'<br>'can be people, authorities, policies, etc.'<br>'living in bad condition, not having a micro system to belong. Living in a poverty-stricken condition or place'<br>'any circumstances that make people be at risk, like HIV/AIDS'<br>'being able to do nothing re: certain circumstances you are in either due to oppression, discrimination or social inequality' |
| Growing up in South Africa – risk and protective factors | 'segregation enhanced domination and subordination'<br>'violence inflicted by the apartheid state demolished families; urban migration left the land and livestock poor and dying as more men migrated to town in search of jobs'<br>'deciding to be passive and accepting the situation – striking back a risk'<br>'forming a community unity to strengthen community resilience'<br>'counselling and the TRC (Truth and Reconciliation Commission) to be able to cope'<br>'people treated badly during apartheid era, still managed to cope'<br>'protective factor was support from their comrades' |

Table 1 (*continued*)

| | |
|---|---|
| Resilience and individual traits and experiences | 'strong emotional bonds, learning and improving from one's mistakes'<br>'patience, goal directedness, and suffering breed character'<br>'ability to believe in themselves and positive self-regard'<br>'level of education' and 'belief system'<br>'perseverance and socialization'<br>'using your experiences or life problems as learning areas' |
| Importance of family and relationships | 'being in a supportive and enhancing relationship'<br>'good interaction with internal and external environment'<br>'the resilience in families pours out into communities' |
| Resilience in community contexts | '*ubuntu* – things are done in a communal and collective manner'<br>'availability of support resources'<br>'the spirit of *ubuntu* where community members support each other' |
| Role of culture and religion | 'most are able to cope/be resilient by performing cultural rituals'<br>'things like circumcision help youth [boys] to be resilient and cope with their difficulties, e.g., they are taught different ways of dealing with their problems'<br>'prayers to cope with problems and ancestral ceremonies'<br>'cultural values, idioms, storytelling' |
| Societal and structural factors in resilience | 'tribal authority help people deal with community problems'<br>'social policies, laws, tribal authorities which hold and guide society about what is acceptable and not'<br>'legislation, policies that support *ubuntu* between different races, ethnic groups' |

understandings of resilience as the ability to cope in the face of adversity. Zide and Gray (2001), for example, state that coping measures include 'efforts to regulate negative feelings' (p. 10). Similarly, Antonovsky (1987) argues that the most basic category of coping resources consists of beliefs and attitudes towards life. Other coping mechanisms include the person's knowledge, successful experiences with life tasks, cognitive capacities and the ability to reason, the ability to control and use emotionally effective responses to stress, and skills to carry out planned action, which usually come from past successful experience. However, we would again like to raise the 'agency' versus 'structure' debate, which examines the dialectic between the ability and freedom of the individual to make choices and those institutional or structural factors that oppress and constrain individual wellness. This dialectic is particularly important in South Africa, where the historical and contemporary structural contexts of poverty and inequality are important factors in resilience and coping.

Students' descriptions of resilience that include references to coping also reflect Ungar's (2004) description of contextual factors that enhance coping, namely social supports, meaningful family relationships (with parents, grandparents, caregivers), and the need for a voice in the political system that controls them.

*Describing Protective and Risk Factors*

Resilience also needs to be understood in terms of risk and protective factors, including personality disposition, supportive family milieu, and external support systems that encourage and reinforce coping efforts while inculcating positive values (Garmezy & Rutter, 1988). As Newman and Blackburn (2002) state, 'the combination of three basic constructs – personality (specifically cognitive skills and styles), social milieu (absence of chronic life stresses and opportunities for meaningful social roles), and family structure (high warmth/low criticism) – has been consistently identified as the key protective factor for children exposed to a wide range of stressors' (p. 6). Ungar (2004) adds to this, describing factors associated with resilience as 'an unwieldy matrix of hundreds of factors that appear in the literature that have been used as indicators of healthy outcomes' (p. 61).

In spite of the diverse views of risk and protective factors, it is important for social workers to be able to identify these factors in order to promote resilience. However, regarding the area of family as a protective factor, it is important to remain critically aware of the potential for 'familism' as a form of cultural racism. Bozalek (2004) argues that the nuclear family as a normative model to be followed holds a range of negative effects, including a devaluation of cultural practices and negative self-conceptions for black women in relation to family forms. It is important, therefore, to understand that when 'family' is described as a protective factor, the term is understood in the broadest possible terms.

Descriptions of protective factors by students reflected those of Newman and Blackburn (2002) and Ungar (2004), echoing the categories described above, including inner qualities such as self-awareness and gaining from past experiences. Students highlighted love and support from family, parent, or significant other. Furthermore, community support, church, spiritual beliefs, cultural values, and human rights were mentioned, as well as a safe community environment. It is interesting to note that these protective factors were viewed in relation to external, concrete forms of threat, injury, harm, or violence, reflecting the South African reality and pointing to the importance of contextual relevance in both understanding and facilitating resilience.

In line with protective factors, students described risk factors as external threats. An absence of support from the family, for example, was seen as a risk factor, and one that could have an impact on inner strength. Such a finding also points to students' awareness that positive support could not be assumed given the presence of a family. Risk factors were also described in terms of other relationship factors, such as peer pressure, relationship violence, and abuse. Additional risk factors listed were HIV/AIDS, poverty, unemployment, malnutrition, and 'deviance' (such as substance abuse, unsafe sexual practices, and crime). Hardships and trauma that posed a risk to coping and resilience were generally described by students in terms of poverty, illness, and loss. Students identified lack of education as a particular risk. Historically, education was viewed as particularly important in South Africa and came to represent a means to liberation. As mentioned earlier, the uprisings of the late 1970s largely centred on education issues.

Additional risks included concrete factors posing real danger or being life threatening, as opposed to internal factors such as personality deficits (this is in keeping with the South African context of violence and extreme poverty; thus the greatest risks often related to basic material and safety needs).

*Growing Up in South Africa*

Historically, South African society has been particularly deleterious for children. Difficulties that children faced in the past, as well as current challenges, affect their development, emphasizing the critical need to explore coping strategies and resilience of children and youth so as to support and promote these strengths.

Students' childhood context is coloured by descriptions of violence, family disintegration, poverty, death and loss, fear, inferiority, real danger to life, and problems resulting from the migrant labour system. Some also viewed resistance, retaliation, and personal or family political involvement as a risk or danger to life and safety due to extreme levels of state repression. Many described having a sense of passivity, silence, fear, and acceptance of the status quo.

Students' experiences underscore the importance of a resilience perspective in approaching this context, with regard to both clients and workers. In the apartheid context, protective or mediating factors for children were severely eroded by years of colonization, apartheid, intra-community warfare, and disintegration of support systems. In this context, Duncan and Rock (1997) describe mediating factors that may in some cases have improved a child's reaction to political violence. These were seen as both intra-individual and situational.

Successful outcomes for youth in these circumstances seemed to depend very much on positive temperament, presence and availability of support systems (especially parents and older siblings), sound relationships with caregivers, and an active versus passive orientation for non-violent activism. Furthermore, being able to 'make sense of' violence, together with a notion of 'required helpfulness,' seemed to act as mitigating factors in the traumatic impact of violence. Student commentary again reflected such literature. Community solidarity, education, support from comrades, a sense of 'we,' and family support were noted and seen as important strengths and protective factors amongst respondents. Although these factors all seemed to enhance resilience, it should be noted that they mediate, rather than protect against, the effects of violence.

*Resilience and Individual Traits and Experiences*

Students showed personality characteristics and inner resources such as hope, assertiveness, patience, a sense of purpose, and the belief that threats can be overcome in their interpretation of resilience. They maintained that learning from difficult experiences as well as socialization processes within the family and community were important in the development of resilience. They also viewed having survived traumatic and difficult experiences as achievements that could develop resilience, and being reminded of coping and overcoming adversities as contributing to present coping and strength. Finally, they perceived a correlation between resilience and levels of education, maintaining that poor levels of education could be seen as a deficit. This is in keeping with the South African discourse around the value of and need for education given the inferior and oppressive nature of apartheid education.

## Resilience: Family and Relationship Factors

Students regard family as an important supportive context in the protection against adversity, stressing, however, that merely being in a family is not sufficient. Support, encouragement, love, and care from family members are required. In general relationships, interdependence and reciprocity are considered to lead to greater resilience. Furthermore, specific values such as respect and good communication result in stronger relationships and therefore greater resilience. The sense of belonging to groups and structures and the sense of 'we' that results from such belonging are also important according to the students. It seems, therefore, that it is what the family and other supportive groups provide rather than the particular form they take that students consider important. Families of various forms could, therefore, provide support for their members.

Similarly, in her study of South African families and how they coped with institutional racism, Bozalek (2004) maintains that the tendency to portray indigenous people as only victims and ignore their agency should be avoided. In her study of students' descriptions of their families she describes various forms of coping tactics in the face of institutional racism. Family members responded positively by supporting each other in day-to-day experiences of exclusion from resources, power, and opportunities; by engaging in collective forms of coping such as activism; or by acts of forgiveness and reconciliation. Alternatively, families responded with resignation in the form of avoidance or acceptance, or even more destructive responses such as alcohol and drug abuse and violence. It can be seen, therefore, that the family in all its forms plays a critical role in terms of support and encouragement in the face of difficulties.

*Resilience in Community Contexts*

Community resilience is built through a process of creating and strengthening personal, familial, social, organizational, and economic systems to resist and cope effectively in times of stress, threats, crises, and emergencies. Sarig (2001) explains that 'building community resilience is a long and constant process that is tested in times of crisis and stress ... often, components of community resilience are keys to individual resilience' (cited in Doron, 2005, p. 184). These include support and empowerment systems that offer a sense of belonging, ability to control crises, adequate formal and informal leadership, adequate skills through training, social solidarity, and a perspective of hope and community vision, values, and beliefs.

Similarly, students in this study emphasize the value or concept of *ubuntu*, a commonly understood and accepted concept in South Africa, explained in the proverb *umuntu ngumuntu ngabantu*. This Xhosa expression, common to all African languages and traditional cultures, means a person is a person through other persons (Shutte, 1994). It is the relationship between oneself and others that defines one as a person.

The students describe 'being community' as relating to and supporting each other. They describe the importance of community cooperation and problem solving, for example, through the utilization of local tribal courts (*makgotla*). Students also highlight the importance of adequate resources at the community level for resilience to be promoted. This view is important in the South African context, where the lack of resources is an immense problem.

*Resilience, Culture, and Religion*

Students described the role of culture in developing resilience as being 'in touch' with, having knowledge of, and practising one's culture and religion. They explained that cultural values, idioms, and storytelling in the oral tradition were important for healthy outcomes in youth. They also expressed their belief that collective values, cultural rituals (such as initiation ceremonies and other rites of passage), and the use of traditional healers were all important protective factors in resilience. The role of ancestors was considered as particularly important. Ceremonies focusing on the acknowledgment and appeasement of ancestors are an important part of family rituals given the deep reverence for, and specifically assigned roles of, ancestors. It can further be argued that these ancestral rituals and ceremonies offer a valuable representation of continuity. Graham (1999) explains that the African world view is a holistic conception of the human condition, reinforced by rituals. Many of these rituals are about promoting family life and structures such as rites of passage, naming ceremonies, child rearing, birth, death, elderhood, and values around governance.

In light of South Africa's history of cultural subjugation and denigration of indigenous practices, students described the importance of freedom to express traditionally held beliefs. In this regard, Freire (1970) describes what he refers to as *cultural invasion*. This occurs when an oppressive group penetrates the cultural context of another group and the creativity of the invaded group is inhibited. Members of the invaded group become convinced of their 'intrinsic inferiority' and become alienated from the values of their own culture. Liberation therefore implies, among other things, the freedom to live and express traditional cultural beliefs.

Many cultural practices that may be of great benefit for coping and resilience, have, however, been affected by 'primitivization' and individualist Western notions. Bozalek (2004) refers to the hegemony of Western views, for example, in relation to African traditional child-rearing practices that may be of great benefit to the growing child. The common practice of keeping a baby in the bed with a mother, for example, to enable attentiveness and constant contact between a baby and caregiver, is contradictory to the generally held Western view of the need for physical separation between the baby and the mother.

Student comments underscore the need for social workers to explore and respect their own cultural context as well as the one within which they work. Graham (1999) maintains that 'to become aware of the cultural self is an important process that connects a person spiritually with others within a culture. Furthermore, self-knowledge within the context of one's authenticity and connection with others provide the basis for transformation, spiritual development and well-being' (p. 259). Similarly, Becvar (1998) describes the spiritual dimension as a valuable resource for many clients, but one that has been neglected by many mental health clinicians. She maintains that 'more and more practitioners and researchers are now exploring how spiritual content can be integrated into a more holistic, collaborative approach to helping clients' (p. 14). In this regard Osei-Hwedi (1996) argues that social work practice must be based on the cultural milieu of the society in which it has evolved and is practised, and must use the model or conceptualization of human beings of that society.

Students' views about the importance of culture are in keeping with the view of both the International Resilience Project (2006) – which describes resilience as relating to culture as one of the four important aspects of individuals' lives – and Ungar (2004), who argues that connection to culture, along with engagement in rituals and rights of passage, is central to the development of resilience.

*Societal and Structural Factors of Resilience*

Students consider the societal or structural level of factors as having a very important impact on resilience. They believe that statutory provision should be made for practices and values supporting *ubuntu* in the form of legislation and policies. In this regard, statutes and adequate supportive structures and resources should acknowledge tribal authorities and traditional healers, thereby allowing factors such as social security to be used in the development of resilience. Students also emphasize the importance of the health care system in the context of HIV/AIDS.

Mirroring student accounts, the International Resilience Project Report (2006) argues that one of the tensions that resilient young people are able to resolve is that of social justice within 'experiences of prejudice and dynamics of socio-political context encountered individually, within one's family, in one's community, and culture, as well as experiences of resistance, solidarity, belief in a spiritual power, and standing up to oppression' (p. 16).

Students also point to the importance of role models and individuals to whom one can look with respect. They mention public figures such as Nelson Mandela, Bishop Desmond Tutu, Winnie Madikizela-Mandel, and Nkosi Johnson (the late young AIDS activist) – individuals who are seen to have demonstrated exceptional resilience. The reason for their choices seems to have been that these individuals were able to overcome traditional South African challenges such as torture, punishment, poverty, abuse, and HIV/AIDS.

## Resilience in Social Workers

By understanding the qualities and skills that promote resilience amongst themselves, social service professionals will be able to consciously develop resistance to the effects of risk. In this regard, the importance of self-awareness cannot be underestimated. Personal traits that facilitate mental health seem to include self-esteem and competence; self-respect and appropriate use of power; introspection, acceptance, and open-mindedness; cultural sensitivity, respect for others, empathy, and tolerance for ambiguity; cognitive complexity and flexibility; a sense of ethics and professionalism; awareness and expression of personal style; respect of personal boundaries; and an ability to delay both gratification of needs and expression of affect (Brems, 2001). Further attributes and skills include assertiveness; an attitude of hope and commitment; being able to deal with disappointment, stress, and change; having a strong value base; motivation; having a support network; and having a sense of humour (Thompson, 2005).

Students described their own strengths as being of both a personal and an academic nature. They noted the importance of self-awareness, goal setting, and a sense of purpose, as well as a commitment to self-care and a willingness to seek professional help. They stressed the need for an appreciation of diversity, together with the ability to deconstruct personal beliefs, in order to engage in critical examination and awareness. They believed that having the emotional strength to cope with difficult situations was correlated with resilience. Ways of building strengths included being self-confident, hopeful, and motivated; valuing 'survival'; and being able to reflect on past coping experiences and previous successes in dealing with adversity.

It is clear, then, that adequate attention during training to issues of resilience and coping is vitally important. As stated by participating students, novice social workers must be provided with the opportunity to reflect critically on their experiences of adversity and coping in order to develop self-awareness and to identify and consolidate these skills. Patel (2005) states that it is essential for social work graduates to be critical thinkers with reflexive competence in order to respond to new realities. Theory and practice need to draw on universal as well as indigenous knowledge systems. In this way, resilience and coping will be promoted among practitioners.

## Conclusion

Although this exploratory study limits generalizations and conclusions, it seems that students were able to articulate their views of resilience, coping, and strengths clearly and that these perceptions were generally in keeping with relevant theory and research findings. Resilience among social work students is critical, as their own resilience will contribute to the adequate and appropriate facilitation of resilience among the youth with whom they work. Their responses not only pointed to the need for an ecological focus on risk and resilience, but emphasized that this focus should also be contextually bound.

For students, ecological factors incorporate individual, relational, community, and cultural factors. Individual factors promoting resilience include personality characteristics, inner resources, learning from difficult experiences, and socialization processes. Family and relationship factors seen to nurture resilience include support from the family in its broadest possible form as well as positive relationships with significant others. Important community factors are seen to be those relating to a sense of belonging, solidarity, and collective action. Strong views were expressed about the importance of traditional cultural and religious beliefs, as well as the role of structural factors in nurturing resilience. In this regard, it was considered important that statutory provision be made for the enablement of supportive environments and factors that promote resilience, such as policies that encourage *ubuntu*, the support of families through social security, recognition of traditional cultural practices, and an adequate health care system.

Students also emphasize that social service professionals should promote and nurture resilience and coping within themselves – especially during their training phase. They believe that this is achieved through critical self-reflection, self-awareness, a commitment to self-care, and a willingness to seek professional help. Furthermore, they emphasize the importance of a strong value base together with an appreciation of diversity.

Questions for further exploration arising from this study include:

- How do students in the helping professions perceive the impact of their own background and context on their views of resilience and coping?

- How do students' perceptions and understandings of resilience connect to the survival and improvement of helping professions such as social work in contexts like South Africa?
- How will students' own resilience and coping skills equip them for the continuing challenges of their future?

## REFERENCES

Antonovsky, A. (1987). *Unravelling the mystery of health: How people manage stress and stay well.* San Francisco: Jossey Bass.

Becvar, D.S. (Ed.). (1998). *The family, spirituality and social work.* New York: Haworth Press.

Bowlby, J. (1979). *The making and breaking of affectional bonds.* London: Tavistock.

Bozalek, V. (2004). *Recognition, resources, responsibilities: Using students' stories of family to renew the South African social work curriculum.* Unpublished doctoral dissertation, Universiteit Utrecht, Netherlands.

Brems, C. (2001). *Basic skills in psychotherapy and counselling.* Pacific Grove, CA: Brooks/Cole and Thomson Learning.

Bulhan, H.A. (1985). *Frantz Fanon and the psychology of oppression.* New York: Plenum Press.

Carter, M. (2004). *Five million new HIV cases in 2004, women and girls bear the brunt.* Aidsmap. Retrieved 15 April 2005 from http://www.aidsmap.com/en/news.

Dawes, A. (2003). Adolescence and youth: Challenges in post-conflict South Africa (HSRC: Child, Youth and Family Development [CYFD] Research Programme). *HSRC Review, 1*(3). Retrieved 16 September 2003 from http://www.hsrc.ac.za/about/HSRCReview/Vol1No3/index.html?adolescence.html~conte nt.

Department of Social Development. (1997). *White paper for social welfare.* Pretoria: DSD.

Department of Social Development. (2000). *Population, poverty and vulnerability: The state of South Africa's population, Report 2000.* Pretoria: DSD.

Department of Social Development. (2005). Address by Zola Skweyiya, Minister of Social Development, to the National Assembly, 1 June 2005, Cape Town, South Africa.

Department of Social Development. (2006). *Draft recruitment and retention strategy for social workers.* 31 March 2006. Pretoria: DSD.

Dominelli, L. (2002). *Feminist social work theory and practice.* Houndmills, Basingstoke, Hampshire: Palgrave Macmillan.

Doron, E. (2005). Working with Lebanese refugees in a community resilience model. *Community Development Journal, 40(2)*, 182–91.

Duncan, N., & Rock, B. (1997). The impact of political violence on the lives of South African children. In C. De La Rey, N. Duncan, T. Shefer, & A. Van Niekerk (Eds.), *Contemporary issues in human development: A South African focus* (pp. 133–58). Johannesburg: Thompson.

Freire, P. (1970). *Pedagogy of the oppressed* (trans. Myra Bergman Ramos). New York: Seabury Press.

Garmezy, N., & Rutter, N. (Eds.). (1988). *Stress, coping, and development in children*. Baltimore: Johns Hopkins University Press.

Graham, M.J. (1999). The African-centred worldview: Developing a paradigm for social work. *British Journal of Social Work, 29*, 251–67.

Helton, L.R., & Smith, M. (2004). *Mental health practice with children and youth: A strengths and wellbeing model*. New York: Haworth Press.

Human Sciences Research Council. (2004). Poor households sink deeper into poverty. *HSRC Review, 2(3)*. Retrieved 15 November 2005 from http://hsrc .ac.za/about/HSRCReview/Vol2No3/index.html?news_roundup.html ~content.

International Resilience Project. (2006). *Project report*. Halifax: Dalhousie University, School of Social Work.

IRIN (Integrated Regional Information Networks). (2004). *South Africa: Child welfare system leaves many AIDS orphans stranded*. United Nations Office for the Co-ordination of Humanitarian Affairs. Retrieved 9 November 2004 from http://irinnews.org.

Lee, J.A.B. (2001). *The empowerment approach to social work practice: Building the beloved community* (2nd ed.). New York: Columbia University Press.

Lombard, A. (1998). Transforming social work education: A contextual and empowerment issue. In F. Kotze & B. McKendrick (Eds.), *Transforming social work education: Proceedings of the Joint Universities' Committee's Annual Conference on Transforming Social Work Education*. Bellville: University of the Western Cape, Department of Social Work.

McKendrick, B. (2001). The promise of social work: Directions for the future. *Social Work/Maatskaplike Werk, 37(2)*, 105–11.

Meintjies, H., Budlender, D., Giese, S., & Johnson, L. (2003). *Children 'in need of care' or in need of cash? Questioning social security provisions for orphans in the context of the South African AIDS pandemic*. Cape Town: Children's Institute and the Centre for Actuarial Research, University of Cape Town.

Newman, T., & Blackburn, S. (2002). *Interchange 78: Transitions in the lives of children and young people: Resilience factors*. Scottish Executive Education

Department, Education and Young People Research Unit. Retrieved 12 May 2005 from www.scotland.gov.uk/insight/.

Noyoo, N. (1998). Transforming social work education for a changing and fluid South African society. In F. Kotze & B. McKendrick (Eds.), *Transforming social work education: Proceedings of the Joint Universities' Committee's Annual Conference on Transforming Social Work Education*. Bellville: University of the Western Cape, Department of Social Work.

Osei-Hwedi, K. (1996). The indigenisation of social work practice and education in Africa: The dilemma of theory and method. *Social Work/Maatskaplike Werk, 32*(3), 215–25.

Patel, L. (2005). *Social welfare and social development in South Africa*. Cape Town: Oxford University Press.

Payne, M. (2005). *Modern social work theory*. Houndmills, Basingstoke, Hampshire: Palgrave Macmillan.

Peirson, L. (2005). Disadvantaged children and families. In G. Nelson & I. Prilleltensky (Eds.), *Community psychology: In pursuit of liberation and wellbeing* (pp. 448 – 467). Houndmills, Basingstoke, Hampshire: Palgrave Macmillan.

Ratele, K. (Ed.) (2006). *Inter-group relations: South African perspectives*. Cape Town: Juta.

Rosenthal, R., & Rosnow, R. (1991). *Essentials of behavioural research: Methods and data analysis*. New York: McGraw-Hill.

Saleebey, D. (2002). *The strengths perspective in social work practice*. Boston: Allyn & Bacon.

Sewpaul, V., & Holscher, D. (2004). *Social work in times of neoliberalism: A postmodern discourse*. Pretoria: Van Schaik.

Sewpaul, V., & Jones, D. (2004). *Global standards for the education and training of the social work profession*. Retrieved on 22 March 2006 from http://www.iassw-aiets.org/en/About_IASSW/GlobalStandards.pdf .

Sheafor, B.W., Horejsi, C.R., & Horejsi, G.A. (1994). *Techniques and guidelines for social work practice* (3rd ed.). Boston: Allyn & Bacon.

Shmukler, K. (1993). *Resilience in children: The role of locus of control and self concept in a sample of township youth*. Unpublished Master of Arts research report. University of the Witwatersrand, Johhanesburg.

Shutte, A. (1994). *Philosophy for Africa*. Rondebosch, South Africa: UCT Press.

Smith, L. (2004). Current challenges for the realisation of human rights in South Africa. *ZEP: Zeitschrift fur internationale Bildungsforschung und Entwicklungspadagogik, 27*(4), 6–11.

*South Africa at a glance*. (2005). Greenside, South Africa: Editors Inc.

Thompson, N. (1998). *Promoting equality: Challenging discrimination and oppression in the human services*. Basingstoke, Hampshire: Palgrave Macmillan.

Thompson, N. (2005). *Understanding social work: Preparing for practice*. Houndmills, Basingstoke, Hampshire: Palgrave Macmillan.

Treatment Action Campaign. (2006). *Report to the National Executive Committee*. Retrieved 15 May 2006 from http://www.tac.org.za/news_2006.html.

Ungar, M. (2004). *Nurturing hidden resilience in troubled youth*. Toronto: University of Toronto Press.

United Nations Development Programme, South Africa. (2003). *South African human development report*. Cape Town: Oxford University Press.

Walsh, F. (1998). *Strengthening family resilience*. New York: Guilford.

Zide, M.R. & Gray, S.W. (2001). *Psychopathology: A competency based model for social workers*. Belmont, CA: Brookes Cole.

# PART TWO

Structuring Services for Youth

# 7 Supporting Resilience among Homeless Youth

NICOLE LETOURNEAU, MIRIAM STEWART,
LINDA REUTTER, AND KRISTA HUNGLER

I'd call it ...'The Hope Program.' 'Cause there's hope for a better future.
— Homeless youth, age seventeen

The Canadian Public Health Association (CPHA) *Position Paper on Homelessness* emphasized the need for health care 'delivery systems that provide care to persons with minimal social support,' including resources to promote resilience among street youth. However, homeless youth report that finding social support is their biggest challenge. Access to appropriate services, supportive individuals, and supportive social organizations that consider youths' social needs is important to enabling homeless youth to make a successful transition to inclusion in mainstream society (Caputo, Weiler, & Anderson, 1997).

This chapter reflects on a program of research designed to assess homeless youths' support needs from their perspectives and the perspectives of their service providers. The aim of the research is to develop an intervention to meet identified support needs, and to pilot the resulting intervention program. Phase 1 of this study revealed social support needs, resources, barriers to support and support preferences of homeless youth. These data were used to develop an innovative intervention that was piloted during phase 2. The phase 2 intervention consisted of a comprehensive mentoring support intervention for homeless youth that was designed to optimize peer influence, reduce isolation, and enhance functioning. Case studies of two home-

This research was funded by the Alberta Heritage Foundation for Medical Research. The authors also thank Catherine Young for her assistance with manuscript revision.

less youth composed of composites of the actual youth in this study are used to illustrate the study's findings.

## Social Support

As a determinant of health (Federal Provincial Territorial Advisory Committee on Population Health, 1998), social support assists homeless youth to attain success (Steinhauer, 1998). Social support is a resource for coping with the abuse, neglect, and poverty associated with homelessness (Ungar, 2004). Consisting of affirmational (e.g., reassurance), emotional (e.g. reliable alliance), informational (e.g., guidance for support seeking) and instrumental support (e.g., transportation to support sources) (Raphael, 2004; Stewart, 1993, 2000), effective social support is characterized as interactions with mentors (peers, volunteers, and professionals) that can improve coping, moderate stresses, and alleviate loneliness and isolation (Gottlieb, 2000, 2002). Social support can moderate the impact of stressful living situations on mental health–related outcomes, such as loneliness, and the emotional distress generated when people feel estranged from or misunderstood or rejected by others (Stewart, Craig, & MacPherson, 2001). Social support may therefore modify the association between health and the stress of homelessness (Caputo & Kelly, 1998), as homeless youth often report conflict within their families, fear of attachment, and inadequate social relationships (Gottlieb, 1998).

## Homelessness

Homeless youth, by definition, range in age from twelve to twenty-four years of age (Caputo & Kelly, 1998) and do not live in family homes or foster care. Rather, they live in unsafe or temporary living arrangements. Given the diversity of their living situations, they have been variously described as 'curbside, entrenched, runaways, throwaways, in and outers, street kids and independently living youths' (McCall, 1992). Estimates of homeless youth in Canada range from 150,000 (Caputo, Weiler, & Anderson, 1997) to 200,000 (Fitzgerald, 1995). In Edmonton, Alberta (a city of one million people), one shelter alone served 640 separate youth between July 1999 and June 2000 (Canada Mortgage and Housing Corporation, 2001).

In Canada, the majority of homeless youth are from 'disrupted' families (Canada Mortgage and Housing Corporation, 2001), and many youth become homeless as a result of life events and circumstances that negatively affect their well-being. Family violence, conflict, and poverty are major contributing factors to leaving home early. Many youth also leave home because of physical and sexual abuse, chemical addiction of a family member, and/or parental neglect (Van Wormer, 2003). Other risk factors associated with homelessness include alcoholism of a family member, ethnic minority status, emotional neglect, and foster care placement. Homeless youth are typically from female-headed, single-parent family backgrounds with elevated poverty levels (Bronstein, 1996).

An Ontario survey revealed that 38% of runaways rated their physical health as fair to poor, versus only 2% of youth enrolled in school (Unger et al., 1998). Prevalent health problems include sexually transmitted diseases, including HIV/AIDS, drug use, and injuries (Dadds, Maujean, & Fraser, 2003). Homeless girls have the highest lifetime rates of pregnancy (Greene & Ringwalt, 1998), often linked to physical and sexual abuse, the exchange of sex for food and shelter, and drug use (Yorden & Yorden, 1995). Drug and alcohol abuse is higher among street youth than domiciled youth (Commander, Davis, McCabe, & Stanyer, 2002) and the longer the duration of homelessness, the more likely youth are to abuse substances (Sibthorpe, Drinkwater, Gardner, & Bammer, 1995) or engage in high-risk sexual behaviour (Clements, Gleghorn, Garcia, Latch, & Marx, 1997). Depression (Unger et al., 1998) and suicidal thoughts and behaviours, prevalent among homeless youth, are often the emotional sequelae of physical, sexual, and substance abuse (Baron, 1999).

Homeless youth have a higher incidence of physical, emotional, and behavioural problems, such as delinquency, than youth who live with their families (Commander et al., 2002; Dadds et al., 2003). Street youth are more likely than domiciled youth to engage in deviant and delinquent behaviours (Baron, 2001; Golden, Currie, Greaves, & Latimer, 1999; Whitbeck & Hoyt, 1999). Homeless youth also experience more violence and abuse than youth who live with families and are more prone to physical and sexual assault (Kipke, Montgomery, Simon, Unger, & Johnson, 1997; Terrell, 1997; Whitbeck & Hoyt, 1999). In a Toronto-based study, Gaetz (2004) found that 82% of street youth reported being assaulted, robbed, and sexually abused.

## Social Support for Homeless Youth

Providing social support to homeless youth is challenging, as they are often unwilling to access mainstream health care and services (Gottlieb, 1998), relying most often on peers for support (Health Canada, 2004; Unger et al., 1998). Moreover, homeless youth are prone to exclusion from mainstream society and isolation from all but their street-youth peers, enhancing their reluctance to seek and access beneficial health and support services (Bronstein, 1996). Most existing programs that are designed to foster youth resilience emphasize social competence, life skills, and social support, but do not focus specifically on homeless youth (Caputo & Kelly, 1998).

With this background, a team of researchers sought to assess homeless youths' and service providers' perspectives of social support and then develop and pilot a social support intervention for homeless youth. In both phase 1 and phase 2 of the research, youth were considered homeless if they (1) had no home at all and were living on the streets (absolute homelessness); (2) were living in a place that was not intended to be housing or was not a suitable long-term residence; or (3) were at risk of becoming homeless through losing their home, being discharged from an institution/facility with nowhere to go, or being threatened with the loss of income support (Olsen & Friedenthal, 2000).

*Phase 1: Assessment Study*

Phase 1 of this study focused on assessment of homeless youths' support needs, resources, barriers to support, and support preferences, from the perspectives of homeless youth and service providers. Methods included in-depth individual interviews with nineteen homeless youth and eighteen service providers from community agencies in Edmonton. In addition, group interviews were with service providers (two groups) and youth (two groups) as well as previously homeless youth who had made the transition from homelessness (one group).

Findings from this exploratory work revealed that homeless youth are particularly interested in accessing a combination of peer and adult mentors from their community. These supports are most helpful when they are perceived to be non-judgmental and caring. Mentors were expected to be able to relate to youth and to be a similar age or only slightly older. Face-to-face support was preferred rather than phone contact. Where mentoring was part of a formal model of service delivery, youth preferred to be given a choice between group and/or one-to-one mentoring. These findings are congruent with other studies of mentoring relationships as part of support interventions that have demonstrated positive changes in the social and emotional development of 'socially excluded' youth (Springer & Basca, 2003).

As an intervention program, mentoring can facilitate the use of active and problem-focused coping behaviours in youth (Springer & Basca, 2003) and enhance intimacy, communication skills, and trust (Rhodes, 2002). Traditionally, mentoring (e.g., guidance, instruction, encouragement) is provided by a more experienced adult to an unrelated, younger person (Rhodes, 2002). Others extend mentoring relationships to include peer mentoring and group mentoring (Bellamy, Springer, Sale, & Espiritu, 2004; Darling, Hamilton, Toyokawa, & Matsuda, 2002). Mentoring programs can involve unstructured and structured activities that are either community based (e.g., going to the movies, museums, zoos, parks, group recreation, community service activities) or site based, such as school (Herrera, 2004) or workplace (Hamilton & Hamilton, 2002) programs.

Mentoring programs have shown that a youth's one-to-one relationship with a supportive adult can lead to a number of positive outcomes, including improved academic achievement, a stronger sense of self-worth, and improved relations with parents and peers, together with decreased alcohol and drug abuse, absenteeism from school, aggressive behaviour, and delinquency (Bellamy et al., 2004; Dubois, Holloway, Valentine, & Cooper, 2002; Grossman & Tierney, 1998; Jucovy, 2002; Novotney, Mertinko, Lange, Falb, & Kirk, 2002). DuBois et al. (2002) concluded from their work that one of the best psychological resources that mentoring promotes is a youth's sense of self-worth.

While there is ample evidence that supportive mentoring relationships have an important and positive formative influence on youth and can promote resilience, there is less evidence of the effect of mentoring on homeless youth (Bellamy et al., 2004). Most existing programs aimed at vulnerable youth exclude homeless youth. Consequently, very little is known about programs that offer social support to these youth (Caputo, Weiler, & Anderson, 1997). Moreover, existing programs have not been based on assessment of homeless youths' preferences for support interventions or comprised of a combination of non-judgmental and caring peer and community mentor supports. One can surmise, however, that mentors can influence health behaviours of homeless youth by providing information, encouragement, or advice; acting as role models; and restraining them from inappropriate and high-risk behaviours. The following case studies demonstrate typical patterns of relationships and behaviour identified among street youth in Edmonton who were the focus of this study.

### CASE STUDY 1: SUE

Sue is a nineteen-year-old aboriginal women. She looks younger than nineteen. She left home for the first time when her mother's latest boyfriend became abusive. Sue says her mother knows about the abuse but cares for the boyfriend more than her. She has been staying with her older sister on and off, and returns home when her mother's boyfriend isn't around. She has been unable to keep up with her schooling since she finished grade 10. Her sister now has a new boyfriend who doesn't like Sue sleeping on the couch. As a consequence, Sue has taken to sleeping in paper recycling bins. She enjoys time with other street youth, who understand what it's like for her and why she is on the street. Whenever she gets money from her family or friends, she spends it on food, alcohol, or drugs. She hasn't had to engage in prostitution for income, but knows of other youth that do.

### CASE STUDY 2: JOEL

Joel is seventeen years old and has been in and out of trouble with the law for fighting, theft, and vandalism over the last couple of years. Most recently he was caught joy-riding 'borrowed' cars and was sent to a juvenile detention centre for the first time. He's had a difficult time controlling his anger for as long as he can remember. He recently returned from Toronto and has been frequenting a youth co-op in Edmonton.

His father left home and moved to Toronto when Joel was fourteen years old. Joel's mother has been off work on a disability allowance since the break-up, and now Joel doesn't think too much of her. After getting out of detention, Joel decided to pay his dad a surprise visit in Toronto. His father was very busy with his work and didn't have much time for Joel, except to lecture him that he'd better change his ways or he'd end up in adult court. His father offered to pay for counselling, but wanted Joel to stay with his mother in Edmonton 'for Joel's sake.' Joel surprised his dad when he left town without warning and went back to Edmonton. He hasn't been to see his mother since returning, preferring to stay with friends.

## Phase 2: Mentoring Support Intervention and Evaluation

Phase 1 findings informed the development of a peer and adult mentor support intervention that was tested during phase 2, the pilot intervention and evaluation phase. A one-group, within-subjects study was employed to evaluate the intervention. Data were collected from participating youth three times. First collection was at the time of their enrolment in the support program. After enrolment, homeless youth participated in the peer and adult mentor support program. Data were collected a second time six weeks after enrolment and a third time upon exit from the program.

## Mentoring Support Intervention

The social support intervention lasted approximately seven months and consisted of three to four hours of weekly support groups facilitated by mentors with opportunities for one-on-one support outside group times. The sample was a convenience sample from agencies that work with homeless youth. Recruitment was conducted with the aid of professionals from partnering agencies. Representatives from these agencies were asked to identify youth as potential participants. Once youth indicated an interest in the study, research assistants approached the youth for recruitment into the study.

Mentors were not matched with youth; instead, youth were free to talk with mentors of their choice. Peer mentors (one or two per group) had previously experienced homelessness or poverty, and the community mentors (two or three per group) demonstrated interest in supporting homeless youth. There were more community mentors (56%) than peer mentors (44%). Mentors' ages ranged from eighteen years to forty-eight years with an average age of twenty-five years. More females (63%) than males (28%) volunteered.

Free recreational activities, nutritious meals, and transportation were provided during each session. Transportation to the support group was offered in the form of bus tickets, and transportation to the site of recreational activities was provided for the entire group. The support intervention included opportunities for both group support and dyadic (one-to-one) support. Given homeless youths' lack of consistent access to telephones and their reported preferences for face-to-face support, this approach was chosen. Four groups ran weekly, one evening a week for three to four hours. Youth chose activities for each week and topics for discussion. The support intervention was flexible and accessible by being offered in the evening, in a location familiar to youth, without restrictive entrance requirements. In each group there were five mentors for approximately ten homeless or at-risk youth. Professional mentors (one per group), recruited from collaborating agencies, had professional experience working with youth and received payment. Peer and community mentors were volunteers recruited from the general population, screened, and trained to work with homeless youth. As noted above, peer mentors (one or two per group) had previously experienced homelessness or poverty, and the community mentors (two or three per group) demonstrated interest in supporting homeless youth.

Recreational activities such as swimming, going to hockey games, and playing pool were chosen by youth in each support group. Professional mentors facilitated the process of selecting activities. Once the activity was chosen, project staff organized the activity for the group with community recreation facilities. A crucially important component of the support intervention was the free nutritious meal that started the evening. During the meal, youth and mentors had the opportunity to sit together and talk. Homeless youth were encouraged to talk about their lives, and mentors were trained to listen attentively and provide emotional, affirmational, and informational support as necessary.

The integrity of the intervention was closely monitored, with professional and volunteer mentors meeting for a debriefing session immediately after each support group. These debriefings served the dual purpose of supporting the volunteer mentors and documenting intervention activities. Moreover, the project coordinator and research assistants communicated with professional mentors on a weekly basis via telephone, email and face-to-face meetings. The project coordinator communicated with all volunteer mentors via email and telephone.

**Data Collection and Measures**

*Data Collection*

Both qualitative and quantitative data collection were a part of phase 2. Qualitative in-depth individual interviews were conducted with participating youth. Interviewers were similar in age to the youth and had experience working with at-risk youth. They were also trained in suicide intervention and non-violent crisis intervention, and had experience in mental health settings. Qualitative interview guide questions focused on elucidating youths' perceived connection with mentors, other sources of support, goal achievement, progress towards personal goals, support-seeking behaviours, strategies to cope with life stressors, markers of intervention success, and the general impact of the intervention. Qualitative interviews were audio-taped for transcription.

In addition to demographic and descriptive data collection, quantitative measures focused on examining depression, health status, social support, loneliness, and social network size. Measures included the Centre for Epidemiological Studies—Depression Scale (CESD; [Radloff, 1977]), The Social Provisions Scale, and the Revised UCLA (University of California, Los Angeles) Loneliness Scale.

Depression was measured by the CESD, a short self-report scale intended for the general population. It lists twenty symptoms of depression that participants are asked to rate on a scale from 1 'rarely or none of the time' to 4 'most or all of the time'. The internal consistency of the CESD ranges from .085 to .90.

The *Social Provisions Scale* is a twenty-four-item self-report instrument. It assesses global perceptions of support (Cutrona & Russell, 1987). Based on the theoretical work of Weiss (1974), six different social functions or 'provisions' are obtained from relationships and are needed for individuals to feel adequately supported, although different provisions may be more crucial in certain circumstances or at different stages of the life cycle. These six social functions include guidance, reliable alliance, reassurance of worth, attachment, social integration, and opportunity for nurturance. Items are rated on a four-point scale to produce a summative score ranging from 24 to 96, with higher scores indicating higher levels of global support. The normative sample mean is 82 (SD = 10), based upon a sample of 1,792 individuals. This measure has well-established reliability and validity, including a valid factor structure.

The Revised UCLA Loneliness Scale consists of twenty statements assessing loneliness, social isolation, and satisfaction and dissatisfaction with social relationships (Russell, 1996). Participants are asked to indicate if they often, sometimes, rarely, or never feel the way described in the statements. Concurrent validity was confirmed by associations between scores on the Revised UCLA Loneliness Scale and other indicators of loneliness, social relationships, and affective states, such as the Beck Depression Inventory (alpha r = .62). In studies using college student samples, high internal consistency coefficients were obtained (.94–.96). The Revised UCLA Loneliness Scale has been used extensively with different populations, including youth. Higher scores indicate a greater degree of loneliness, social isolation, and dissatisfaction with social relationships. A score of 40 is the norm, and the maximum possible score is 80.

Health status questions were taken from the World Health Organization's *Health Behaviour in School-Aged Children (HSBC)* cross-national study (Currie et al., 2004). Youth were asked to indicate whether or not they experienced any of a list of chronic health conditions (e.g., asthma, allergies), psychological health conditions (e.g., attention deficit disorder, schizophrenia), and high-risk health behaviours (e.g., tobacco use, drug use). Youths were also asked to respond to the question 'Overall, how healthy are you?' with possible answers ranging from 1 (not healthy at all) to 5 (very healthy).

Social network size was assessed by youths' answers to the question 'How many friends (including peers and people you "hang out with") do you have?'

*Sample*

Seventy homeless youth who did not participate in phase 1, were recruited into the study and completed pre-test measures at enrolment into phase 2. At pre-test, the mean age was nineteen years (SD = 2.5; *n* = 70), with ages ranging from sixteen to twenty-four years. Slightly more males (54%; *n* = 38) were recruited than females (46%; *n* = 32). Sixty percent of the sample were Aboriginal/Metis/First Nations, with Caucasian youth making up the next-largest cultural group at 27% (*n* = 19), followed by 13% (*n* = 9) visible minority youth. Fifteen percent (*n* = 11) of the youth were parents, of whom most had one child (11%; *n* = 8) and a few (4%; *n* = 3) had two children. However, only four participants lived with their children. These children ranged in age from two months to seven years.

Participants' level of education ranged from grade 5 to those who had graduated high school (M = Grade 10; SD = 1.3; $n$ = 70): 19% ($n$ = 13) were high school graduates; 31% ($n$ = 22) had completed grade 11, 26% ($n$ = 18) grade 10, 21% ($n$ = 15) grade 9. One youth had only completed grade 5, another grade 8. Fourteen percent of youth ($n$ = 10) were still in school, 42% ($n$ = 29) had dropped out, and 16% ($n$ = 11) had been expelled. Thirty percent ($n$ = 21) of the youth were employed. Twenty seven percent ($n$ = 19) of participants claimed employment as their main source of income, while parents were a main source of income for 23% ($n$ = 16) and 10% ($n$ = 7) reported no income. Tables 1, 2, and 3 summarize the characteristics of the sample at the time the pre-test was administered.

Most youth had been in their current living arrangement for less than six months (36%, $n$ = 25). The transitory nature of their housing arrangements was reflected by the fact that 20% of the youth had been at their current arrangement for less than one month, 11% for only one to two weeks, and 4% less than one week. Keeping in mind that the definition of homelessness used in this study includes youth at risk for homelessness, only two participants had been in their current arrangement their whole life (3%). Nine percent had been living in their current arrangement for six months to one year, while 10% had been there for over a year. Forty-five percent reported that they were continuously moving or transient.

The CES-D was used to measure symptoms of depression in the last seven days. Participants in this study had a mean score of 23 ($n$ = 68; SD = 11), where scores above 16 may be indicative of clinical depression. However, to reduce interview burden, the CES-D scale was removed from the interview guide at mid- and post-test. The majority of youth (59%; $n$ = 41) believed that they were 'somewhat healthy,' while 29% (n = 20) reported that they were very healthy. Nevertheless, half of the sample (51%; $n$ = 36) reported a chronic illness; 30% ($n$ = 22) had psychological problems, and 41% ($n$ = 33) had physical conditions. Some had more than one chronic illness.

*Attrition*

From the seventy youth recruited to take part in the intervention at pre-test, twenty-nine participated in the midpoint interviews (41%) and fourteen participated in the post-test interviews and attended

Table 1: Participant school, work, and behaviours

| Characteristics | Yes | | No | |
|---|---|---|---|---|
| | % | n | % | n |
| Go to school | 34 | n=24 | 64 | n=45 |
| Work full time | 27 | n=19 | 71 | n=50 |
| Work part time | 47 | n=33 | 50 | n=35 |
| History of arrest | 77 | n=54 | 20 | n=14 |
| Incarcerated | 57 | n=40 | 40 | n=28 |
| Do drugs frequently | 69 | n=48 | 29 | n=20 |
| Get drunk frequently | 63 | n=44 | 34 | n=24 |
| Makes Money illegally | 40 | n=28 | 57 | n=40 |
| Gets into fights frequently | 40 | n=28 | 56 | n=39 |

Note: Percentages do not add up to 100 as a result of missing values.

Table 2: Participant income source

| | % | n |
|---|---|---|
| Employment | 27% | (n=19) |
| Mom/dad | 23% | (n=16) |
| No income | 10% | (n=7) |
| SFI | 13% | (n=9) |
| AISH | 6% | (n=4) |
| Illegal activity | 6% | (n=4) |
| Relatives | 2% | (n=3) |
| KITH | 2% | (n=3) |
| Aboriginal funding | 1% | (n=1) |
| Métis association | 1% | (n=1) |
| Panhandling | 2% | (n=3) |
| Family allowance | 1% | (n=1) |
| 'Found' | 1% | (n=1) |

the peer and adult mentor support intervention ten or more times (24%). Of the youth who participated in the intervention and had mid-point interviews (n=29), 41% (n=12) did not attend every session; of those, five moved away from Edmonton and one had a chronic health condition that reduced his participation.

Table 3: Participants' living arrangements at pre-test

| Current Living Arrangement | % | (n) |
|---|---|---|
| Mother or father | 29 | (n=20) |
| Relatives | 17 | (n=12) |
| Absolute homeless | 14 | (n=10) |
| Friends | 9 | (n=6) |
| Boy/girlfriend | 9 | (n=6) |
| Alone | 7 | (n=5) |
| Group homes | 6 | (n=4) |
| Shelters | 4 | (n=3) |
| Semi-independent living | 3 | (n=2) |
| Independent living | 1 | (n=1) |
| Roommates | 1 | (n=1) |
| Total | 100 | (n=70) |

## Data Analysis

Quantitative data were analysed with measures of central tendency and parametric statistics (paired $t$-tests and repeated measures analysis of variance). Non-parametric statistics were used as appropriate. While quantitative analyses attempted to include as much data as possible, repeated measures analysis of variance were conducted on only the fourteen participants who completed all pre-, mid-, and post-testing. Qualitative data were analysed via thematic content analysis. Coding created categories for data that were mutually exclusive and exhaustive. Coding and analysis of data was facilitated by Statistical Package for the Social Science (SPSS) version 9 or greater (Norusis, 1992) and QSR NUD*IST qualitative data management software.

## Quantitative Findings

Differences between mean pre-test, mid-point, and post-test scores for the Social Provisions Scale were examined with paired $t$-tests. A repeated measures analysis of variance (ANOVA) was also used to examine differences over time, using Greenhouse-Geiser values due to significant sphericity. No significant differences were observed in any of the analyses over time. However, the scale score remained below the normative mean of 82 in all analyses, with an average score of 75 over time indicating less than optimal support.

The mean pre-test, mid-point, and post-test scores for the UCLA Loneliness Scale were examined with repeated measures ANOVA. Since the test for sphericity was significant, the Greenhouse-Geiser values were used. The repeated measures model was significant ($F = 4.6_{(2,26)}$, $p = .05$; $n = 14$). Figure 1 illustrates decrease evident over time.

Youth were asked to describe how many friends (including peers and people they 'hang out with') they had at pre-, mid-, and post-test. At pre-test ($n = 70$), youth had an average of twenty-five people in their support networks. A mean increase of eleven persons was found from pre- to mid-point for the twenty-nine youth interviewed at mid-point. For the sample of fourteen that provided data at all three data points, the mean increase in social network size was nineteen from pre-test to mid-point, and this increase was maintained to post-test (see figure 2). However, repeated measures ANOVA did not reveal any statistically significant difference over time for this group; however the small sample size likely reduced the ability to determine significant differences.

## Qualitative Findings

Qualitative data analysis, based on interviews with youth at mid-point ($n = 29$) and post-test ($n = 14$) revealed several themes, including enhanced social networks, enhanced social skills, increase in mental and emotional well-being, and an improved coping repertoire. Figure 3 depicts the interactions among these themes.

*Enhanced Social Networks*

Youth reported that the intervention affected their lives by expanding their social networks. Furthermore, some youth commented that these expanded social networks contained new people who cared. They reported that new-found friends lessened time spent with the 'wrong crowd.' Thus, the support intervention affected relationships external to the program. Youth also observed differences in the behaviours of friends in the support intervention versus those outside of the intervention. Specifically, their friends in the program discussed new topics and acted differently. For example, youth were pleased to see

Figure 1: Estimated marginal means of UCLA Loneliness Scale ($n$ = 14)

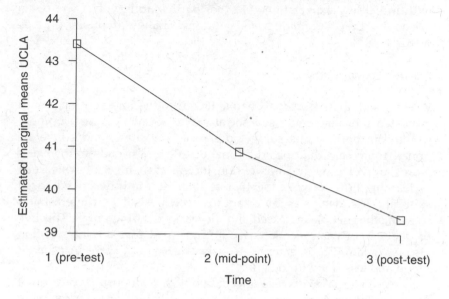

Figure 2: Estimated marginal means of social network size ($n$ = 14)

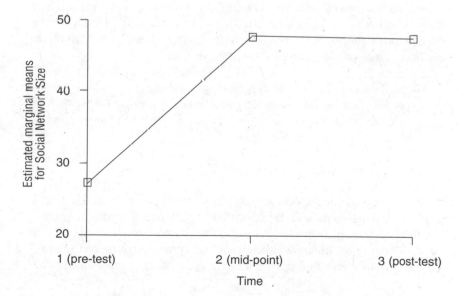

their friends being active instead of just 'hanging out.' Participants with initial low expectations of other participating youth were surprised that they had made friends and saw changes in other youth as well.

## Enhanced Social Skills

When asked about personal change linked to the intervention, youth indicated they had increased social skills. Social skill development resulted in participants being more social, talkative, and conversational. Youth said that the additional people and friends in their networks, provided by the intervention, increased their social skills, such as learning how to work together as a team. Youth described social skills and friendships as important to success. Also, their interest and trust in other people increased and they gained a different perspective of people. For example, some youth indicated that the intervention affected relationships external to it because youth were in a better mood and less shy with others.

Increased social skills also affected youths' relationships outside of the intervention. At post-test, youth specifically mentioned being more positive in their relationships, perhaps as a result of being more positive about themselves. Youth recounted changes to their existing social networks (inclusion of some and exclusion of others) and reported that their families also perceived the intervention positively. However, some youth mentioned conflicts with friends/family pertaining to absence while participating in the intervention:

> All you need to do is show them you do care, and they're not alone; there are people out there that are in the same situation, and they're trying to turn their lives around too. Best thing is to support them and guide them. (Homeless youth, age eighteen years)

## Increase in Mental/Emotional Well-Being

Youth described increased confidence, self-esteem, personal strength and assertiveness gained from participation. In addition to greater confidence, youth discussed relaxation and stress relief derived from respite from street life and through the positive environment the intervention created. Youth reported a sense of equality, increased satisfaction, and overall mood enhancement. They said that intervention activities offered entertainment and the opportunity to relax, forget about problems, and recollect positive memories.

*Improved Coping Repertoire*

Youth reported an increased repertoire of coping strategies, mood enhancement, and stress relief due to the intervention. They contended that the emotional and informational support derived from mentors created a safe place to discuss problems and provided a different perspective on their situation. This, in turn, helped them to cope with relationship challenges, in particular family-related issues, and to gain perspective on their life situations. Youth said they had a greater ability to cope with problems in their lives because the intervention served as a drug/alcohol-free option, which helped them avoid negative influences, remain 'off the streets,' and manage boredom.

Youth also identified increased coping skills because the intervention supported their personal goals such as continuing with school and finding housing. The intervention supported youth in moving towards personal goals, including acceptance into college, completing a course, and being a better parent. Housing was also considered a means of achieving success, with some youth reporting a place to stay at mid-point and post-test. Intervention aided them to achieve personal goals of sobriety. They stated that having something fun to look forward to each week alleviated the need for drugs/alcohol, or at least provided a distraction:

> Yeah. I had a hard time with drugs, and after I started this program, it helped me. It gives me something to do and something else to think about. (Homeless youth, age nineteen years)

**Discussion**

In spite of ascertaining homeless youths' preferences regarding support intervention, it was extremely challenging to engage homeless youth for the duration of the planned intervention, likely due to their transience and distrust of mainstream services and authority figures. As such, it was nearly impossible to follow up with youth who discontinued their participation, to examine possible reasons for attrition. While seventy participants enrolled in the program, only twenty-nine completed midpoint data collection and fourteen completed post-test data collection. It is impossible to rule out sample bias due to this high rate of attrition, but findings reveal that the mentoring intervention was beneficial for those who participated.

A significant difference was observed in scores on the UCLA Loneliness Scale, suggesting that participants were less lonely, less isolated, and more satisfied with their social relationships over time. Observing this significant difference over time, in such a small sample, suggests that the intervention had a large effect on the fourteen participants (Borenstein, Rothstein, & Cohen, 2001). Qualitative data validated these observations. Thematic analysis revealed enhanced social networks, social skills, mental and emotional well-being, and coping. These findings are consistent with other research demonstrating the positive impact of mentoring relationships on youth (Dubois et al. 2002). Our findings, while tentative, are a first step towards extending that research to examine the impact of social support, including mentoring, on homeless youth.

Youth also reported that their social networks grew in size. However, this finding was not observed in the quantitative multivariate analyses of the fourteen participants who completed data collection at each time point. Moreover, the impact of the intervention on the Social Provisions Scale did not reveal statistically significant changes. At all three time points, homeless youth unexpectedly reported social support that was only slightly below, and within one standard deviation of, the normative mean of 82.

These inconsistent findings deserve further study and may be explained by a combination of factors including measurement design, small effect sizes, and attrition. Given the large effect observed on the UCLA Loneliness Scale and the qualitative findings, the intervention likely had an effect on social support, needs, resources, and satisfaction. The Social Provisions Scale may, however, be inappropriate to accurately measure the support homeless youth receive. Instruments used in future studies should be adapted to the realities of homeless youths' life contexts.

Maintaining the participation of homeless youth in the mentoring support intervention was difficult. Attrition from the sample influenced the findings. Even more importantly, infrequent attendance may have reduced intervention impact. Support relationships that

Figure 3: Key themes derived from qualitative analysis

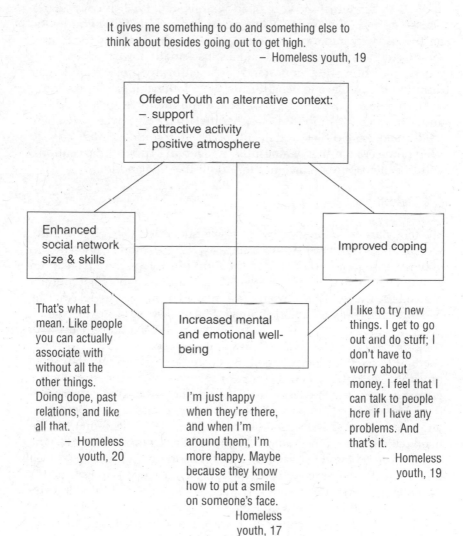

strengthen beneficial outcomes are dependent on frequency of contact between mentors (support intervention agents) and mentees (partici-pants) (Springer & Basca, 2003), duration of the relationship (Grossman & Rhodes, 2002), and perception of the quality of the mentor-and-youth relationship (Grossman & Johnson, 1999; Jucovy, 2002). Grossman and Johnson's (1999) evaluation concluded that youth who participated in mentoring relationships that lasted less than three months felt less confident and had a substantially lower sense of self-worth, indicating the importance of mentoring projects of longer duration if youth are to benefit from the relationships. Support intervention research also suggests that the minimally sufficient dosage and duration of support is approximately twelve weeks (Cohen, Underwood, & Gottlieb, 2000). Future research could address ways to keep homeless youth meaningfully engaged in support interventions, and to foster optimal outcomes for youth like Sue and Joel.

### Sue: Case Study 1

Sue took part in the program when it was suggested to her by her case-worker at the youth co-op. It was Tuesday, she was hungry, and she had nowhere else to go, so why not? She found it was great to have a fun activity to do that didn't involve drugs and alcohol. She couldn't remember how long it had been since she had been to a movie! And she had the chance to try rock climbing. She looked forward to coming every week, and only missed a few times when she hooked up with some friends from her native band and they got partying. Later, she checked to see if her party friends could come to group with her some time. She was glad when the answer was yes. She was also relieved when she was welcomed back even though she had missed group meetings. Marian (a community mentor in her twenties) remembered her and said how glad she was to see Sue again. Sue noticed that Marian liked talking to the other kids and to the other mentors like Sandy, who used to live on the street like Sue. Marian hadn't been homeless herself but was really interested in Sue's thoughts and opinions and seemed to like talking to Sue. Marian encouraged Sue to try the rock climbing and noticed how athletic Sue was. It made Sue think that maybe she was good at stuff, like sports, after all. It was good to be active and to talk to new people. Sue knew that she could talk to Marian about her problems if she wanted to. It was good just knowing that.

### Joel: Case Study 2

Joel showed up at the program when he heard there was free food and some of the other kids said the program was okay. A few of them went together the first time. The food was good, and it was 'pretty sweet,' the youth said, to go bowling for a change. Joel mostly talked to his friends during the group and couldn't wait to get stoned after group. The mentors wanted to plan activities with the kids for the next week, so Joel suggested basketball, and the other kids agreed. He used to be good at basketball so attended for that, but skipped when the activity was painting. His mother showed up crying at his girlfriend's apartment that week, looking for him. He said his mom had been a mess, as usual. How much of this did he have to take, he'd wondered? How many times was she going to show up and ruin his life? Later that week, he got into a fight and beat up another kid. After that, Joel thought that maybe he wouldn't be welcomed back to the group. His friends were going to the movie night and persuaded him to come along. Some of the mentors talked to him, asked him where he'd been. He didn't feel like talking and just ate his pizza instead. They didn't need to know that his dad didn't want him and his mom was a wreck. He didn't feel like talking about all that. He didn't think he would go back home.

As the case studies demonstrate, and in spite of a small sample size, significant differences were observed over time in relation to loneliness outcomes for those youth who participated in the intervention. Furthermore, quantitative findings were validated by the qualitative findings. Innovative, engaging research is needed, however, to determine the barriers that prevented greater participation of youth in the intervention. The key to successfully supporting homeless youth may lie in finding innovative ways to connect and maintain positive engagement with them. Peer mentoring may be part of the solution, but more research is needed to understand the specific aspects of programming most likely to engage street youth in positive peer and adult relationships. The mixed methods employed in this study, phased to encourage participation by the youth themselves and community partners, seems to be an important part of study design and implementation.

## REFERENCES

Baron, S.W. (1999). Street youth and substance abuse: The role of background, subculture, and economic factors. *Youth and Society, 31,* 3–26.

Baron, S.W. (2001). Street youth labor market experiences and crime. *Canadian Review of Sociology and Anthropology, 38,* 189–225.

Bellamy, N.D., Springer, U.F., Sale, E.W., & Espiritu, R.C. (2004). Structuring a multi-site evaluation for youth mentoring programs to prevent teen alcohol and drug use. *Journal of Drug Education, 32*(2), 197–212.

Borenstein, M., Rothstein, H., & Cohen, J. (2001). Power and precision. Englewood Cliffs, NJ: Biostat.

Bronstein, L.R. (1996). Intervening with homeless youths: Direct practice without blaming the victim. *Child and Adolescent Social Work Journal, 13*(2), 127–38.

Canada Mortgage and Housing Corporation. (2001). *Inventory of projects and programs addressing homelessness.* Ottawa: CMHC.

Canadian Public Health Association. (1998). *1997 position paper on homelessness and health.* Retrieved 27 January 2005 from www.cpha.ca.

Caputo, T., & Kelly, K. (1998). Canada Health Action: Children and youth. Papers Commissioned by the National Forum on Health. Quebec: Editions MultiModes.

Caputo, T., Weiler, R., & Anderson, J. (Eds.). (1997). *The street lifestyle study.* Prepared for Office of Alcohol, Drugs, and Dependency Issues, Health Canada, Ottawa.

Clements, K., Gleghorn, A., Garcia, D., Latch, M., & Marx, R. (1997). A risk profile of street youth in Northern California: Implications for gender-specific human immunodeficiency virus prevention. *Journal of Adolescent Health, 20*(5), 343–53.

Cohen, S., Underwood, L., & Gottlieb, B. (Eds.). (2000). *Social support measurement and intervention: A guide for health and social sciences.* New York: Oxford University Press.

Commander, M., Davis, A., McCabe, A., & Stanyer, A. (2002). A comparison of homeless and domiciled young people. *Journal of Mental Health, 11*(5), 557–64.

Currie, C., Roberts, C., Morgan, A., Settertobulte, W., Samdal, O., & Rasumussen, V. (2004). *Young people's health in context: Health behaviour in school-aged children (HSBC) study* (No. 4). Geneva: WHO.

Cutrona, C., & Russell, D. (1987). The provisions of social relationships and adaptation to stress. In W. Jones & D. Perlman (Eds.), *Advances in personal relationships* (Vol. 1, pp. 37–67). Greenwich, CT: JAI Press.

Dadds, M.R., Maujean, A., & Fraser, J.A. (2003). Parenting and conduct problems in children: Australian data and psychometric properties of the Alabama Parenting Questionnaire. *Australian Psychologist, 38*(3), 238–41.

Darling, N., Hamilton, S., Toyokawa, T., & Matsuda, S. (2002). Naturally occurring mentoring in Japan and the United States: Social roles and correlates. *American Journal of Community Psychology, 30*(2), 245–70.

Dubois, D., Holloway, B., Valentine, J., & Cooper, H. (2002). Effectiveness of mentoring programs for youth: A meta-analytic review. *American Jounal of Community Psychology, 30*(2), 157–97.

Federal Provincial Territorial Advisory Committee on Population Health. (1998). *Building a national strategy for healthy child development.* Ottawa: Health Canada.

Fitzgerald, M. (1995). Homeless youths and the child welfare system: Implications for policy and service. *Child Welfare, 74,* 717–30.

Gaetz, S. (2004). *Understanding research on homelessness in Toronto: A literature review.* Toronto: York University.

Golden, A., Currie, W.H., Greaves, E., & Latimer, E.J. (1999). *Taking responsibility for homelessness: An action plan for Toronto.* Report of the Mayor's Homelessness Action Task Force. Retrieved 27 January 2005 from www.city.toronto.on.ca/mayor/homelessnesstf.htm

Gottlieb, B. (1998). *Support groups.* San Diego: Academic Press.

Gottlieb, B. (2000). Accomplishments and challenges in social support research. In M. Stewart (Ed.), *Chronic conditions and caregiving in Canada: Social support strategies.* Toronto: University of Toronto Press.

Gottlieb, B. (2002). Coping research: The road ahead. *Canadian Journal of Nursing Research, 34*(1), 13–27.

Greene, J.M., & Ringwalt, C.L. (1998). Pregnancy among three national samples of runaway and homeless youth. *Journal of Adolescent Health, 23*(6), 370–77.

Grossman, J., & Johnson, A. (1999). Assessing the effectiveness of mentoring programs. In J.B. Grossman (Ed.), *Contemporary issues in mentoring* (pp. 25–47). Philadelphia: Public/Private Ventures.

Grossman, J., & Rhodes, J. (2002). The test of time: Predictors and effects of duration in youth mentoring relationships. *Amercian Journal of Community Psychology, 30*(2), 199–219.

Grossman, J., & Tierney, J. (1998). Does mentoring work? An impact study of the Big Brothers Big Sisters program. *Evaluation Review, 22*(3), 403–26.

Hamilton, M.A., & Hamilton, S.F. (2002). Why mentoring in the workplace works. *New Directions for Youth Development, 93,* 9–20.

Health Canada. (2004). *Young people in Canada: Their health and well-being.* Ottawa: Minister of Health.

Herrera, C. (2004). School-based mentoring: A closer look. Philadelphia: Public/Private Ventures.

Jucovy, L. (2002). Measuring the quality of mentor-youth relationships: A tool for mentoring programs. Retrieved 26 January 2005 from www.nwrel.org /mentoring/pdf/packeight.pdf.

Kipke, M., Montgomery, S., Simon, T., Unger, J., & Johnson, C. (1997). Homes less youth: Drug use patterns and HIV risk profiles according to peer affiliation. *AIDS & Behavior, 1*(4), 247–59.

McCall, K. (1992). *Support services to homeless/street youth: A needs assessment and plan for action.* Ottawa: Regional Municipality of Ottawa-Carleton.

Norusis, M. (1992). *Statistical Package for the Social Sciences.* Chicago: SPSS Inc.

Novotney, L.C., Mertinko, E., Lange, J., Falb, T., & Kirk, H. (2002). Juvenile Mentoring Program (JUMP): Early evaluation results suggest promise of benefits for youth. *Juvenile Justice Bulletin.* Retrieved 26 January 2005 from http://www.itiincorporated.com/assets/pdf%20files/bulletin.pdf.

Olsen, B., & Friedenthal, S. (2000). *Housing and homelessness: Edmonton Social Plan – Release 3.* Edmonton Community Services: Edmonton.

Radloff, L.S. (1977). The CES-D scale: A self-report depression scale for research in the general population. *Applied Psychological Measurement, 1*(3), 385–401.

Raphael, D. (2004). *Social determinants of health: Canadian perspectives.* Toronto: Canadian Scholar's Press.

Rhodes, J.E. (2002). *Stand by me: The risks and rewards of mentoring today's youth.* Cambridge, MA: Harvard University Press.

Russell, D.W. (1996). UCLA Loneliness Scale (Version 3): Reliability, validity, and factor structure. *Journal of Personality Assessment, 66*(1), 20–40.

Sibthorpe, B., Drinkwater, J., Gardner, K., & Bammer, G. (1995). Drug use, binge drinking and attempted suicide among homeless and potentially homeless youth. *Australian and New Zealand Journal of Psychiatry, 29*(2), 248–56.

Springer, F., & Basca, B. (2003). *Effective youth and adult partnerships mentoring strategies.* San Francisco: California Department of Alcohol and Drug Programs.

Steinhauer, P. (1998). Developing resiliency in children from disadvantaged populations. In *Determinants of health: Children and youth* (pp. 47–102). Sainte-Foy, QC: Editions MultiMondes.

Stewart, M. (1993). *Integrating social support in nursing.* New York: Sage.

Stewart, M. (2000). *Chronic conditions and caregiving in Canada: Social support strategies.* Toronto: University of Toronto Press.

Stewart, M., Craig, D., & MacPherson, K.E.A. (2001). Promoting positive affect and diminishing loneliness of widowed seniors through a support intervention. *Public Health Nursing, 18,* 59–63.

Terrell, N.E. (1997). Street life aggravated and sexual assaults among homeless and runaway adolescents. *Youth and Society, 28*(3), 267–91.

Ungar, M. (2004). *Nurturing hidden resilience in troubled youth.* Toronto: University of Toronto Press.

Unger, J., Kipke, M., Simon, T., Johnson, C., Montgomery, S., & Iverson, E. (1998). Street-coping and social support among homeless youth. *Journal of Adolescent Research, 13*(2), 134–57.

Van Wormer, R. (2003). Homeless youth seeking assistance: A research-based study from Duluth, Minnesota. *Child & Youth Care Forum, 32*(3), 89–103.

Weiss, R. (1974). The provisions of social relationships. In Z. Rubin (Ed.), *Doing unto others* (pp. 17–26). Englewood Cliffs, NJ: Prentice-Hall.

Whitbeck, L., & Hoyt, D. (1999). *Nowwhere to grow: Runaway and homeless adolescents and their families.* New York: McGraw-Hill.

Yorden, E.E., & Yorden, R.A. (1995). Problems associated with homelessness and young pregnant teenagers. *Adolecent & Pediatric Gynecology, 8*, 135–9.

# 8 The Impact of an Informal Career Development Program on the Resilience of Inner-City Youth

KATHRYN LEVINE AND DAWN SUTHERLAND

Current theories associated with career development are applicable to only a small percentage of the population – those who can realistically expect employment and have the freedom to choose a preferred career (Chartrand & Rose, 1996). In other words, the people who most need assistance with career development are the ones about whom the least is known. This is particularly true for at-risk youth from marginalized and under-represented groups who have limited opportunity to explore a variety of occupations due to limited career exposure, access to post-secondary education, and social factors related to family, school, and community relationships. This chapter reports on the findings of one study that focused on identifying the resilience-enhancing factors children and their families demonstrated while participating in a community-based career intervention program.

Career Trek is an early intervention program located outside of the formal education system. It is designed to expose academically at-risk, inner-city children aged ten and eleven to a variety of potential careers that are accessible as a function of post-secondary education. The primary objective of Career Trek is to minimize children's future risk of living in poverty by reinforcing the connection between completing high school and moving on to post-secondary education. This goal is partially accomplished by strengthening participants' relationships with family and school using the vehicle of career exploration. The present study examined the short-term impact of the program on participants' academic resilience within a relational framework.

This research examines how a career development program can strengthen the relationships that foster career decision making by interviewing participants, parents, and school staff involved in the

Career Trek program. The program is well suited to the examination of the relational factors that contribute to career development in children. First, it actively involves families and schools in program activities and therefore encourages collaborative relationships between participants' family members and school staff. Second, it acts as a catalyst to foster dialogue between children and their families about career aspirations, personal likes and dislikes, and career-specific abilities. Third, it facilitates positive interactions between children and school staff and contextualizes program content within an academic context. All of these relationships have been identified as factors that contribute to children's academic resilience (Brooks, 2006).

## Ecological Model of Social Interaction

Bronfenbrenner's (1979) ecological model of human development and social interaction provides a conceptual framework for understanding interactions between individuals, their families, and their communities. Development is recognized as a process in which the individual is shaped by the complex interplay of biological, genetic, psychological, social, and cultural forces within the individual and the environment. Research incorporating this perspective moves from a focus that is directed solely towards the individual to a focus on the individual embedded within the context of the surrounding systems. These include the *macro* system, encompassing the natural environment and social, economic, and cultural constraints; the *exo system*, which describes how an individual may be influenced by legislation and policies at an institutional level; the *mezzo* system, which describes an individual's relationships with groups, organizations, informal networks, and their extended family; and the *micro system*, represented by parent–child relationships and individual biological, psychological, emotional, and cognitive factors within the child.

## Resilience

The construct of resilience, from the Latin *resilire* for 'leap back,' is derived from two bodies of literature: the physiological aspects of stress and the psychological aspects of coping (Tusaie & Dyer, 2004). The introduction of resilience within the discipline of developmental psychopathology refers to children who exhibited positive developmental outcomes in spite of exposure to adverse and negative circumstances (Howard, Dryden, & Johnson, 1999; Waller, 2001). One of two major concepts in the resilience model is risk, originally developed within the epidemiological literature to refer to 'any influence that increases the probability of onset, digression to a more serious state, or maintenance of a problem condition' (Kirby & Fraser, 1997, p. 23). The construct of risk is assessed through factors ordinarily associated with a high probability of undesirable outcomes, difficulties, and problems for individuals and groups.

Exposure to risk factors can be readily assessed within an ecological framework, identifying factors at the individual, family, community, social, and cultural levels. Individual risk factors can include demographic variables, including age, gender, and ethnicity, or genetic/biological factors, including the presence of disabling conditions; family-level factors may include parental conflict, marital violence, or mental health disorders; community factors can include inadequate educational opportunities or chronic poverty; and social or cultural factors can include discrimination based on gender, class, race, sexual orientation, or perceived ability.

The additive model of risk suggests that the number of risk indicators is positively correlated with the likelihood of negative outcomes (Landry & Tam, 1998). Sameroff, Seifer, and Bartko (1997), for example, demonstrated that development is most compromised when several risk factors occur together. This is supported by Rutter's (1979) finding that the presence of one isolated risk factor does not raise the likelihood of poor outcomes for children. Within this framework, inner-city youth, particularly those from lower income or racially/ethnically diverse families, may be exposed to clusters of risk factors that have a negative impact on academic success

However, not all individuals who are exposed to risk exhibit negative outcomes. Rutter (1985) found that 'even with the most severe stresses and the most glaring adversities, it is unusual for more than half of children to succumb' (p. 600). This introduced the second major concept in the resilience literature: protective factors. These are defined as individual or environmental characteristics that enhance one's ability to resist stressful events and promote adaptation and competence (Garmezy & Rutter, 1983).

Protective factors are similarly situated within an ecological framework, and may be internal, including personality types, or external, such as a supportive family environment, strong social support, and social and economic resources. Taken together, two key components of resilience are (a) the individual's demonstrating a positive response to an adverse situation and (b) the individual's emerging feeling 'strengthened, more resourceful, and developmentally advanced' (Simon, Murphy, & Smith, 2005, p. 427).

## Academic Risk and Resilience

The concept of 'academically at risk' refers to students who, by virtue of factors in their background or environment, are at higher risk of educational failure or early school leaving. Factors associated with academic risk include poverty, family structure and instability, and residential mobility (Wang, Haertel, & Walberg, 1997, 1998; Wang & Kovach, 1995; Wang & Walberg, 1996). For these very reasons, the inner city of Winnipeg, Manitoba, Canada, is a challenging social, economic, and educational environment for children and families. In 2001, the majority of households in Winnipeg's inner city had incomes below the poverty line (Institute of Urban Studies, 2005). Aboriginal, visible minorities, and immigrant children, many of whom reside within the inner city, are disproportionately impacted by poverty (Social Planning Council of Winnipeg, 2004). Silver (2000) states that currently 'at each and every one of Winnipeg's 15 inner-city elementary schools, more than 50 percent of families with children have incomes below the low income cut-offs' (p. 36). Furthermore, 'more than one in every four inner-city households in 1996 was headed by a single parent' (p. 29). While he cautions against unwarranted extrapolations, he also points out that 'there is a higher probability that inner-city single-parent families will have incomes below the poverty line' (p. 31).

The link between community characteristics and children's educational outcomes is increasingly accepted. High-poverty neighbourhoods are strongly associated with residential mobility due to the poor quality and limited availability of housing. In 2001, the inner city of Winnipeg had the highest proportion of houses that required major repairs of all neighbourhoods in Winnipeg (Jacobucci, 2005). The absence of quality housing that is affordable for low-income families typically results in short-term residential occupation, necessitating frequent school moves that have a negative impact on children's academic achievement (Crowley, 2003; Offenberg, 2004).

Additionally, children living in inner-city neighbourhoods may not have opportunities to interact with people who are employed or reside in families that have a consistent income earner. When this is the case, the relationship between schooling and post-schooling employment takes on a different meaning (Wilson, 1987). The cumulative effect of poverty, inadequate housing, school transience, and limited exposure to career opportunities means that Winnipeg's inner-city children are less likely to develop the cognitive, academic, and motivational skills necessary for the transition to post-secondary education. Additionally, they are less likely to have access to high-earning employment opportunities. Consequently, inner-city children are at greater risk of being caught in a cycle of poverty that is increasingly difficult to extricate oneself from.

Although past literature has focused on identifying risk and protective factors that contribute to school achievement (Borman & Overman, 2004; Bryan, 2005), there has been much less attention directed towards understanding the transactional relationship between risk and protection. The question arises as to how knowledge of academic resilience can be enhanced through investigating the simultaneous, interactive, and continuously evolving relationships between risk and protective factors. The primary purpose of this study was, therefore, to assess the impact of a career exploration program on children's academic resilience, and how this was impeded or facilitated within their multiple relational contexts of family, school, and community.

**The Career Trek Program**

Career Trek, Inc. is a not-for-profit organization that provides a range of comprehensive career-related educational programs for youth with perceived barriers to entering post-secondary education. Career Trek was prescient in its recognition that social barriers, and not financial factors, are more powerful determinants of whether at-risk children will advance to post-secondary education. The participants may be considered at risk for any number of internal or external challenges, including socio-economic status, gender, disability, family structure, and membership in a marginalized group. The core program of Career Trek is directed towards children in grades 5 and 6 who are perceived to be at risk for not completing secondary school and, consequently, not advancing to post-secondary education. Based on the recognition that career development is a process, not an outcome, upon successful completion of the core program participants are invited back to phase 2, which provides an intensive focus on one career (selected by participants) for youth entering grade 9. Moreover, when program participants enter post-secondary schooling, they are offered part-time employment as instructors or group leaders in the Career Trek program.

Each year, 240 youth identified as academically at risk by their teachers and school administrators participate in the Career Trek core program held on Saturdays for twenty weeks during the academic year. Participant nominations are based on two criteria: (*a*) the individual has, in the estimation of teachers and administrators from the sponsoring school, the academic potential to pursue and complete post-secondary education (which Career Trek interprets as being any child), and (*b*) nominated participants and their families must be in a position to attend and commit to completing the program. Career Trek is performance based, and both children and their families contract for commitment. Expectations for children include regular attendance (program participants are allowed no more than three absences), and expectations for parents or family members are to facilitate their children's attendance (e.g., preparing lunch, ensuring that children are at the pick-up site on time) and to fully participate on family days.

Participants rotate through four to eight career modules held at one of Winnipeg's three participating post-secondary institutions: the University of Manitoba, Red River College, and the University of Winnipeg. A variety of departments and faculties have participated within each institution, including native studies, engineering, building construction, graphic arts, criminal justice and law, education, aeronautics, physical education and recreational studies, and political science. In total, the participants receive ninety-five hours of programming (eighty hours in class). At the conclusion of a five-week block, each group rotates to a new set of departments or faculties.

Career Trek educates participants on two levels of awareness, post-secondary admission requirements and career trajectories, and on personal and social skills development. Each module informs participants about the post-secondary admission requirements of a given career path. For example, in order to enter the Department of Biology at the Faculty of Science at the university level, a student must have completed high-school chemistry and math. This alerts participants at the elementary school level to the importance of specific subject areas for any given career, as well as the importance of future course selection at the secondary school level. Secondly, each module exposes participants to the wide range of career opportunities within a specific field. For example, in the module associated with biology, participants would complete activities that encompass a range of biology-related careers, such as zoologist, botanist, pathologist, medical doctor, and veterinarian. Similar information is provided regarding careers accessible through college education. For example, although building construction may be perceived to require only physical ability, participants are also informed about the necessity of skills in mathematics in order to be successful within that career. Participants are also made aware of the range of opportunities within different trades. The experiential nature of the program further ensures that participants do not merely learn about a career, but have the opportunity to physically engage in the tasks associated with it. One example of careers accessible through college-level studies is in the field of aeronautics. Career Trek has partnered with a private aeronautical engineering firm that provides an aircraft to help participants to learn and practise the skills of mechanical diagnostics.

The modules are further designed to develop team building and problem solving skills among participants. Career Trek endeavours to build an awareness of the importance of interpersonal skills within a workplace setting. The importance of the relational component is emphasized, as participants are deliberately grouped with students from different schools and geographic locations. The rural/urban dynamic is one example that contextualizes how participants learn to negotiate with others, mediate conflict, and become less fearful/judgmental of diversity. Over the course of the program and through lessons that require collaboration, participants develop a network of support in their peer groups. Continuing with the example of biology, during the class on pathology participants would complete a problem-based learning activity related to the dispersal of a pathogen from a restaurant buffet. Working in teams and assuming the different roles required to solve this problem, some participants would determine the source of a particular pathogen by collecting samples, others would be responsible for the analysis, others would determine how it was transmitted, and still others would present the findings to the larger group for discussion.

Family involvement occurs through four family days held throughout the program year. Participants are encouraged to invite parents, guardians, siblings, and other significant individuals to participate in the program, and the participants act as instructors for the day. Given that the family structures of academically at-risk children vary considerably, it is important to note that participants define 'family' in terms of who they see as supportive. Additionally, parental or guardian involvement is encouraged through program-based information sessions that focus on central issues related to post-secondary education, including the differences between university and college programs, admission requirements, accessibility, and financial costs. One issue to emerge has been that low-income families typically overestimate the cost of post-secondary education and thus interpret cost as the primary barrier that will prevent their children from accessing it. Therefore, all families are offered free financial counselling through the local credit union and are provided with information regarding actual costs; potential subsidies, including bursaries, student loans, and scholarships; and registered educational savings plans. Parents are also provided with information about the importance of secondary school course selection as an enabling factor to access post-secondary education, as well as the availability of non-financial supports for at-risk students at the post-secondary level. These include specialized services for aboriginal students and students with disabilities, peer counselling services, and other student supports that are directed towards ensuring accessibility.

## Theoretical Framework of Career Trek

The primary mandate of Career Trek is poverty prevention through career exploration. The relationship between poverty and education is well established. In Canada, low education is linked with elevated risk for poverty (Valetta, 2005). Additionally, parental educational level is a significant predictor of post-secondary participation (Frenette, 2005). Taken together, these suggest a cyclical effect wherein children in poor families with low educational attainment are less likely to advance to post-secondary education and thus are more likely to continue to live in poverty as adults. Parental knowledge is also known to influence children's post-secondary participation. Previous research has suggested that low-income families generally believe access to post-secondary education is limited, completing a post-secondary degree is difficult, and post-secondary education is primarily limited to the disciplines of medicine and law (Sandefur, Meier, & Campbell, 2005; Sutherland & Levine, 2004; Usinger, 2005).

Career Trek structures its program and develops learning opportunities to mitigate risk and enhance protective factors within an ecological framework. For example, within the inner city, lack of supervised and/or structured activities during the weekends and evenings increases children's risk of engaging in delinquent activities (Hay, Fortson, Hollist, Altheimer, & Schaible, 2006). Given that the Career Trek program occurs on Saturdays, children are provided with the opportunity to engage not only in structured activities, but in meaningful activities with positive role models, as the majority of program staff are themselves graduates of the Career Trek program. Additionally, a protective factor found to contribute to academic engagement is peer relationships (Zimmer-Gembeck, Chipuer, Hanisch, Creed, & McGregor, 2006). The Career Trek program provides ample opportunity for participants to make positive peer associations, specifically with children from other schools and school divisions, as they are deliberately grouped with children from different areas.

In summary, Career Trek focuses on (1) increasing self-confidence through recognizing and celebrating success, (2) increasing social and independent problem-solving skills through problem-based learning within collaborative groups, (3) encouraging the active involvement of parents via family days and information sessions, and (4) fostering greater connections between the participant, the family, the school, and post-secondary institutions. All of these foci are considered to be protective factors that contribute to positive life trajectories.

## Methods

The focus of this study is academically at-risk students aged ten to eleven from Winnipeg's inner city and enrolled in grades 5 and 6. The study sample included thirty-one Career Trek (CT) participants and eighteen students as part of the control group. Upon completion of the Career Trek program, a total of twenty-two boys (fourteen CT and eight controls) and twenty-seven girls (seventeen CT and ten controls) from eight different inner-city elementary schools formed the research group. The study incorporated both quantitative and qualitative components. Participants were administered a series of pre- and post-program measures that examined factors of self-esteem, perceptions of abilities, intrinsic motivation, and relationships with family members, friends, and school staff. These are the Family, Friends, and School Scale (Hater & Simpson, 1981), the Perception of Ability Scale for Students (PASS) (Boersma & Chapman, 1992), and the Children's Academic Intrinsic Motivation Inventory (Gottfried, 1985). Full results of the quantitative analysis are reported elsewhere (Sutherland & Levine, 2004).

All participants were interviewed prior to the start of the Career Trek program and again approximately two months after program completion. The majority of these interviews were audiotaped and transcribed for analysis. Several of the students chose not to be audiotaped; their responses were recorded in written form by the research assistant. In addition to student interviews, parents and teachers of both participant and control cohort students were interviewed pre- and post-program. A total of forty-nine interviews (thirty-one participant and eighteen control students) form the basis of the content analysis.

The interview questions were based on an ecological framework and explored issues related to the student's perceived school performance, school satisfaction, peer relationships, family relationships, extracurricular activities, and career development. The interview guide was designed to be sufficiently detailed to allow for focused discussion of career knowledge and planning, but sufficiently open to allow for examination of emerging themes and constructs. Examples of career-related questions are: What would you describe as your career goal at this time? Describe what you think are some of the roadblocks you may come across while trying to meet your career goal. Describe what you think are some of the factors that will contribute to your success in pursuing your career goal. What are your friends doing when it comes to pursuing a career? How would you describe your family's ideas about having a career?

The foundation of the first level of analysis consisted of classifying each interview according to the components of the theoretical framework. This is conceptually similar to template analysis (Crabtree & Miller, 1992), which involves using an *a priori* codebook developed from predetermined concepts based on existing theory. Therefore, coding consisted of identifying relational constructs at each ecological level that were perceived by students, parents and guardians, and teachers to act as risk or protective factors in terms of career exploration. The second level of analysis was completed by examining the interview data as they pertained to the impact of Career Trek on participants' academic resilience.

## Results

### Child/Family Risk and Protection

Students in both control and participant groups resided within similar family structures ranging from foster families to separated, divorced, two-parent, single-parent, and grandparent families. The majority of students had siblings or foster siblings. Career Trek participants described their relationships with parents or caregivers as generally positive and reported that family members and peers were their most important supports. They further described positive relationships with their teachers and schools. All were able to identify a favourite subject – predominantly math, science, and social studies. The majority of Career Trek participants described their grades as 'better than last year' (prior to participation in Career Trek) and their current grades as average to good. They reported positive relationships with peers, and many indicated they had made new friends, compared to their last school year. The quantitative analysis examining the perceptions Career Trek participants had of their family, peer group, and school environments, compared to students who did not participate in Career Trek, confirmed that in general Career Trek fostered more positive attitudes towards these aspects of an individual's environment. In contrast, non-participants' perspectives changed more negatively over the same period of time, and, in the case of their views regarding family and friends, these changes were significant.

The interview data revealed that Career Trek participants described their personal strengths – including confidence and ability to make people laugh – and determination as factors that would help them become successful in achieving their career goals. Regarding perceived ability, Career Trek participants had a more positive self-perception after program completion, whereas non-participant's perceived abilities had decreased, although neither change was significant.

*Family Factors*

Although the majority of parents were employed, most had not completed high school. Only three of the twenty-four parents interviewed reported that they had attended a post-secondary educational institution. Parents perceived the key protective factors influencing whether their children remained in school and advanced to post-secondary education were the individual characteristics of perseverance and academic ability. Comments from parents of Career Trek participants about their children's strengths included, 'Once he gets his head set on something, there is no stopping him,' 'When she cannot do something, that's when she tries harder,' and 'She's bound and determined to pass grade 12 and make something of herself.'

Parents also identified family support as a contributing factor related to children's remaining in school and advancing to post-secondary education. Family support is a multidimensional concept that is significantly associated with children's academic resilience and advancement (Dubow, Arnett, Smith, & Ippolito, 2001; Hebert, 1999). Within educational settings, support may reflect concepts of family cohesion, emotional bonding, and parent/family involvement in school-related activities. In this study, parents of Career Trek participants referenced family cohesion factors of emotional support more frequently. Parents described themselves as being proud of their children, encouraging them to choose careers perceived to be enjoyable, 'staying behind their children no matter what,' and helping their children with their homework.

*Teachers*

Academic capability, positive work ethic, leadership qualities, and maturity emerged as the predominant protective factors identified by the teachers of Career Trek participants. Teachers used descriptors in their interviews about Career Trek participants such as 'independent,' 'optimistic,' 'consistent,' 'responsible,' and 'well-balanced.'

*Family/School Risk and Protection*

All Career Trek participants had a significant history of school transience, and the majority of students had changed schools at least once in the previous twelve-month period. Several families had relocated from rural areas to the city, others had moved to different neighbourhoods while remaining within the inner city, and some families had recently immigrated to Canada. Several participants had also changed schools due to parent–school conflict or negative peer interactions.

Parents believed that protective factors within schools included actively 'recruiting family involvement,' having a 'good/great teacher,' and 'keeping the kids challenged.' Parents did not, however, perceive their personal involvement in school-related activities as important to their children's academic success, and felt that their participation in parent-teacher meetings, on parent councils, or as a volunteer in the classroom was most often initiated by school staff.

In contrast, teachers identified family involvement in school, family functioning, family–school communication, and boundary maintenance as key protective factors for Career Trek participants. Teachers spoke of the need for parents to take a proactive role in creating a positive future orientation and ensuring a structured home environment.

Families were perceived to be the primary factor in controlling negative peer influences. As one teacher noted,

> Support is the biggest thing with him. With any student ... [what will] help them is support at home ... he's in grade six, goes to grade seven next year. If he gets caught up with the wrong crowd, starts hanging around with the wrong people, you know, let's be realistic, if that starts happening, and parents don't intervene right away, graduation day will be non-existent.

### Family, School, and Community Risk and Protection

Parents identified a number of risk factors at the community level. One mother stated that 'lots of poverty, theft, and bullying' had occurred in her child's school as a function of being in an inner-city neighbourhood. Aboriginal parents believed that their children were less likely to obtain a good job in the absence of an education due to their status, and recognized that having an education was especially important for their children. Interestingly, several parents stated that the cultural diversity of their neighbourhood was a protective factor, as it exposed their children to a range of cultures.

### Career Trek

Parents described Career Trek as a mechanism that instilled a sense of future orientation within their children regarding potential careers. One father stated that Career Trek provided his daughter with the opportunity for 'diversification, so she'll have a variety of choice and hopefully find something that she'll like.' Another parent explained that through participation in Career Trek, his child was 'seeing all the options and being exposed to the variety of careers.'

Analysis of the qualitative data further indicated that children's participation in Career Trek functioned as a catalyst to initiate career-related conversations between parents and children. Parents described how their children would routinely return from Career Trek and report on their activities for the day, discuss how a particular career was or was not exciting, and generally express positive self-perceptions about their abilities to advance to post-secondary education. As one mother stated, 'Whenever she's finished on Saturdays, she'll tell me what she's done and how she likes it.' Other parents took the initiative to discuss

Career Trek activities with their children. One father indicated that he and his son engaged in a weekly discussion upon the child's return from the program, 'We ask him what he did in CT and then he goes into lots of detail and tells us about everything that he does.'

Career Trek participants were identified by teachers as being better able to connect with the classroom curricula as a result of their experiences with similar material within the Career Trek program. Several schools instituted weekly 'debriefing' sessions with participants as a means of consolidating their knowledge. Teachers further identified that the physical exposure to post-secondary institutions was influential for Career Trek participants and their families. As one teacher noted, this is particularly relevant for inner-city students because they do not have the financial means to attend 'mini-university' summer programming. It was also found that Career Trek provides a focus to education. As one teacher reported,

> I think it gives the kids focus, so that if the kids know that they've got a career that they're looking forward to it can help them focus a lot more. It can help them focus a lot more on their jobs in school because they know it's going somewhere.

## Career Decision Making and Planning

In terms of career aspirations, both control and participant groups were able to identify specific career goals. However, there were distinct differences noted between the two groups. The majority of Career Trek participants identified career goals that required post-secondary education, including scientist, animator, nurse, veterinarian, teacher, and social worker. Additionally, they were able to identify specific careers that did not interest them. With some exceptions, the control group identified careers that did not necessarily require post-secondary education or training. The most significant difference between the Career Trek participants and control students was in terms of educational completion and career planning. When asked what they needed to do in order to achieve their career goals, regardless of whether they had named a specific goal, the Career Trek participants overwhelmingly referenced the concept of 'finishing' high school and 'finishing' college. Conversely, members of the control group did not make reference to the idea of completion. The salient difference was revealed by the Career Trek participants being able to describe in detail the educational pathway that is necessary to achieve their career goals. This is highlighted by the responses of two students, one control and one participant, both of whom stated that their career goal was to become a lawyer. When asked what they thought they would need to do in order to achieve their goal, the control student stated that one needs to 'go to the school where lawyers, police and judges go to learn.' In contrast, the Career Trek participant responded, 'You have to go to high school and get a diploma and you have to go to university for a long time and then you have to go to law school for around seven years or something.'

## Discussion

As a community-based program that partners with both the elementary and post-secondary educational systems, Career Trek extends the capacities of families and schools to foster academic resilience in children. Results of the interviews with Career Trek participants, parents, and teachers are congruent with previous findings that school-based initiatives directed towards academically at-risk children within their homes, schools, and communities are more likely to foster successful academic outcomes (Borman & Overman, 2004). More importantly, the results provide clear direction on how family, school, and community collaboration is best achieved. School staff work together with parents at the point of students' nomination to the program, family members participate through family days and graduation ceremonies, and students and families become more familiar with the variety of educational and career options available at different post-secondary institutions within the community. First, from an ecological perspective, the Career Trek program is a comprehensive initiative that provides opportunities for positive interactions and knowledge building between students, families, schools, and the post-secondary community. This is particularly important for at-risk students, as poverty, discrimination, and limited exposure to post-secondary institutions restrict minority children from learning about the broad range of educational and vocational options (Kozol, 1997).

Second, Career Trek adopts a developmental perspective in career decision making that recognizes the importance of beginning career exploration activities at the elementary school level. Although children at this age are routinely advised that 'school is important,' they are generally unclear why formal education is essential and likely do not have the capacity to make the links between specific subject areas and particular careers. Further, career development content tends to be scattered throughout the elementary school curriculum. Therefore, there are no clear opportunities for students to investigate possible career options during these formative years. The Career Trek program builds on many of the previously established resilience-enhancing factors for children and families by exposing them to future educational opportunities at a stage when at-risk children begin to exhibit school-related problems. In the absence of comprehensible links between education and future aspirations, elementary to middle-school transitions for academically at-risk youth precipitate increasing disengagement from school (Eccles & Midgley, 1989). This challenges existing curriculum guidelines that introduce content on formal career exploration toward the beginning of senior years. At this point, youth who are not already academically engaged are significantly less likely to become so, and are therefore at increased risk of not graduating.

Academic resilience may develop through intrinsic motivation, wherein education becomes important to the student personally, or extrinsically, in terms of their future career opportunities. Either way, it is important to provide students with meaningful experiences that will assist them with decisions regarding future accomplishments and means to these goals. Clearly, career development programs need to include strategies that build on students' beliefs in the importance of education. However, in order to accomplish this, children need the opportunity to actively define and develop their skills and talents. Generally, children living in at-risk situations have exposure to a narrowly defined future. Career Trek broadens children's aspirations beyond the expectations of their social context by developing their problem-solving skills and exploring how their talents fit within a career. Additionally, resilience may be further enhanced when the links between remaining in school and achieving future opportunities for career satisfaction are strongly reinforced. Although high-school completion may be personally important for many students, others will graduate as a means of establishing the foundation for future post-secondary exploration.

Informal career education positively contributes to academically at-risk students' perceptions of their own abilities and their attitudes towards school compared to students in the general population (Sutherland & Levine, 2004). Upon completion of the Career Trek program, participants described personal attributes and career aspirations in much greater detail, than did the control students. Additionally, interviews with participants and family members provide some support for the idea that creating new learning opportunities outside of the school setting enables and encourages participants to access learning in new and different ways. Therefore, Career Trek offers a medium that is more congruent with the developmental and learning needs of the participants and their families.

Previous research has also identified the positive influence of parental involvement in the career development of their children (Downing & D'Andrea, 1994). However, when parents feel helpless or uninformed, their capacity to influence their children's career exploration activities is limited. The majority of Career Trek parents have not completed high school, and for many of them, this is the first opportunity to be exposed, via their children, to a post-secondary institution. Parents reported that as a result of their children's involvement in Career Trek, they have an increased awareness of the range of career paths that are possible within post-secondary institutions.

## Implications for Practice

Findings from this study have useful implications for educators, administrators, and school social workers. First, academic resilience is facilitated through academic institutions and community-based programs that translate the ecological perspective into actual practice. Family-centred collaboration suggests that all family members benefit from involvement in children's education. However, fostering positive family–school involvement remains a challenge. Low-income parents have less involvement in school-related activities than do middle-class parents (McNeal, 1999), and parents, particularly aboriginal parents, continue to struggle with the historical legacy of highly conflictual or negative relationships with schools (Neegan, 2005). Inner-city schools continue to reflect cultural and economic disparities between families and school staff, and this study indicated that parents and teachers have disparate ideas regarding how family–school connections are best facilitated. Our findings suggest that community-based career education programs can act as interfaces in which to reinforce the links between family, school, and post-secondary communities that are critical to children's academic resilience.

At the individual level, academic resilience is associated with social competence. Based on the belief that learning is facilitated by the quality of personal relationships, Career Trek ensures that students from different schools are grouped together. This provides opportunities for students to interact with children from a range of geographically, ethnically, culturally, and linguistically diverse groups. Particular attention is given to ensuring that groups have a mix of rural and urban as well as suburban and inner-city students. These experiences create the context in which children may develop alternative viewpoints to some stereotypical beliefs about 'difference' that remain embedded within school systems, and are encouraged to develop larger friendship and social networks. Further enhancing these relationships is a curriculum designed to foster essential skill development in the areas of team work, problem solving, decision making, assertiveness, peer relationships, and conflict resolution. Working with other students on group projects provides participants with opportunities to develop positive relationships with a variety of individuals, share new ways of thinking, and develop new ways of behaving. These are skills that are critical for the twenty-first-century workplace.

Second, findings from this study suggest that formal career development programs can promote academic resilience by creating opportunities for children to experience the wide variety of careers that are possible within post-secondary institutions. Many career exploration activities are based on personality inventories or other paper-based measures that do not allow children to experience the actual tasks and activities associated with different careers. The experiential format of Career Trek encourages children to assess for themselves which careers may and, perhaps just as importantly, may not fit.

Academic resilience is associated with direct experience compared to other forms of knowledge transmission, and at-risk youth learn more effectively through kinaesthetic experiences. Therefore, Career Trek ensures that all career-related activities are experiential and hands-on. Participants become more knowledgeable regarding the specific types of tasks and activities associated with different careers and increasingly aware of which types of activities they excel at or enjoy. For example, many children express the desire to be veterinarians because of their love of animals. When 'veterinarian' is translated into performing surgeries on animal cadavers, children recognize that becoming a veterinarian requires a strong knowledge of the sciences as well as a love of animals. At the same time, resilience is further facilitated when participants are encouraged to challenge themselves, and thus the activities are designed to be somewhat complex in order to encourage critical thinking skills.

At the family level, findings reinforce the importance of collaboration between family, school, and community-based programs and the association with academic resilience. School staff – including administrators, educators, and social workers – need to reinforce with parents the critical association between family involvement and children's career exploration activities. Although perseverance is a key personality trait that contributes to children's academic success, parents need to be aware of their own influence in promoting career exploration. Children's participation in informal career exploration activities can act as the catalyst to spark career-related discussions between parents and children. This supports emerging literature that suggests that career development is enhanced through the 'family push' or when career exploration becomes a family project (Whiston & Keller, 2004). Moreover, in order to successfully engage with their children, families need to be informed about the content of their children's education. Many parents will recognize themselves in the image of a parent who is unable to assist his or her child with math homework. For families who are marginalized on the basis of language, socio-economic status, family structure, or ethnicity, feelings of shame are only intensified. In order to counteract these effects, it is critical for school staff to make concerted efforts to provide information in a manner that parents can accept without fear of being perceived as inadequate. Building on this, educators can then develop school-based initiatives that will encourage parents and children to undertake career exploration activities together and engage in career-related discussions. Although these occurred spontaneously in the context of Career Trek, similar discussions may be facilitated through structured activities initiated at the school level that involve meaningful family participation.

That community involvement targeted towards improving educational outcomes for marginalized youth is essential to sustain the long-term efforts to develop and maintain career exploration opportunities is a position that needs to be further entrenched. Building relationships between elementary school systems and post-secondary institutions is an important component of creating a future orientation within children and their families, particularly those from inner-city communities. Furthermore, it is these types of family–school–post-secondary initiatives that are more likely to result in successful educational outcomes for academically at-risk students. In a manner that parallels the career-related discussions that occur between participants and their families, the Career Trek program has facilitated ongoing dialogue between communities of practice regarding the career development needs of marginalized children and youth, through encouraging greater involvement at the private-sector level as well as expanding the program to northern and First Nation communities.

The connection between elementary school systems and post-secondary institutions meshes with the ongoing issue of funding that impacts career development programs at several levels. The need to extend resources to develop promising demonstration projects into sustainable initiatives that target larger numbers of children and youth is well demonstrated. For example, children with disabilities, youth located in remote northern communities, adolescent mothers, and aboriginal youth from both urban and rural communities are often socially isolated and lack the resources to access career development information or programs. All of these communities would benefit from career exploration programs that target their unique needs.

We conclude, therefore, that Career Trek is an innovative program that provides educators, social workers, and other professionals concerned about poverty reduction with ideas about how to promote resilience in academically at-risk youth. It begins from a position that all children are capable of completing school and advancing to post-secondary education if presented with the appropriate information and opportunities. Research continues to indicate that teachers tend to deprive students of a meaningful or motivating context for learning or for using skills that are taught. They also postpone more challenging and interesting work for too long and underestimate what disadvantaged students are capable of doing (Knapp & Turnbull, 1990). Career Trek engages children in meaningful career exploration activities that encourage them to actively think, grow, experience, change, and develop by creating the life they want to live, the work they want to do, and the means by which to achieve their goals.

## REFERENCES

Boersma, F.J., & Chapman, J.W. (1992). *Perception of Ability Scale for students manual.* Los Angeles: Western Psychological Services.

Borman, G., & Overman, L. (2004). Academic resilience among poor and minority students. *Elementary School Journal, 104,* 177–96.

Bronfenbrenner, U. (1979). *The ecology of human development.* Cambridge, MA: Harvard University Press.

Brooks, J.E. (2006). Strengthening resilience in children and youths: Maximizing opportunities through the schools. *Children & Schools, 28,* 69–76.

Bryan, J. (2005). Fostering educational resilience and achievement in urban schools through school-family-community partnerships. *Professional School Counselling, 8,* 219–31.

Chartrand, J.M., & Rose, M.L. (1996). Career interventions for at-risk populations: Incorporating social cognitive influences. *Career Development Quarterly, 44,* 341–53.

Crabtree, B., & Miller, W. (1992). *Doing qualitative research.* Newbury Park, CA: Sage.

Crowley, S. (2003). The affordable housing crisis: Residential mobility of poor families and school mobility of poor children. *Journal of Negro Education, 72,* 22–39.

Downing, J., & D'Andrea, L.M. (1994). Parental involvement in children's career decision making. *Journal of Employment Counseling, 3,* 115–26.

Dubow, E.F., Arnett, M., Smith, K., & Ippolito, M. (2001). Predictors of future expectations of inner-city children: A 9-month prospective study. *Journal of Early Adolescence, 21,* 5–29.

Eccles, J.S., & Midgley, C. (1989). Stage/environment fit: Developmentally appropriate classrooms for early adolescents. In R.E. Amos & C. Amos (Eds.), *Research on motivation in education* (Vol. 3, pp. 139–86). San Diego: Academic Press.

Frenette, M. (2005). *Is post-secondary access more equitable in Canada or in the United States?* Analytical Studies Branch Research Paper Series. Ottawa: Statistics Canada.

Garmezy, N., & Rutter, M. (1983). *Stress, coping, & development in children.* New York: McGraw-Hill.

Gottfried, A. (1985). Academic intrinsic motivation in elementary and junior high school students. *Journal of Educational Psychology, 77,* 631–45.

Hater, J.J., & Simpson, D.D. (1981). *The PMES information form on family, friends and self: A report on scale construction.* (Technical Report no. 81–17). Fort Worth: Texas Christian University, Institute of Behavioural Research.

Hay, C., Fortson, E.N., Hollist, D.R., Altheimer, I., & Schaible, L.M. (2006). The impact of community disadvantage on the relationship between the family and juvenile crime. *Journal of Research in Crime and Delinquency, 43,* 326–56.

Hebert, T. (1999). Culturally diverse high-achieving students in an urban high school. *Urban Education, 34,* 428–58.

Howard, S., Dryden, J., & Johnson, B. (1999). Childhood resilience: Review and critique of literature. *Oxford Review of Education, 25,* 307–23.

Institute of Urban Studies. (2005). *Physical activity and the inner city: The case of West Central Neighbourhood* (Student Paper 22), Institute of Urban Studies II, University of Winnipeg.

Jacobucci, C. (2005). *A central housing registry: Recommendations for Winnipeg.* Unpublished master's thesis, University of Winnipeg.

Kirby, L.D., & Fraser, M.W. (1997). Risk and resilience in childhood. In M.W. Fraser (Ed.), *Risk and resilience in childhood: An ecological perspective* (pp. 10–33). Washington, DC: NASW Press.

Knapp, M.S., & Turnbull, B.J. (1990). *Better schooling for children of poverty: Alternatives to conventional wisdom,* Vol. 1: *Summary.* Washington, DC: US Department of Education, Office of Planning, Budget and Evaluation.

Kozol, J. (1997). Reflections on resiliency. *Principal, 77,* 5–6.

Landry, S., & Tam, K.K. (1998). Understanding the contribution of multiple risk factors on children's development at various ages. (Report no. W-98-22E). Ottawa: Human Resources Development Canada.

McNeal, R. (1999). Parental involvement as social capital: Differential effectiveness on science achievement, truancy, and dropping out. *Social Forces, 78,* 117–44.

Neegan, E. (2005). Excuse me: Who are the first peoples of Canada? A historical analysis of aboriginal education in Canada then and now. *International Journal of Inclusive Education, 9,* 3–15.

Offenberg, R.M. (2004). Inferring adequate yearly progress of schools from student achievement in highly mobile communities. *Journal of Education for Students Placed At-Risk, 9,* 337–55.

Rutter, M. (1979). Protective factors in children's responses to stress and disadvantage. In M.W. Kent & J.E. Rolf (Eds.), *Primary prevention in psychopathology, Vol. 3: Social competence in children* (pp. 49–74). Hanover, NH: University Press of New England.

Rutter, M. (1985). Resilience in the face of adversity: Protective factors and resistance to psychiatric disorder. *British Journal of Psychiatry, 147,* 598–611.

Sameroff, A.J., Seifer, R., & Bartko, W.T. (1997). Environmental perspectives on adaptation during childhood and adolescence. In S.S. Luthar, J.A. Burack, D. Cicehetfi, & J. Weisz (Eds.), *Developmental psychopathology: Perspectives on adjustment, risk, and disorder* (pp. 507–26). New York: Cambridge University Press.

Sandefur, G.D., Meier, A.M., & Campbell, M.E. (2005). Family resources, social capital, and college attendance. *Social Science Research, 35,* 525–53.

Silver, J. (2000). Persistent poverty in Canada. In J. Silver (ed.), *Solutions that work: Fighting poverty in Winnipeg* (pp. 1–12). Halifax: Fernwood.

Simon, J., Murphy, J., & Smith, S. (2005). Understanding and fostering family resilience. *Family Journal, 13,* 427–36.

Social Planning Council of Winnipeg. (2001). A community plan on homelessness and housing in Winnipeg ( A report prepared by The Community Partnership for Homelessness and Housing and the Aboriginal Reference

Group on Homelessness and Housing). Winnipeg: Social Planning Council of Winnipeg.

Sutherland, D.L., & Levine, K.A. (2004). *Addressing risk factors and building resilience through protective mechanisms in a weekend career exploration program.* Paper presented at the Canadian Association for Studies in Education, Winnipeg, MB.

Tusaie, K., & Dyer, J. (2004). Resilience: A historical review of the construct. *Holistic Nursing Practice, 18*(1), 3–8.

Usinger, J. (2005). Parent/guardian visualization of career and academic future of seventh graders enrolled in low-achieving schools. *Career Development Quarterly, 53,* 234–45.

Valetta, R. (2005). *The ins and outs of poverty in advanced economies: Poverty dynamics in Canada, Germany, Great Britain, and the United States.* Ottawa: Statistics Canada.

Waller, M.A. (2001). Resilience in an ecosystemic context: Evolution of the concept. *American Journal of Orthopsychiatry, 71,* 290–97.

Wang, M.C., Haertel, G.D., & Walberg, H.J. (1997). *Fostering educational resilience in inner-city schools* (Publication Series no. 4). Washington, DC: Office of Educational Research and Improvement.

Wang, M.C., Haertel, G.D., & Walberg, H.J. (1998). *Educational resilience.* (Publication Series no. 11). Washington, DC: Office of Educational Research and Improvement.

Wang, M.C., & Kovach, J.A. (1995). *Bridging the achievement gap in urban schools: Reducing educational segregation and advancing resilience-romoting strategies.* (Publication Series no. 95–9). Paper presented at a Conference of the Urban Education National Network of the Regional Educational Laboratories, Washington, DC.

Wang, M.C., & Walberg, H.J. (Eds.). (1996). *Strategies for improving education in urban communities: A collection of articles in honor of Edmund W. Gordon and Maynard C. Reynolds.* Washington, DC: Office of Educational Research and Improvement.

Whiston, S.C., & Keller, B.K. (2004). The influences of the family of origin on career development: A review and analysis. *Counseling Psychologist, 32,* 493–568.

Wilson, W.J. (1987). *The truly disadvantaged: The inner-city, the underclass, and public policy.* Chicago: University of Chicago Press.

Zimmer-Gembeck, M.J., Chipuer, H.M., Hanisch, M., Creed, P.A., & McGregor, L. (2006). Relationships at school and stage-environment fit as resources for adolescent engagement and achievement. *Journal of Adolescence, 29,* 911–33.

# 9  Resilience as Process: A Group Intervention Program for Adolescents with Learning Difficulties

LINDA THERON

The study of resilience endeavours to understand what makes it possible for youth who have the odds stacked against them to succeed. By understanding why some youth thrive despite the adversity they confront, we may be better able to assist those youth who continue to be vulnerable in situations where they face considerable risk (Masten, 1999). This chapter reports on the pilot phase of an experimental intervention program with vulnerable youth who have learning disabilities. The program is aimed at engendering resilient functioning in participating youth. The intervention was based on lessons learned from the observation of youth with learning disabilities who demonstrate resilience despite their handicaps.

In order to critique this intervention meaningfully, it needs to be positioned within a framework of recent resilience theory. The intervention took place in late 1999–2000 and reflected the earlier assumptions of resilience researchers that resilience is dependent on, amongst others, protective individual traits (Schoon, 2006). More recent research has moved beyond this: currently, the complex interaction between context-specific risk and protective processes is emphasized (Schoon, 2006). With hindsight, the pilot phase of the group intervention program discussed in this chapter had only limited success because it failed to look at the broader context of the participants and failed to acknowledge resilience as a multifactor process.

Some of the data in this chapter were previously published in, and are reproduced by kind permission of, the *South African Journal of Education, 26,* 199–214.

## Learning Difficulty as a Risk Factor

Whilst protective factors decrease the likelihood of hardship resulting in dysfunctional patterns, risk factors increase such likelihood (Mash & Wolfe, 2005). A learning difficulty is equivalent to a risk factor: traditionally, adolescents with learning difficulties were thought to have insufficient strengths to cope with their disability (Bauer, Keefe, & Shea, 2001; Lerner, 2003). Learning difficulties prevent a learner from achieving optimal learning and development and are not the result of physical, visual, auditory, or sensory handicaps (Donald, Lazarus, & Lolwana, 2002). Although the learner's innate potential to learn is adequate, his/her ability to progress scholastically is inadequate (Dednam, 2005; Empson & Nabuzoka, 2004). A specific learning difficulty includes trouble in using spoken or written language and may manifest itself as difficulty with listening, speaking, reading, writing, spelling, or mathematical calculations (Bauer et al, 2001). This implies that the learner who experiences a learning difficulty will be familiar with failing and struggling within the academic arena. Given the cycle of perpetual failure that many youngsters with learning difficulties experience, they are more vulnerable and frequently lacking in protective strengths (Dednam, 2005; Donald et al., 2002).

Persistent failure takes its toll on emotional and social functioning (Mash & Wolfe, 2005) and sets the stage for non-resilient outcomes. A learning difficulty creates a stressful life-situation both during and after school. Associated emotional and social problems regularly persist into adulthood and limit the potential for future success on intellectual, social, and emotional fronts (Bauer et al., 2001; Cordoni, 1990; Mash & Wolfe, 2005). The interaction of this stressful life-situation with other common life stresses often leads to poor mental health and behavioural outcomes (Empson & Nabuzoka, 2004; Keogh & Weisner, 1993; Spekman, Goldberg & Herman, 1993). Nevertheless, within the population of individuals with learning difficulties, researchers have also found successful, well-adjusted individuals (Mash & Wolfe, 2005; Miller, 1996).

## Personal Protective Factors Associated with Adolescents with Learning Difficulties

Traditionally, resilience was narrowly defined in terms of the factors associated with positive development under stress (Masten, 1999).

The capacity for resilience was thought to be anchored by a triad of protective factors. This triad included a cohort of personal protective factors (intrinsic factors such as temperament, goal orientation, flexibility), familial protective factors (such as nurturing parents, consistent parenting, a positive support network, and advantageous socio-economic resources), and extra-familial protective factors (environmental factors such as involvement in pro-social organizations, a good school, supportive educators, and attachment to pro-social adults) (Ross & Deverell, 2004). While these protective factors are still acknowledged in resilience research, the interaction of this protective triad with risk factors is now emphasized (Schoon, 2006).

In line with the earlier lack of focus on the interaction of protective factors within a given context, a South African study (MacFarlane, 1998) identified nine personal factors, each with a potential buffering effect, associated with resilient adolescents who have been identified as having learning difficulties. These include:

- *Positive attitude*, suggesting the ability to remain cheerful and optimistic
- *Moderately positive self-concept*, suggesting an affirmative relationship to the self, and positive self-talk
- *Positive future orientation*, suggesting tenacity, orientation towards achievement, and optimism
- *Assertiveness*, suggesting autonomous functioning, independent-mindedness, and the ability to fight for deserved personal rights in a socially appropriate manner
- *Enthusiasm*, suggesting a tendency towards excitability and spontaneity
- *Drive*, suggesting tenacity, creative problem-solving ability, a curiosity about life, and attention to goals
- *Moderate anxiety*, suggesting sensitivity and a sense of obligation, which translates into increased drive and a sense of responsibility
- *Internal locus of control*, suggesting a sense of authorship or choice over one's destiny, even if such choice only pertains to attitude
- *Good interpersonal relationships*, suggesting positive social orientation and the ability to derive optimal benefit from social interaction, as well as empathy and a desire for love

## Intervention Framework for Assessing the Intervention Program

The lessons learned from studying resilience resulted in three broad approaches to intervention design: risk-focused, asset-focused and process-focused strategies.

*Risk-focused strategies* specifically aim to reduce the number of risks that vulnerable youth face (Masten & Reed, 2005). For example, in the context of youth with learning difficulties, a risk-focused strategy might include genetic counselling to parents with learning difficulties to anticipate their child's potential for problems, or preschool interventions for early identification of learning difficulties.

*Asset-focused strategies* have a very specific agenda: to encourage resilient functioning among vulnerable youth. These youth need to be ensured of increased access to resources that foster competence (Masten & Reed, 2005). For example, in the context of youth with learning difficulties, an asset-focused strategy might include access to remediation services. In such an approach, assets include skills, social resources, and strengths and are found in individuals and their communities (Ebersöhn & Eloff, 2006).

*Process-focused strategies* go beyond limiting exposure to risks or amplifying assets; they target processes that enhance resilient functioning (Masten & Reed, 2005). For example, in the context of youth with learning difficulties, a process-focused strategy might include programs that target adaptive social behaviours.

For the purposes of this chapter, process-focused strategies will be favoured as the framework from which to critique the intervention program that is being reported on. Resilience denotes the dynamic interaction between an individual, a given milieu, and accessible opportunities (Mampane & Bouwer, 2006; Powers, 2002; Richman & Fraser, 2001), rather than a fixed attribute or personal trait (Rutter, 2001; Ungar, 2005). As such, resilient functioning is considered to be a process or multitude of processes that vary according to the context in question (Rutter, 2001; Ungar, 2005).

Kumpfer (1999) views the components of the multifaceted process of resilience as follows:

1  A stressor or risk factor threatens the well-being of an individual and activates the resilience process.
2  The stressor is found within a context. Within this context risk and protective factors interact. This interaction is fluid and variable over time.

3 Simultaneously, the individual interacts with his or her environment. This person–environment interaction can be in response to
perceived or experienced risk factors.
4 Individuals possess internal factors that buffer them against risk.
These internal protective factors form part of the process of
resilience.
5 The individual learns coping processes over time as she is exposed
to challenges. These processes enable her to bounce back and continue to develop adaptively despite risk.
6 Finally, a positive outcome in response to the stressor is achieved,
which bodes well for future outcomes.

An optimal process-focused strategy should seek to generate adaptive
behaviour that will facilitate all of the above.

## The Group Intervention Program

In the light of Kumpfer's model, the major stressor for youth in this
study was a learning difficulty. The adolescents at the school where the
program was implemented needed intervention to cope resiliently
with the impacts of their learning difficulty. The group intervention
program was aimed at augmenting their potential for resilience by
enhancing personal protective factors that characterize other resilient
adolescents with learning difficulties (MacFarlane, 1998; Theron,
2004).

For an intervention to function optimally it needs to be tailored to
the target group (Mash & Wolfe, 2005). For this reason a group intervention program was designed based on MacFarlane's (1998) nine
factors associated with resilience among adolescents with learning difficulties. As such, only personal protective factors characteristic of
resilient adolescents with learning difficulties were targets of this
intervention. Furthermore, because the pilot program was implemented at a school for learners with special educational needs, it also
allowed for the multidisciplinary support participating adolescents
were already receiving as part of varied remedial and scholastic interventions. Thus, the program limited its focus to inculcating skills that
would most affect the nine personal protective factors. The program
themes that facilitated these factors are indicated in Table 1.

Although the program was directive, the approach was still flexible:
methods were adapted to suit the temperament and needs of the participating experimental group. As a broad range of strategies is recom-

Table 1: Program themes

| Session | Focus |
| --- | --- |
| 1 | Introductory session: The need for resilience |
| 2 | Self-knowledge |
| 3 | Internal locus of control and choices |
| 4 | Attitude & anxiety |
| 5 | Assertiveness skills |
| 6 | Faulty thinking |
| 7 | Personal bill of rights |
| 8 | Empowerment |
| 9 | Future orientation and drive |
| 10 | Social orientation |
| 11 | Self-concept |
| 12 | Closure |

mended for successful interventions (Nastasi & Bernstein, 1998), the method of presentation varied and included art therapy, music therapy, gestalt work, visualization techniques, cognitive therapy, role play, and cognitive-behavioural therapies.

The program was constructed to facilitate interactive small-group activity. A small six-member group (four boys and two girls) was preferred in order that every group member have the chance to actively participate (Spitz & Spitz, 1999). The groups contained more boys as this reflected the school's demographics. The program ran for twelve sessions (each at least an hour long) during the learners' non-academic activity periods of regular school hours. Continuity was disrupted by scheduled exams and a holiday period.

## Research Design

To assess the effectiveness of the intervention, a mixed-methods assessment study incorporating both quantitative and qualitative data was designed in order to determine the effectiveness of the intervention. Quantitative instruments used in the study included three structured questionnaires: the Adolescent Self-Concept Scale (Vrey & Venter, 1983), the Emotional Profile Index (Roets, 1997), and the High School Personality Questionnaire (Madge & Du Toit, 1989). These questionnaires were used to evaluate levels of the nine personal protective factors. Given that there was no South African instrument for measuring resilience among adolescents with learning difficulties at the time of this study, the quantitative instruments were varied. This replicated the data collection used in MacFarlane's (1998) original study, which had identified personal protective factors in adolescents with learning difficulties (see also Theron, 2004).

Qualitative methods included frequent semi-structured inter-views with participating adolescents, prolific process notes from the actual group sessions, and psychological projection techniques. The projection techniques included Draw-a-Person-in-the-Rain (Brink, 2005), Kritzberg's Three Animal Technique (Brink, 2005), the Three Wishes Technique (Brink, 2005), Incomplete Sentences Question-naire (MacFarlane, 1998), and The Forest Adventure Metaphor (MacFarlane, 1998). These projection techniques were used to verify the levels of personal protective factors identified in the quantitative data collection.

Because the study was experimental, a pre-test and a post-test (using the above data collection techniques) were also conducted, incorporating an experimental and control group. The experimental group participated in the intervention program, while the control group did not. The members of each group were not randomly assigned, but rather placed in accordance with feedback from staff. Youth whom staff regarded as most vulnerable were assigned to the experimental group (see discussion below for selection criteria), result-ing in a quasi-experimental research design (Leedy & Ormrod, 2005). Both participants and their parents gave verbal informed consent to participation. Comparisons between pre- and post-test results were used to determine whether the intervention program was effective in promoting resilient functioning.

**The Research Groups**

Each of the research groups, the control group and the experimental group, consisted of six senior-phase high-school learners identified as having special educational needs. The groups were culturally similar in that all were English mother-tongue speakers. The study took place in a school for learners with special educational needs during the weekly activity period (a period in which learners choose to partici-pate in recreational, sporting, or cultural activities).

Purposive selection was used to identify participants. As there was no other South African instrument to rate resilience and vulnerability levels among adolescents with learning difficulties at the time this research was undertaken, staff assessment informed the identification procedure. Selection was therefore facilitated by asking school guidance teachers and psychologists to complete a questionnaire consisting of four open-ended questions concerning the vulnerable learner's typical functioning and nine closed items relating directly to personal attributes associated with resilient adolescents with learning difficulties. The questionnaire was based on prevailing literature (Garmezy & Rutter, 1983; Loesel & Bliesener, 1994; O'Leary, 1998; Werner & Smith, 1992). The suitability of identified participants was verified by using background history, behaviour reports, and discussions with members of the school's psychology department together with an independent assessment of the data by a practising psychologist.

Both groups of participating youth contained comparable risk factors, including exposure to parental pathology, severe marital discord, parental rejection, financial difficulties, and abuse. The open-ended questions completed by the school's guidance teachers and psychologists reported incidence of depression, drug and alcohol abuse, and aggressive and antisocial behaviour as manifestations of non-resilient behaviour (e.g., poor academic achievement, involvement in age-inappropriate activities) by participating youth.

## Data Collection

Quantitative data were collected during four three-hour sessions, during regular school hours. A school psychologist was present throughout these sessions to ensure that the data were gathered in an unbiased manner. Because participation was voluntary, the participants were generally cooperative.

Collection of this data was followed up by lengthy, individual, semi-structured interviews to verify results. As previously mentioned, qualitative data were also collected in the form of process and observation notes made during the twelve group sessions. Each session was tape recorded so that the independent psychologist, with whom conclusions (based on the process notes) were debated, had objective data to assess.

## Pre-test Data Analysis

Data obtained from the projective techniques were assessed interpretatively (Brink, 2005) in terms of factors pointing towards resilience.

For example, the extent of protection illustrated against the rain in Brink's draw-a-person-in-the-rain technique provided some clues about the adolescent's need for protection against life's difficulties and hence the degree of resilience. Here, the absence of protective measures such as an umbrella combined with a small human figure denoted vulnerability. Similarly, in Kritzberg's three animal technique, the animals chosen were appraised as metaphorical clues in terms of the degree of resilience. So, choosing to be a little mouse, for example, denoted vulnerability. The same pertained to findings in the three wishes technique. In the Forest Adventure Metaphor technique, the metaphor of an adventure in a forest served to symbolically represent the degree of resilience in the adolescent's functioning. These interpretations were verified in interviews with the adolescents.

Structured questionnaires were marked according to test specifications. Data were used to formulate a composite description of preliminary levels of resilience relating to the nine personal protective factors hypothesized to have a buffering effect on risk associated with learners experiencing learning difficulties. For example, the Adolescent Self-Concept Scale was used to determine self-concept. The High School Personality Questionnaire was used to determine the degree of ego-strength (specifically factor C) and the traits (such as drive, assertiveness, enthusiasm, attitude) contributing to, or detracting from, resilience. The Emotions Profile Index was used to determine basic emotional dimensions, such as levels of aggression, anxiety, distrust, and depression. The Incomplete Sentences Questionnaire was used to evaluate the degree to which personal protective factors, not measured by the above tests, affected an adolescent's ability to demonstrate resilience.

Each participant was also interviewed using semi-structured interviews, yielding data that facilitated discussion and verification of findings. As previously stated, these discussions included an independent psychologist as well as the school's psychologists.

On the basis of all of the above data, each participant could be described in terms of self-concept, positive attitude, future orientation, assertiveness, enthusiasm, drive, good interpersonal relationships, and internal locus of control and anxiety. Traits were considered lacking when quantitative data showed below-average scores in accordance with test norms and when qualitative data could be interpreted to show vulnerability. When these traits were lacking, the individual was described as vulnerable. An example of such a description is provided in Table 2.

Table 2: Example of pre-test composite description of Subject B, experimental group

| Vulnerable Trait | Yes/No | Confirmation |
| --- | --- | --- |
| Negative attitude, suggesting loneliness, rejection, and depression, as well as emotional vulnerability. | Yes | −0 Incomplete sentences: dominant theme is rejection<br>−1 Low gregarious score and high distrust score (EPI)<br>−2 Forest metaphor<br>−3 Teachers' reports emphasize her propensity to whine and complain |
| Poor self-concept, suggesting emotional instability and negative self-talk. | Yes | −0 Self-concept questionnaire suggests poor self-concept (stanine of 1)<br>−1 Incomplete sentences<br>−2 Follow-up interview confirms poor self-concept |
| Poor future orientation, suggesting negative orientation to achievement, and pessimism. | Yes | −0 Follow-up interview reveals negative orientation towards being able to succeed |
| Hostility, suggesting aggressive, angry functioning, and low frustration tolerance. | Yes | −0 HSPQ (extreme sten of 10 for Factor E, suggesting aggression) |
| Excitability, suggesting a tendency towards impulsiveness, recklessness, and rebelliousness. | Yes | −0 HSPQ (sten of 10 for excitability and 2 for opportunism, suggesting impulsiveness and some recklessness) |
| Evasiveness, suggesting a lack of drive and an avoidance of responsibility. A tendency to quit is also present. | Moderate | −0 Some teachers report a tendency to quit when things are difficult<br>−1 Follow-up interview indicates quitting with regard to school tasks only |
| External locus of control, suggesting a sense of hopelessness over one's destiny. Affinity for victim identity is noted. | Yes | −0 Metaphor exercise<br>−1 Incomplete sentences<br>−2 HSPQ (sten of 4 for being uncontrolled and for going with the group decision) |

Table 2 (continued)

| | | |
|---|---|---|
| Inadequacy, suggesting a sense of personal dissatisfaction and a critical attitude. This inadequacy does not translate into motivation to change. | Yes | −0 High distrust score on the EPI suggests experience of inadequacy<br>−1 Three wishes<br>−2 HSPQ (sten of 3 for emotional vulnerability)<br>−3 Draw-a-person<br>−4 Follow-up interview confirms personal dissatisfaction |
| Poor interpersonal relationships, suggesting negative social orientation and reservation. A lack of empathy is noted. | Yes | −0 HSPQ (extreme sten of 1 for factor A, suggesting extreme reservation, and 2 for shyness)<br>−1 Three wishes<br>−2 Teachers' reports |

## Post-test Data Analysis

The post-test was conducted approximately five and a half months after the pre-test. For both groups, the same procedure was followed as with the pre-test. Although the sixth member of the experimental group agreed to the post-testing, he was in the process of leaving school, primarily because of an escalating substance abuse problem. His results were used in overall consideration of the efficacy of the program.

The post-test data were triangulated with written and oral reports from the educators who interacted with the learners in the research groups on a daily basis. Educators were asked to comment on attitude, interpersonal relationships, assertiveness, enthusiasm, drive, and sense of responsibility.

The pre- and post-test composite descriptions of the experimental and control group members were then compared and debated: psychologists from the school's psychology department and an independent, practising psychologist deliberated on the composite descriptions compared to a profile of resilient adolescents with learning difficulties as gleaned from literature (MacFarlane, 1998). The post-test composite descriptions were triangulated with educator reports that attested to generally improved levels of resilience for the members of the experimental group and a lack of resilient functioning for members of the control group.

## Findings of the Study

Table 3 summarizes the incidence of the factors associated with resilience before and after the intervention for both the experimental and control groups.

Prior to the intervention, the degree of resilience in the functioning of control and experimental group members was equally low. No member of either group was considered resilient when compared with identified functional characteristics of resilient adolescents with learning difficulties (MacFarlane, 1998). No member in either group demonstrated a positive self-concept, positive attitude, internal locus of control, or anxiety. Two members of the experimental group showed more positive social relationships, compared to one member of the control group. Two members of the control group evidenced drive and assertiveness, compared to only one in the experimental group. One

Table 3: Comparison of resilience factors in experimental and control groups, pre- and post-test

| Resilience factor | Experimental Group | | Control Group | |
|---|---|---|---|---|
| | Number of participants to demonstrate this trait *pre-test* | Number of participants to demonstrate this trait *post-test* | Number of participants to demonstrate this trait *pre-test* | Number of participants to demonstrate this trait *post-test* |
| Positive attitude | 0 | 4 | 0 | 0 |
| Positive self-concept | 0 | 3 | 0 | 0 |
| Positive future orientation | 0 | 5 | 1 | 2 |
| Assertiveness | 1 | 5 | 2 | 1 |
| Enthusiasm | 2 | 6 | 2 | 3 |
| Drive | 1 | 5 | 2 | 2 |
| Anxiety | 0 | 4 | 0 | 1 |
| Internal locus of control | 0 | 3 | 0 | 0 |
| Good interpersonal relationships | 2 | 6 | 1 | 1 |

Table 4: Percentage of improvement per factor

| Resilience factor | Pre-test experimental group numbers | Post-test experimental group numbers | Percentage of improvement (%) |
|---|---|---|---|
| Positive attitude | 0 | 4 | 66 |
| Positive self-concept | 0 | 3 | 50 |
| Positive future orientation | 0 | 5 | 83 |
| Assertiveness | 1 | 5 | 66 |
| Enthusiasm | 2 | 6 | 66 |
| Drive | 1 | 5 | 66 |
| Anxiety | 0 | 4 | 66 |
| Internal locus of control | 0 | 3 | 50 |
| Good interpersonal relationships | 2 | 6 | 66 |

member of the control group showed positive future orientation, compared to none in the experimental group. In both groups two members displayed enthusiasm.

Following the experimental group's participation in the intervention program, dissimilarities regarding protective factors connected to resilience were noted when comparing the composite descriptions of the members of the experimental and control groups. Every one of the nine attributes associated with buffering risk and augmenting resilience was improved in at least half of the experimental group members. Enthusiasm and positive interpersonal relationships were projected by all experimental group members during the post-test. In the control group only two attributes buffering risk showed improvement (two members as compared to the initial one): positive future orientation and enthusiasm.

A comparison of the experimental and control group's post-test composite descriptions suggests that the intervention program succeeded in augmenting attributes associated with resilience in the experimental group. The degree of success, though, is not uniform. Table 4 summarizes the experimental group's improvement per attribute.

The ability to view the future more positively was the most augmented attribute in the experimental group – five of the six members projected positive future orientation during the post-test. Assertiveness and drive were enhanced in four of the six members, suggesting that these adolescents acquired the psychological vigour necessary to persevere.

Using Table 4 to comment on the effectiveness of the intervention program, it is clear that components of the intervention need to be reviewed. The attributes least affected on were an internal locus of control and a positive self-concept. In both instances only 50% of the group members demonstrated improvement in these attributes. In particular, sessions 3 and 11 need to be adapted, as these sessions deal with an internal locus of control and self-concept (see Table 1). Furthermore, the length of these sessions should be examined – it is quite possible that two sessions of an hour each are inadequate to address the complex issues of self-concept and locus of control, implying that additional sessions should be added so that the program consists of more than twelve sessions. A trial program of fourteen to sixteen sessions needs to be piloted.

In reviewing the remaining seven personal protective factors targeted by this intervention program, we noted a success rate of 66% improvement in six of the seven factors. In other words, the program was constructive two thirds of the time only and thus only partially successful. Whilst this is encouraging groundwork, it does suggest that the program's suitability to the culture of the adolescent with learning difficulty needs further refinement.

### Implications of the Findings

The experimental group was too small to allow generalizations to the broader population of adolescents with learning difficulties, but a direct implication of this study is that the intervention program could develop personal attributes associated with resilience among adolescents with learning difficulties. The partial success of this program must be seen in the light of its attempt to be contextually suitable. The program themes related specifically to attributes associated with resilience in adolescents with learning difficulties, and the facilitation of the program was flexible enough to allow adaptation to group members' context.

Nevertheless, not all attributes associated with resilience in adolescents with learning difficulties were equally well augmented by the program, and not all the participants benefited equally. The program also failed the sixth group member. The fact that this member quit school could be seen as affirmation that intervention occurred too late in his/her school career and was also too one-sided. At the outset of this program, educator reports highlighted a range of risk behaviours

Table 5: The intervention program's ability to facilitate the process of resilience

| Resilience Process (Kumpfer 1999) | Intervention Tool |
|---|---|
| A stressor or risk factor(s) threaten(s) the well-being of an individual and activates the resilience process. | All participants were formally identified with specific learning difficulties and considered vulnerable by their school community. The intervention program was designed in response to this activated process. |
| The stressor is found within a context. Within this context risk and protective factors interact. This interaction is fluid and variable over time. | The context in which the participants functioned, and in which the intervention occurred, was a South African government school for learners with special needs. Such schools are exclusive, accommodating only learners who have been formally recognized as being learning disabled. The school functions within a multidisciplinary framework: learners attending the school receive remedial and psychological intervention, speech and occupational therapy where necessary, and supportive familial intervention in addition to regular teaching. All of the afore-mentioned function protectively. |
| | Although the program was implemented within the above context, it did not address the role of the context in resilient functioning sufficiently. The multidisciplinary framework of the school was seen to operate protectively, and consequently the intervention did not include asset-focused strategies. However, no effort was made to address the risks inherent to the above context (e.g. social stereotyping of learners attending a special school) or to address further risk behaviours highlighted by staff. |
| Simultaneously the individual interacts with her environment. This person–environment interaction can be in response to perceived and experienced risk factors. | The interaction of the individual within her environment was not directly addressed. Although the program used group therapy as a medium, and although factors that impact on social and contextual functioning were included, no parts of the program encouraged interaction in order to engender support from the environment. The program failed to specifically address:<br>1 Youth–parent interaction<br>2 Youth–educator interaction<br>3 Youth–sibling interaction<br>4 Youth–environment interaction<br>The program also did not invite participation by environmental role players. |

Table 5 (continued)

| | |
|---|---|
| Individuals possess internal factors that buffer them against risk. These internal protective factors form part of the process of resilience. | Internal factors typically found in resilient youth who have learning difficulties formed the focus of this program. The program focused on inculcating:<br><br>1 Positive self-concept<br>2 Positive attitude<br>3 Positive future orientation<br>4 Assertiveness<br>5 Enthusiasm<br>6 Drive<br>7 Good interpersonal relationships<br>8 Internal locus of control<br>9 Moderate anxiety (MacFarlane, 1998; Theron, 2004) |
| The individual learns coping processes over time as she is exposed to challenges. These processes enable her to bounce back and continue to develop adaptively, despite risk. | The intervention program consisted of 12 weekly sessions, which taught coping by focusing on individual protective factors. If the program had focused more specifically on coping processes greater levels of resilient functioning might have been achieved. The period of intervention (five and a half months) is relatively brief. |
| Finally, a positive outcome in response to the stressor is achieved that bodes well for future outcomes. | A semi-positive outcome was achieved.<br><br>This study failed to indicate whether the augmented strengths of the experimental group remained intact – a follow-up study is needed to determine whether the initial positive outcomes were maintained. |

that group members were engaging in. The intervention should have addressed these behaviours specifically in addition to promoting resilience skills – further suggesting that the program was not sufficiently context specific for the sixth group member. The implication for future interventions is that they need to be contextually multifaceted and multidisciplinary.

The non-involvement of parents and educators in this program must also be reconsidered. It is very possible that an intervention program that included parents and educators would have been more effective, as systemic elements that reinforce or corrode personal protective factors could then have been addressed.

The shortcomings of the program, considered from the perspective of a process-focused strategy, are summarized in Table 5.

Overall, the program achieved partial success because it was tailored to suit adolescents with learning difficulties, but this success was limited because the greater environmental context of these adolescents, and their interaction within it, was ignored.

## Implications for Practitioners

The limited success of this intervention is linked to the program's attempt to be contextually suitable, implying that programs designed for a specific population cannot be generically applied. Being designed from the outset for adolescents with learning difficulties, program themes were based on attributes associated with resilience in adolescents with learning difficulties, and the facilitation of the program was flexible. Because learning difficulties are commonly associated with poorer concentration spans (Dednam, 2005), short sessions (no longer than an hour each) were designed. The sessions were designed to be active and interactive, incorporating role playing, art, and visualization activities in order to keep adolescents focused and engaged. Prior to the design of this program, an attempt at understanding these adolescents' level of language, typical metaphors, and energy levels was made through interaction with them during school hours. All of this information informed program design. For example, the Forest Adventure Metaphor was adapted from a popular quiz enjoyed by the adolescents of the school at that time. All handouts used in the program were written in simple English to accommodate participants' limited levels of English mastery (given their learning difficulties). Music with empowering words was incorporated into the sessions.

Songs such as Mariah Carey's 'Hero' were chosen because of their popularity among adolescents of this school at the time.

The content of each session was adapted to embrace the issues raised by participants during the session. For example, in the fourth group session focusing on attitude and anxiety, participants spoke of their anxiety surrounding academic failure. Of the six participants, five had failed and repeated a grade. The use of a common group-specific experience proved very uniting and empowering for the group. Participants shared feelings of stupidity, embarrassment, and a belief that nothing would ever be easy for them. One participant who had scarcely participated in the previous three sessions began to participate freely, identifying strongly with content of which he had ownership. Similarly, during the tenth session, which occurred just after the school had elected new youth leaders (prefects), participants expressed their frustration with their new leaders, feeling generally browbeaten by them. As a result of participants' disgruntled mood, the theme for the session (social orientation) was immediately altered to include an explanation of transactional analysis and the roles from which participants themselves were transacting. Group members were astounded and determined to transact from the adult state during the following week. The repertoire of assertiveness skills dealt with in session five was then also revised as part of the repertoire of adult skills.

The implication for practice is twofold: (1) for a program to suit participants, participants need to be free to introduce content, and (2) the program facilitator needs to be flexible enough to deal with new content and to adapt it to overall goals. To do so she needs to be well trained in group facilitation and have a sound grasp of overarching theory.

The group resilience program was implemented at a special school as part of the school's curricular program. This suggests that given suitable programs and training, schools can function as agents of primary intervention, thereby facilitating learner wellness and forestalling attrition. This is especially important in the current day and age when psychotherapy is beyond the fiscal reach of many learners (Heard, 2000). However, for greater success to be achieved, the program should not be implemented as a stand-alone program. It needs to actively address risk factors within the school environment and participants' greater environment (i.e., home and community), and it needs to encourage participation from role players within these environments.

In instances where practitioners work with youth who have learning difficulties but who are not accommodated in schools that specifically cater to special educational needs, it would be especially important to include stakeholders such as staff and peers from the youths' schools. The latter is to ensure that stakeholders do not inadvertently function as risk factors through their misunderstanding of, and bias against, youth with learning difficulties. Furthermore, in such instances the intervention program would also need to include asset-focused strategies (e.g., ensuring access to remediation) in order to encourage resilient functioning.

The partial success of this program could be related to the fact that it used group therapy and a facilitator (the researcher in this instance). Being part of a group for five and a half months could be partly responsible for the growth in the members of the experimental group. Quite possibly, associated aspects such as relationship building, positive expectations, and adult availability, and not the program per se, could explain the heightened incidence of resilience factors. Intervention with adolescents should therefore preferably occur within a group setting.

The downfall of this program (from a process perspective; see Table 5) needs to be addressed. Practitioners who wish to encourage resilient functioning among youth with learning difficulties need to emphasize resilience as a process. If this program were to be used again, the content and program participants would need to be enlarged accordingly.

## Conclusion

To encourage resilience among adolescents with learning difficulties is possible. This provides hope for adolescents with learning difficulties and for their families and educators. To encourage resilience does, though, require more than program-based intervention – even when (as in this research) the program is tailored to suit the profile and needs of resilient adolescents with learning difficulties. For resilient functioning to be encouraged, the focus should be on resilience as a process. As such, practitioners need to facilitate intervention that acknowledges that the individual is part of a larger, unique context and that addresses the dynamic demands of this context whilst inviting program participation from role players in the given context. For the adolescent with learning difficulties this implies that teachers, local mental health professionals (who are knowledgeable about learning difficulties), peers, and parents need to be included in program planning as sources of information regarding contextual demands, and also as program participants, encouraging them to buffer adolescents with learning difficulties against such contextual demands. In this way intervention is not implemented as a stand-alone program, but rather actively tackles risk factors within both the school and the broader environment (i.e., home and community). To succeed, interventions ultimately need to be multifaceted and must facilitate adaptive interaction between youth and multiple contextual stakeholders. Only when intervention is process oriented and cognizant of the dynamic, interactive nature of adolescents and their contexts will practitioners be in a position to truly empower adolescents with learning difficulties.

## REFERENCES

Bauer, A.M., Keefe, C.H., & Shea, T.M. (2001). *Students with learning disabilities or emotional/behavioural disorders*. Upper Saddle River, NJ: Merrill Prentice Hall.

Brink, M. (2005). *Projective techniques*. Unpublished workshop notes.

Cordoni, B. (1990). *Living with a learning disability* (rev. ed.). Carbondale: Southern Illinois University Press.

Dednam, A. (2005). Learning impairment. In E. Landsberg (Ed.), *Addressing barriers to learning: A South African perspective* (pp. 363–79). Pretoria: Van Schaik.

Donald, D., Lazarus, S., & Lolwana, P. (2002). *Educational psychology in social context*. Cape Town: Oxford University Press.

Ebersöhn, L., & Eloff, I. (2006). Identifying asset-based trends in sustainable programmes which support vulnerable children. *South African Journal of Education, 26*(3), 457–72.

Empson, J.M., & Nabuzoka, D. (2004). *Atypical child development in context*. New York: Palgrave McMillan.

Garmezy, N., & Rutter, M. (Eds.). (1983). *Stress, coping and development in children*. New York: McGraw-Hill.

Heard, C. (2000). Psychotherapy and the consumption principle. *New Therapist*, May/June, 23–7.

Keogh, B.K., & Weisner, T. (1993). An ecocultural perspective on risk and protective factors in children's development: Implications for learning disabilities. *Learning Disabilities Research and Practice, 8*, 3–10.

Kumpfer, K.L. (1999). Factors and processes contributing to resilience: The resilience framework. In M.D. Glantz & J.L. Johnson (Eds.), *Resilience and development: Positive life adaptations* (pp. 179–224). New York: Kluwer Academic/Plenum.

Leedy, P.D., & Ormrod, J.E. (2005). *Practical research: Planning and design.* Upper Saddle River, NJ: Pearson Merrill Prentice Hall.

Lerner, J. (2003). *Learning disabilities: Theories, diagnosis and teaching strategies.* Boston: Houghton Mifflin.

Loesel, F., & Bliesener, T. (1994). Some high-risk adolescents do not develop conduct problems: A study of protective factors. *International Journal of Behavioral Development, 17*(4), 753–77.

MacFarlane, L.C. (1998). *An educational-psychological perspective of the personal attributes which serve to anchor resilience.* Unpublished MEd thesis, University of South Africa, Pretoria.

Madge, E.M., & Du Toit, L. (1989). *Manual for the JR.–SR. High School Personality Questionnaire.* Pretoria: HSRC.

Mampane, R., & Bouwer, C. (2006). Identifying resilient and non-resilient middle-adolescents in a formerly black-only urban school. *South African Journal of Education, 26*(3), 443–56.

Mash, E.J., & Wolfe, D.A. (2005). *Abnormal child psychology* (3rd ed.). Belmont, CA: Thomson Wadsworth.

Masten, A.S. (1999). Resilience comes of age: Reflections on the past and outlook for the next generation of research. In M.D. Glantz & J.L. Johnson (Eds.), *Resilience and development: Positive life adaptations* (pp. 281–96). New York: Kluwer Academic/Plenum.

Masten, A.S., & Reed, M.J. (2005). Resilience in development. In C.R. Snyder & S.J. Lopez (Eds.), *Handbook of positive psychology* (pp. 74–88). New York: Oxford University Press.

Miller, M. (1996). Relevance of resilience to individuals with learning disabilities. *International Journal of Disability, Development and Education, 43*(3), 255–69.

Nastasi, B.K., & Bernstein, R. (1998). Executive summary: Resilience applied: The promise and pitfalls of school-based resilience programmes. *School Psychology Review, 27*(3). Retrieved 1 June 2005 from http://www.nasp online.org/publications.

O'Leary, V.E. (1998). Strength in the face of adversity: Individual and social thriving. *Journal of Social Issues, 54*(2), 425–46.

Powers, G.T. (2002). Towards a resilience-based model of school social work: A turnaround mentor. In R.R. Greene (Ed.), *Resiliency: An integrated approach to practice, policy and research* (pp. 153–70). Washington, DC: NASW.

Richman, J.M., & Fraser, M.W. (2001). Resilience in childhood: The role of risk and protection In J.M. Richman & M.W. Fraser (Eds.), *The context of youth violence: Resilience, risk and protection* (pp. 1–12). London: Praeger.

Roets, H.E. (1997). *EPI: Unpublished lecture notes.* University of South Africa, Pretoria.

Ross, E., & Deverell, A. (2004). *Psychosocial approaches to health, illness and disability.* Pretoria: Van Schaik.

Rutter, M. (2001). Psychosocial adversity: Risk, resilience and recovery. In J.M. Richman & M.W. Fraser (Eds.), *The context of youth violence: Resilience, risk and protection* (pp. 13–41). London: Praeger.

Schoon, I. (2006). *Risk and resilience. Adaptations in changing times.* Cambridge, MA: Cambridge University Press.

Spekman, N.J., Goldberg, R.J., & Herman, K.L. (1993). An exploration of risk and resilience in the lives of individuals with learning disabilities. *Learning Disabilities Research and Practice, 8*(1), 11–18.

Spitz, H.I., & Spitz, S.T. (1999). *A pragmatic approach to group psychotherapy.* Philadelphia: Brunner/Mazel.

Theron, L.C. (2004). The role of personal protective factors in anchoring psychological resilience in adolescents with learning difficulties. *South African Journal of Education, 24*(4), 317–21.

Ungar, M. (2005). Introduction: Resilience across cultures and contexts. In M. Ungar (Ed.), *Handbook for working with children and youth. Pathways to resilience across cultures and contexts* (pp. xv–xxxix). Thousand Oaks, CA: Sage.

Vrey, J.D., & Venter, M.E. (1983). *Manual to the Adolescent Self-Concept Scale.* Pretoria: UNISA.

Werner, E.E., & Smith, R.S. (1992). *Overcoming the odds: High risk children from birth to adulthood.* Ithaca: Cornell University Press.

# 10 Youth Expedition Programming in Singapore: Building Resilience and Positive Personal Development

MAH-NGEE LEE AND SIEW-LUAN TAY-KOAY

Fostering positive development among youth by instilling in them the values and strength of character to face the future with confidence remains a very important goal of Singapore's education system (Ministry of Education, 2004). The aim is to help Singapore's students develop the motivation to successfully navigate their way around problems even when they lack the skills and knowledge they need to do so. In line with this, the Youth Expedition Project (YEP) provides opportunities for all youth to participate in overseas community service learning experiences through which they can develop valuable, life-long skills, become confident of their identity, and develop a desire to create a better future for the society in which they live (Singapore International Foundation, 2002).

Such a focus follows on recent developments in psychological research. Increasingly, researchers (Garmezy, 1990; Masten, 2001; Seligman, 2002; Ungar, 2005) are shifting their professional paradigm away from a narrow focus on pathology, victimology, and mental illness (Rutter, 1985) to positive emotion (Fredrickson, 2001), virtue and strength (Masten, Hubbard, Gest, Garmezy, & Ramirez, 1999), academic resilience (Finn & Rock, 1997), and positive youth development (Larson, 2000; Lerner, Almerigi, Theokas & Lerner, 2005; Roth & Brooks-Gunn, 2003).

By way of illustration, Larson (2000) posits that during youth activities, youth experience a unique combination of intrinsic motivation and concentration that is rarely present during their daily experience. These two components of experience are hypothesized to occur during the overseas community service learning that is part of YEP. YEP activities are intended to foster positive outcomes such as greater achievement and increased self-control and self-efficacy. Thus, in the overseas community service learning expeditions, the process of personal integration should provide a rich context for the development of other positive qualities such as altruism and a secure identity.

During the overseas expedition, there is consistent communication (both direct and indirect) from program staff indicating that youth participants can succeed when acting responsibly (WestEd, 2002). Opportunities are continuously provided for meaningful participation. For example, youth are invited to involve themselves in relevant and engaging activities before, during, and after the expedition. These activities include marine and terrestrial conservation, cottage industry development, sharing knowledge and skills in such areas as primary health-care and information technology, and infrastructural development such as the constructing and upgrading of schools, nurseries, and community facilities (Singapore International Foundation, 2002). These opportunities help youth realize their value for both the responsibility they take and the decisions they make (Larson, 2000; Lerner, 2003).

The overseas expeditions provide opportunities for youth to develop a shared set of beliefs, especially a commitment to serve others and to be lifelong learners. Through the project's organization, youth develop a sense of belonging to a team along with the social supports they need from adults to succeed. Specifically, this is done through the structure and programming of the YEP.

This chapter presents an evaluation of YEP as it is carried out with youth from Singapore. The chapter sets out an explanation of YEP and relevant connections with research exploring similar programs with youth. This study, couched within the terms of the resilience and positive development literature, and its findings are then presented, focusing especially on the factors that contribute to the development of tenacity and resilience in youth involved in YEP. These factors include the intersection of personal attributes and social support and its relationship to positive outcomes such as civic attitudes and personal competence skills. The chapter concludes with a discussion about learning experiences through the Youth Expedition Project, particularly their ability to provide rich opportunities for youths to build their capabilities and develop resiliency.

## An Overview of the YEP

In the pre-expedition phase of YEP, participants are involved in site survey, fund-raising, and team-bonding activities. The central goal of the team building is to develop a social support system for participants in anticipation of their coming work in unfamiliar conditions. During the actual expedition, project services such as infrastructure development and knowledge sharing, interaction with locals, and nightly facilitation and reflection sessions are carried out. Team leaders and facilitators help group members understand their experiences through a process of individual reflection and collective discussion. There are also opportunities for youth input and decision making about their onsite work. These work to facilitate youths' encounters with difficulties or challenges that require them to learn to cope and adapt while working in their host communities. Educational visits and recreational activities are carried out upon completion of the project service. Once the participants come back from the expedition, post-program activities such as exhibitions and evaluation may be carried out.

A common tenet of adventure learning, service learning, or community service is the belief that youth are more capable than we generally believe them to be. Recent research (Batchelder & Root, 1994; Eyler, Root, & Giles, 1998; Giles & Eyler, 1994; Ikeda, 1999; Lund, 1998; Markus, Howard, & King, 1993; Reeb, Sammon, & Isackson, 1999) has documented a wide range of positive personal, attitudinal, moral, social, and cognitive outcomes related to service learning, including improved critical thinking skills (Jacoby, 1996). Service learning also helps youth understand the importance of their involvement in addressing the needs of their communities (Bringle & Duffy, 1998; Ferrari & Chapman, 1999; Jacoby, 1996; Mullins, 2003), enhancing aspects of citizenry.

Combined, YEP activities emphasize students' civic-mindedness and life skills. Such goals seem attainable based on research in other contexts. Moely, Mercer, Ilustre, Miron, and McFarland (2002) contend, for example, that service-based learning can help youth to enhance their sensitivity and to develop competencies such as interpersonal, problem-solving, and leadership skills. Civic attitudes, such as a desire to participate in civic action, political awareness, a willingness to promote social justice, and tolerance for diversity, may also be developed through service learning. As suggested by Larson (2000), structured youth activities, such as the Youth Expedition Project, can create a context in which there is a higher density of growth experiences than young people may normally experience.

## Resilience Factors and Positive Personal Development

The meaning of resilience and its operational definition have been the subject of considerable debate and controversy over the years

(Luthar, Cichetti, & Becker, 2000; Masten et al., 1999; Wang & Gordon, 1994). This study takes the perspective that resilience is a multidimensional construct, consisting of traits, processes, and outcomes associated with successful adaptation despite exposure to challenging conditions.

Longitudinal studies (Garmezy, Masten, & Tellegen, 1984; Rutter, 1985; 1987; Werner & Smith, 1982, 1992) have identified personal characteristics and traits that elicit a positive response or an active approach towards problem solving. Such traits include even temperament, optimism, determination, and perseverance in overcoming adversity. Resilient individuals tend to be socially competent, autonomous, optimistic, and able to elicit positive attention and support (Masten & Coatsworth, 1998; Werner & Smith, 1982, 1992; Wyman, Cowen, Work, & Kerley, 1993). They have good problem-solving skills, self-efficacy, future goal-orientation, and high self-esteem (Werner & Smith, 1982; 1992).

Resilience may also be seen as the process of building the capacity for, or the outcome of, successful coping and adaptation under threatening conditions (Maluccio, 2002; Masten, Best, & Garmezy, 1990; Wang & Gordon, 1994). Coping and adaptation are the processes through which individual potentialities develop in response to environmental challenges and opportunities. Studies conducted by Chan (2000), Holahan, Holahan, Moos, and Cronkite (1999), Jew, Green, and Kroger (1999), Kobasa (1979), Khoo (2002), and Lim (2002) have all focused on the adaptive value of effective coping strategies and improvement in psychological functioning that result when children and adults overcome challenges. Thus, successful adaptation or coping may result in positive outcomes such as improved personal competence and sense of civic responsibility (Bringle & Duffy, 1998; Moely, Mercer, Ilustre, Miron, & McFarland, 2002).

In this chapter, resilience refers operationally to traits, processes, and positive outcomes that are indicative of youth who have the ability and tenacity to fight against the odds and not quit. Positive personal development is the ongoing process in which young people engage, investing their time and energies positively to meet their basic personal and social needs. A focus on resilience is synonymous, then, with a focus on a youth's capacities, strengths, and ability to meet developmental needs (Larson, 2000; Luthar & Cichetti, 2000), and is reliant upon contextual factors, including relationships and community supports.

Research also supports the importance of positive relationships for youth resilience. Longitudinal studies, for example, provide compelling evidence of family characteristics that help raise resilient children (Rutter, 1985, 1987; Werner & Smith, 1992) and establish the importance of family support as a predictor of positive outcomes in children (Egeland, Carlson, & Scroufe, 1993; Huan, 1998; Rutter, 1985, 1987; Werner & Smith, 1982, 1992).

Also consistent amongst findings in the literature is that of teacher–student relationships, which enhance achievement through high expectations for students coupled with a classroom climate characterized by encouragement and support (Chong, 2000; Roeser, Midgley, & Urdan, 1996; Wang & Gordan, 1994). An influential factor also seems to be children's perceptions of the support they receive from peers. A number of studies have demonstrated a link between children's perception of peer support and children's positive outcomes, including a better self-concept (Hauser, 1999; Mau & Seng, 1997).

Community resources and opportunities have been identified as one constellation of resilience factors that contribute to positive development in youth. Researchers have agreed that individuals who have more personal and social resources are more likely to make use of active forms of coping (Ungar, 2005; Wang & Gordon, 1994; Werner & Smith, 1982, 1992). Findings suggest that building upon people's strengths in their communities can promote feelings of efficaciousness and competence. It can also foster a commitment to ensure that positive changes endure within their communities (Luthar & Cicchetti, 2000).

Constantine and Benard (2001) posit that individuals can create environments that promote positive development and successful learning for young people, such as that achieved through adventure learning and community service. Resilience research has highlighted the importance of tracking the effectiveness of functioning in major developmental tasks and the assessment of qualities in relationships, schools, and communities or organizations that appear to make a difference (Masten & Powell, 2003). Particular attention has been given to the power of belief systems that facilitate meaning making, positive outlooks, and transcendence or spirituality (Walsh, 2003). Larson (2000) believes that initiative and resiliency are components for positive development, contributing to problem-solving abilities, leadership, altruism, and civic engagement.

## A Study to Test the Effectiveness of YEP

In order to evaluate the effectiveness of YEP, we conducted a study focusing on resilience factors and opportunities for meaningful civic participation by Singapore youth who participate in overseas community service expeditions. The study is organized around Marzano's (1998) self-system approach and Bronfenbrenner's (1979, 1993) ecological-transactional theory in order to explore how particular individual and environmental factors serve to promote resilience and personal development in YEP participants. Specifically, the study explores resilience factors such as personal attributes and social supports that distinguish resilient and non-resilient YEP participants. In this study, a resilient youth is one who possesses a positive outlook on life, engages in problem-focused coping, and has a higher level of self-esteem, self-efficacy, and goal mastery orientation. Such youth also possess ego-resilient personality characteristics. As well, the study sought to assess the impact of the overseas service learning experience on participants' development of tenacity, civic attitude, and personal competence skills. These skills include interpersonal and problem-solving skills, leadership skills, and sensitivity. We hypothesized that how well the participants cope with the stress of YEP, together with how they use their individual competencies, will affect the degree of positive outcomes they experience. Personal attributes such as coping abilities, self-esteem, efficacy, goal orientation, ego-resiliency and ego-under-control, and demographic characteristics were suggested as resilience-related factors that would be developed through the capacity-building activities that are part of YEP. Additionally, social support variables such as contact with family members, teachers, and group leaders, peer relationships, and involvement with community members were all hypothesized to be influential in these young people's lives and were therefore part of this investigation.

### Objectives of the Study

By exploring the service learning experience provided by YEP, this study helps to fill a void in the resilience and service learning research literature to date. This research strives to uncover processes that enhance positive outcomes as identified by participants, comparing findings to those found by other researchers (Batchelder & Root, 1994;

Eyler et al., 1998; Giles & Eyler, 1994; Ikeda, 1999; Lund, 1998; Markus et al., 1993).

Two questions were used to guide this study. First, what are the personal characteristics and resilience factors that distinguish resilient participants of YEP from non-resilient participants in this study? Second, what positive outcomes can be attributed to participation in the overseas community service expedition for (*a*) the group as a whole and (*b*) sub-groups of resilient and non-resilient youth?

*Research Design*

This study included both quantitative and qualitative approaches to data collection. Hill, Grange, and Newmark's (2003) argument that quantitative and qualitative approaches are complementary rather than incompatible is strengthened by Ungar and Liebenberg (2005), who identify the need for a combination of methods in the study of resilience and positive development in youth. The intention is to weave a rich tapestry of detail in order to capture youth's learning experience and personal growth through service learning. Thus, a mixed-methods approach may ensure a better grasp of resilience factors that contribute to positive personal development of YEP participants who were involved in overseas community service learning from November to December 2004.

Using a pre- and post-test design, we administered a survey questionnaire and interviews with participants prior to the overseas community service learning expedition and after the youth returned. Focus group interviews with some of the community members, team leaders, and facilitators were conducted in January and February 2005.

*The Participants*

Participants in this study were drawn from the 3,979 participants of YEP that were sent out by the Singapore International Foundation for overseas community service learning in various Asian countries during 2004. The 347 participants (135 males, 212 females; M = 20.79 years old, SD = 2.77) in this study represented 8.7% of the youths involved in the 2004 overseas service learning projects. Participants were randomly selected based on their being spread across different schools or organizational groups, gender, race, age, and level of education. The Singapore International Foundation encourages participants between the age of seventeen and twenty-five to join the Youth Expedition Projects, although those who are younger or older may also volunteer (Singapore International Foundation, 2002).

The majority of YEP participants were students who went for their expeditions during their November–December school holidays. Out of the twenty project teams in this study, seven went to Cambodia, one to China, six to India, two to Indonesia, one to the Philippines, and three to Thailand, with teams comprising eleven to thirty-five youth volunteers (M = 21.4 participants, SD = 5.31), one team leader, and one facilitator. Expeditions ranged from thirteen to twenty-two days (M = 17.6 days, SD = 2.60)

*The Instruments*

Several measures associated with resilience were included in the analyses, including the *Coping Abilities Scale*, the *Self-Esteem Scale*, the *Efficacy and Mastery Goal Orientation Measure*, and the *ego-resiliency* and *ego-undercontrol* measures, as well as the *Civic Attitudes and Skills Questionnaire*. The *Coping Abilities Scale*, the *Self-Esteem Scale*, and the *Efficacy and Mastery Goal Orientation Measure* have all been adapted from existing measures.

The Coping Abilities Scale was adapted from the short-form of the *Adolescent Coping Scale* (ACS) (Frydenberg & Lewis, 1993). These items, which were empirically derived by means of conceptual grouping and factor analyses, assess a comprehensive range of coping strategies of adolescents on a five-point Likert-type scale, ranging from 1 (didn't do it) to 2 (used a great deal). Cronbach alpha reliability coefficients for the subscales problem-focused coping, non-productive coping, and social support, were .66, .54, and .70 respectively, and the coefficient for the overall total scale was .69.

The Self-Esteem Scale derived from Rosenberg (1965) is a ten-item scale with items that assess general self-esteem. Typical items are 'I feel that I am a person of worth, just like other people' and 'I am able to do things as well as most other people.' It incorporates a four-point Likert-type scale, ranging from 1 (strongly disagree) to 4 (strongly agree). Coefficient alpha reliability for the measure obtained in this study was .87.

The Efficacy and Mastery Goal Orientation measure is a twelve-item scale and is based on subscales from the *Patterns of Adaptive Learning Survey* (PALS) (Midgley et al., 2000). Typical items include 'It's important to me that I learn a lot of new concepts this year' and 'I'm certain that I can master the skills taught this year.' The respondent rates the items on a five-point Likert-type scale, ranging from 1 (not at all true) to 5 (very true). Coefficient alpha reliability for the measure was .73.

*Ego-Resiliency* (ER) (Block & Kremen, 1996) and *Ego-Undercontrol* (UC) (Letzring, Block, & Funder, 2005) are both personality scales. Typical items are 'I am generous with friends' and 'I tend to buy things on impulse' and are based on a four-point Likert-type scale, ranging from 1 (does not apply at all) to 4 (applies very strongly). Coefficient alpha reliabilities for both measures obtained were .81 and .82 respectively.

For measuring positive outcomes, the locally constructed *Civic Attitudes and Skills Questionnaire* (CASQ) yields scores on six scales developed through factor analysis (Moely et al., 2002). The subscales measure civic action (plans for future involvement in the community), political awareness (knowledge of current and local and national politics), social justice attitudes (awareness of the importance of social institutions in determining the fate of the individual), and diversity attitudes (appreciation and valuing of friendships with persons of diverse backgrounds and characteristics). These subscales make up the civic attitudes scale. Interpersonal and problem-solving skills (the ability to communicate and work effectively with others), leadership skills (the ability to guide others), and sensitivity (the ability to empathize with people) constitute the personal competence skills. Items are scored on a five-point Likert-type scale, ranging from 1 (strongly disagree) to 5 (strongly agree). Coefficient alpha reliability for the full measure was .87.

The structured interview schedules for the participants consisted of seven main open-ended questions that elicited their reflections and evaluations on the following: their expedition activities, their contributions to service learning, the achievement of their objectives, and their personal growth and insights into the connection between resiliency development and service learning. The questions also asked about their critical evaluations of the extent to which the expedition made a difference in their lives, in the lives of the community that they served, and in their relationships with friends, families, and program leaders, as well as their plans for future community volunteerism. All interviews were tape recorded and later transcribed. Content analysis was used to analyse the qualitative interview data using a systematic stage-by-stage process so as to be able to better understand the perceptions and difficulties of the interviewees.

**Results**

*The Youth Expedition Project Participant Profile*

Table 1 summarizes some of the characteristic differences between resilient and non-resilient participants of YEP. Participants were categorized into two groups, based on ther self-report and description of whether they belong to the resilient or non-resilient group. Classification of resilient and non-resilient groups was based on the questions: 'Before the overseas community service-learning expedition, do you think you were a resilient person?' and 'Do you think this overseas expedition has made you into a more resilient person?' The participants' positivity, coping abilities, self-esteem, self-efficacy, mastery goal orientation, and ego-resiliency total scores, which were validated by the quantitative data, were also taken into consideration. There were 233 'resilient' participants (male = 94, 27.1%; female = 139, 40.1%) and 114 'non-resilient' participants (male = 41, 11.8%; female = 73, 21.9%). Results in Table 1 show that the groups differed significantly by race ($\chi^2_{(3)}$ = 8.06, $N = 347$, p < .05), religion ($\chi^2_{(5)}$ = 11.05, $N = 347$, p < .05), educational level ($\chi^2_{(5)}$ = 24.08, $N = 347$, p < .001), and leadership role ($\chi^2_{(1)}$ = 9.10, $N = 347$, p < .01). There was no significant difference in gender.

It is interesting to note that a number of the YEP participants were actively involved in extra-curricular activities such as clubs or societies ($n$ = 119; 34.3%) and games or sports ($n$ = 96; 27.7%) and a small number ($n$ = 19; 5.5%) were members of groups such as Girls' Brigade, Boys' Brigade, Scouts, or Guides. Of these, ninety participants (25.9%) were involved in leadership roles such as being house captains, presidents, vice-presidents, student councillors, secretaries, or committee members. In terms of leadership roles, resilient youth constituted 20.7% ($n$ = 72) of the sample, compared to just 5.2% of the non-resilient youth ($n$ = 18) ($\chi^2_{(1)}$ = 9.10, $N = 347$, p < .01).

*Comparison of Personal Resilience Factors Scores by Resilient Types*

Table 2 compares the mean scores of the resilient and non-resilient groups on the Coping Abilities, Self-Esteem, Efficacy and Mastery Goal Orientation, Ego-Resiliency, and Ego-Undercontrol measures.

Table 1: Characteristics of participants in YEP teams by youth types

| | Youth Type | | | | | | |
| | Resilient (n = 233) | | Non-resilient (n = 114) | | Total (n = 347) | | |
| | n | % | n | % | n | % | p[a] |
|---|---|---|---|---|---|---|---|
| Gender | | | | | | | |
| Male | 94 | 27.1 | 41 | 11.8 | 135 | 38.9 | |
| Female | 139 | 40.1 | 73 | 21.9 | 212 | 61.1 | |
| Race | | | | | | | .05* |
| Chinese | 198 | 57.1 | 85 | 24.5 | 283 | 81.6 | |
| Malay | 23 | 6.6 | 22 | 6.3 | 45 | 13.0 | |
| Indian | 5 | 1.4 | 5 | 1.4 | 10 | 2.9 | |
| Other | 2 | .6 | 7 | 2.0 | 9 | 2.6 | |
| Religion | | | | | | | .05* |
| Buddhism | 62 | 17.9 | 33 | 9.5 | 95 | 27.4 | |
| Christianity | 66 | 19.0 | 30 | 8.7 | 96 | 27.7 | |
| Hinduism | 2 | .6 | 2 | .6 | 4 | 1.2 | |
| Islam | 27 | 7.8 | 24 | 6.9 | 51 | 14.7 | |
| No religion | 76 | 21.9 | 25 | 7.2 | 101 | 29.1 | |
| Educational Level | | | | | | | .001*** |
| Secondary school | 13 | 3.7 | 21 | 6.1 | 34 | 9.8 | |
| Junior college | 19 | 5.5 | 9 | 2.6 | 28 | 8.1 | |
| ITE/Polytechnic | 14 | 4.0 | 13 | 3.7 | 27 | 7.8 | |
| University | 107 | 30.8 | 50 | 14.4 | 157 | 45.2 | |
| National institute of education | 39 | 11.2 | 14 | 4.0 | 53 | 15.3 | |
| Working/graduates | 41 | 11.8 | 7 | 2.0 | 48 | 13.8 | |
| Co-Curricular Activity | | | | | | | |
| Club/society | 75 | 21.6 | 44 | 12.7 | 119 | 34.3 | |
| Games/sports | 67 | 19.3 | 29 | 8.4 | 96 | 27.7 | |
| Uniform group | 11 | 3.2 | 8 | 2.3 | 19 | 5.5 | |
| Leadership Role | | | | | | | .01** |
| Leader | 72 | 20.7 | 18 | 5.2 | 90 | 25.9 | |
| Non-leader | 161 | 46.4 | 96 | 27.7 | 257 | 74.1 | |
| Home Background | | | | | | | |
| Living with both parents | 200 | 57.6 | 97 | 28.0 | 297 | 85.6 | |
| Parents with post-secondary education | 78 | 22.5 | 36 | 10.4 | 104 | 32.9 | |
| Family income > S$3000 | 145 | 41.8 | 53 | 15.2 | 198 | 57.0 | |

[a]Significance level for chi-square statistics for two-way tables of percentages.
*p < .05. **p < .01. ***p < .001.

Table 2: Comparison of personal resilience factor scores of participants by youth types

| | Youth Types | | | | | | |
| | Resilient ($n$ = 233) | | Non-resilient ($n$ = 114) | | | | |
| Measures | M | SD | M | SD | $t$-value | df | $p$-value |
|---|---|---|---|---|---|---|---|
| Coping Abilities[a] | 3.33 | .40 | 3.28 | .41 | .91 | 345 | .36 |
| Problem-Focused Coping | 4.07 | .53 | 3.93 | .60 | 2.13 | 203 | .03 |
| Non-productive Coping | 2.86 | .59 | 3.07 | .67 | -2.94 | 345 | .01** |
| Social Support | 3.05 | .62 | 3.14 | .62 | -1.26 | 345 | .20 |
| Self-Esteem | 3.16 | .47 | 2.93 | .46 | 4.34 | 345 | .001*** |
| Efficacy and Mastery | 3.81 | .44 | 3.68 | .49 | 2.45 | 345 | .02* |
| Goal Orientation[b] Efficacy | 3.74 | .50 | 3.57 | .52 | 2.79 | 345 | .01** |
| Mastery Goal Orientation | 3.87 | .49 | 3.78 | .57 | 1.60 | 345 | .11 |
| Ego-Resiliency | 3.16 | .39 | 3.05 | .39 | -3.27 | 426 | .001*** |
| Ego-Undercontrol | 3.16 | .47 | 2.93 | .46 | -.76 | 345 | .44 |
| Personal Resilience Factor Total Score[c] | 180.61 | 16.19 | 174.37 | 16.32 | -3.36 | 345 | .001*** |

[a]Coping Abilities Scale consists of Problem-Focused Coping, Non-Productive Coping, and Social Support subscales. When summing up for Coping Abilities scale, items in Non-productive Coping are reversed-scored. [b]Efficacy and Mastery Goal Orientation Scale consists of Efficacy subscale and Mastery Goal Orientation subscale. [c]Personal Resilience Factor Total Score is the sum of all the total scores of Positivity, Coping Abilities, Self-Esteem, Self Efficacy & Mastery Goal Orientations, and Ego-Resiliency. *$p$ < .05. **$p$ < .01. ***$p$ < .001.

Each comparison between the groups is tested for statistical significance of mean score differences using $t$-tests. All mean scores on positive characteristics that differed significantly between resilient and non-resilient youth were indicative of higher mean scores for resilient youth, while negative characteristics differed in the opposite direction.

Resilient youth (M = 4.07, SD = .47) used problem-focused coping strategies more than non-resilient youth (M = 3.16, SD = .47; $t_{(202)}$ = 2.15, p < .05). Conversely, non-resilient youth scored significantly higher on Non-Productive Coping (M = 3.07, SD = .67) than resilient youth (M = 2.86, SD = .59; $t_{(345)}$ = −2.94, $p$ < .01). Results indicate that the coping abilities of resilient youth are higher than those of non-resilient youth.

Self-esteem mean scores show the strongest statistically significant difference between the resilient group (M = 3.16, SD = .47) and non-resilient group (M = 2.93, SD = .46; $t_{(345)}$ = 4.34, p < .001). Similarly, mean scores on the Efficacy and Mastery Goal Orientation show statistically significant differences between resilient (M = 3.81, SD = .44) and non-resilient youth (M = 3.68, SD = .49; $t_{(345)}$ = 2.45, p < .05). The mean scores on the Ego-Resiliency scale show also meaningful differences between resilient youth (M = 3.16, SD = .47) and non-resilient youth (M = 2.93, SD = .46; $t_{(345)}$ = 2.77, $p$ < .01). These results indicate that resilient participants have higher self-esteem and self-efficacy and that they are more goal oriented than non-resilient participants.

*Resilience Factors and Civic Attitudes and Skills Measures*

Correlations among the resilience factor measures and civic attitudes and skills measures are given in Table 3. Most of these correlation coefficients are modest. Variables in this study can, for the most part, be considered independent enough to be used in later analyses. The majority of the intercorrelations between dimensions of resilience factors and positive outcomes are significant and are in a positive direction. Coping abilities and competence skills were weakly but significantly correlated to each other ($r$ = .27, $p$ < .01). Coping abilities were modestly and significantly correlated with self-esteem ($r$ = .41, $p$ < .01), efficacy and mastery goal orientation ($r$ = .31, $p$ < .01), and ego-resiliency ($r$ = .31, $p$ < .01). However, coping abilities and competence skills were negatively correlated with ego-undercontrol ($r$ = -.11, $p$ < .05) and subscale civic action ($r$ = -.17, $p$ < .01).

Self-esteem was correlated with positive outcomes such as competence skills ($r$ = .30, $p$ < .01), civic attitudes ($r$ = .16, $p$ < .01), efficacy and mastery goal orientation ($r$ = .37, $p$ < .01), and ego-resiliency ($r$ = .34, $p$ < .01), but negatively correlated with ego-undercontrol ($r$ = -.21, $p$ < .01). Among the resilience factors, ego-resiliency has modest and significant correlation with positive outcomes such as competence skills ($r$ = .41, $p$ < .01), while efficacy and mastery goal orientation has a modest but significant correlation with civic attitudes ($r$ = .32, $p$ < .01).

Table 3: Correlations of Personal Resilience Factors Measures and Civic Attitudes and Civic Attitudes and Skills Measures (N = 347)

| Measures | 1 | 2 | 3 | 4 | 5 | 6 | 7 | 8 | 9 | 10 | 11 | 12 | 13 | 14 | 15 | 16 | 17 | 18 | 19 | 20 |
|---|---|---|---|---|---|---|---|---|---|---|---|---|---|---|---|---|---|---|---|---|
| 1 Coping Abilities[a] | — | | | | | | | | | | | | | | | | | | | |
| 2 Problem-focused | .59** | — | | | | | | | | | | | | | | | | | | |
| 3 Non-productive coping | .42** | .11** | — | | | | | | | | | | | | | | | | | |
| 4 Social support | .85** | .27** | -.01 | — | | | | | | | | | | | | | | | | |
| 5 Self-Esteem | .41** | .46** | -.49** | .09 | — | | | | | | | | | | | | | | | |
| 6 Efficacy & mastery goal orientation[b] | .31** | .37** | -.19** | .15** | .37** | — | | | | | | | | | | | | | | |
| 7 Efficacy | .50** | .33** | -.13** | .18** | .28** | .90** | — | | | | | | | | | | | | | |
| 8 Goal orientation | .26** | .32** | -.22** | .09 | .38** | .89** | .60** | — | | | | | | | | | | | | |
| 9 Ego-resiliency | .31** | .38** | -.14** | .16** | .34** | .39** | .32** | .37** | — | | | | | | | | | | | |
| 10 Ego-undercontrol | -.11* | -.08 | .31** | .04 | -.21** | -.05 | -.07 | -.02 | .19** | — | | | | | | | | | | |
| 11 Civic attitudes[c] | .08 | .15** | -.15** | -.02 | .16* | .32** | .29** | .28** | .29** | -.01 | — | | | | | | | | | |
| 12 Civic action | .12* | .14** | -.08 | .05 | .08 | .30** | .28** | .25** | .34** | .06 | .76** | — | | | | | | | | |
| 13 Political awareness | .06 | .10 | -.09 | -.01 | .15** | .17** | .14** | .17** | .24** | .06 | .67** | .42** | — | | | | | | | |
| 14 Social justice | .01 | .08 | -.01 | -.03 | .09 | .16* | .16** | .13* | .03 | -.03 | .65** | .24** | .22** | — | | | | | | |
| 15 Diversity attitude | -.01 | .08 | -.07 | -.09 | .10 | .23** | .20** | .21** | .13** | -.14** | .55** | .26** | .10 | .29** | — | | | | | |
| 16 Competence[d] | .27** | .31** | -.20** | .12** | .30** | .36** | .35** | .30** | .41** | -.17** | .50** | .48** | .39** | .12* | .34** | — | | | | |
| 17 Interpersonal & problem-solving | .23** | .24** | -.19** | .10 | .24** | .35** | .33** | .30** | .38** | -.10 | .58** | .52** | .39** | .21** | .41** | .88** | — | | | |
| 18 Leadership skills | .11** | .17** | -.16** | -.02 | .26** | .22** | .18** | .21** | .29** | .04 | .37** | .29** | .32** | .14** | .23** | .61** | .47** | — | | |
| 19 Social desirability | .26** | .08 | -.11** | .15** | .20** | .24** | .26** | .18** | .26** | -.28** | .19** | .25** | .19** | -.07 | .12** | .76** | .46** | .15** | — | |
| 20 CASQ TOTAL[e] | .20** | .27** | -.17** | .06 | .26** | .40** | .37** | .34** | .40** | -.10 | .86** | .72** | .61** | .44** | .51** | .87** | .84** | .57** | .55** | — |

[a]Coping Abilities Scale consists of Problem-Focused Coping, Non-productive Coping, and Social Support subscales. [b]Self-Efficacy and Mastery Goal Orientation Scale consists of Efficacy subscale and Mastery Goal Orientation subscale. [c]Civic Attitudes Scale consists of Civic Action, Political Awareness, Social Justice, and Diversity Attitude subscales. [d]Personal Competence Skills Scale consists of Interpersonal and Problem-Solving Skills, Leadership Skills, and Social Desirability subscales. [e]CASQ total mean score consists of Civic Attitudes and Personal Competence Skills.

* $p < .05$. ** $p < .01$.

*Perceived Resilience of Participants after the YEP Experience*

In response to the questions on their perceived resilience before and after the overseas community service-learning expeditions ('Before the overseas community service-learning expedition, do you think you were a resilient person?' and 'Do you think this overseas expedition has made you into a more resilient person?), 198 participants (57%) who had considered themselves as resilient indicated that they became even more resilient after the expedition. On the other hand, 102 participants (29.4%) who felt they were not resilient before the expedition actually became more resilient after their participation in YEP. In other words, 300 of the participants (86.4%) perceived themselves to be more resilient after their overseas community service learning expeditions. The chi-square test results showed that there were no significant gender differences in perceived resilience of participants ($\chi^2_{(3)} = 4.61$, $N = 347$, $p < .20$).

In explaining how the recent overseas expedition had helped enhance their resilience, many participants indicated that they were now able to deal with problems and were much stronger. An example of such a response included:

> [The expedition] has taught me to work through difficulties and to be strong for the team when they need someone to be strong.

Participants also talked about persevering in their shared activities in order to achieve their goals of completing their projects, and becoming more resilient:

> I do not give up easily when I'm not good at doing a certain task. For example, I wasn't good at mixing the cement but I persevere until I finally perfect it.

Participants also learned about interpersonal relationships, how to be socially competent. and how to resolve conflicts:

> My unhappy experience working with one of my food team members in the first three days of the expedition made me really accept her as she is and thus, I am better able to work with her for the rest of the trip.

Participants learned to be more empathetic towards people around them. A participant explained that the experience made me aware that the problems these people were facing were probably far worse than mine. I should be even stronger to overcome the minor problems I face.

Because resilience represents the dynamic person-environment interaction, it is never the same episode that is being assessed moment by moment. Thus, many of the participants viewed themselves as 'more resilient' after the expedition. An example of such a response is:

The Youth Expedition Project allows me to see things from a different perspective. It allows me to see the importance of being more disciplined with myself, and more grateful with what I have now. And hence, these two elements made me a more resilient person.

### Comparison of Positive Outcomes by Resilient Types

In terms of positive outcomes, $t$-tests were conducted on the mean scores of civic attitudes and skills measures (CASQ) so as to compare resilient with non-resilient youth. For civic attitudes, resilient youth (M = 3.70, SD = .34) scored higher than non-resilient youth (M = 3.62, SD = .33; $t_{(345)}$ = 2.12, $p < .05$). Although only the subscale of political awareness yielded significant differences in the mean scores between resilient (M = 3.41, SD = .60) and non-resilient youth (M = 3.23, SD = .52; $t_{(345)}$ = 2.75, $p < .01$), the mean scores for the rest of the subscales were generally higher for resilient than non-resilient youth.

For competence skills, significant differences in mean scores were found in the subscales Interpersonal and problem-solving skills, and leadership skills. Interpersonal and problem-solving skills show higher scores for resilient youth (M = 4.05, SD = .39) than non-resilient youth (M = 3.93, SD = .44; $t_{(345)}$ = 2.58, $p < .01$). Similarly, resilient youth (M = 3.43, SD = .54) scored higher on leadership skills than non-resilient youth (M = 3.20, SD = .55; $t_{(345)}$ = 3.74, $p < .001$). Mean scores on the overall competence skill measure also yielded statistically significant differences between resilient (M = 3.66, SD = .31) and non-resilient youth (M = 3.57, SD = .34; $t_{(345)}$ = 2.26, $p < .05$).

### Outcome Differences of Participants by Resilient Type
### Using Qualitative Data

Further investigation of outcome differences of 'non-resilient' and 'resilient' participants of YEP was examined using qualitative analyses.

Table 4:   Comparison of Scores on Civic Attitudes and Competence Skills Measure by youth types

| | Youth Types | | | | | | |
| | Resilient ($n = 233$) | | Non-resilient ($n = 114$) | | | | |
| Measures | M | SD | M | SD | $t$-value | df | $p$-value |
|---|---|---|---|---|---|---|---|
| Civic Attitudes[a] | 3.70 | .34 | 3.62 | .33 | 2.12 | 345 | .03* |
| Civic action | 3.98 | .49 | 3.89 | .53 | 1.53 | 345 | .12 |
| Political awareness | 3.41 | .60 | 3.23 | .52 | 2.75 | 345 | .01** |
| Social justice | 3.66 | .44 | 3.58 | .43 | 1.57 | 345 | .12 |
| Diversity attitude | 3.69 | .50 | 3.73 | .57 | -.63 | 200 | .53 |
| Competence skills[b] | 3.66 | .31 | 3.57 | .34 | 2.26 | 345 | .02* |
| Interpersonal and problem-solving skills | 4.05 | .39 | 3.93 | .44 | 2.58 | 345 | .01** |
| Leadership skills | 3.43 | .54 | 3.20 | .55 | 3.74 | 345 | .001*** |
| Sensitivity | 3.36 | .37 | 3.37 | .36 | .39 | 345 | .69 |
| Civic attitudes and skills measure (CASQ)[c] | 3.68 | .24 | 3.60 | .30 | -2.54 | 345 | .01** |

[a]Subscale Civic Attitudes consists of Civic Action, Political Awareness, Social Justice, and Diversity Attitude. [b]Subscale Competence Skills consists of Interpersonal and Problem-Solving Skills, Leadership Skills, and Sensitivity. [c]Civic Attitudes and Skills Measure consists of Civic Attitudes subscale and Competence Skills subscale.
*$p < .05$. **$p < .01$. ***$p < .001$.

Statements made by participants exemplify differences between the two groups. For example, a 'non-resilient' individual remarked at the end of the trip that 'I don't know what it meant to me after the trip; I felt it seems to become worse. I felt annoyed whenever I think of the trip. The team left me with an impression that I can't sense any belonging to the team' (ID 422). Another 'non-resilient' participant from the same youth group found that the community service was 'tough.' Although he found that he had not changed much, and that he was still 'hyperactive' and easily 'excited,' he also found that he had 'learnt to be more independent and appreciate everything I have and also learnt that if I want something, I have to work hard to achieve it.' This particular participant found that the expedition was 'meaningful' and even stated that he had plans to join future expeditions 'anywhere to help people' (ID 420). His comments point to benefits of the service learning experience.

Perceptions and attitudes of 'resilient' participants were markedly different from those of their counterparts. In one particular report submitted to the Singapore International Foundation after the expedition by a 'resilient' team leader, self-efficacy, goal orientation, personal responsibility, and optimism were clearly reflected in his remarks:

'The idea for this follow-up project kept ringing in my mind the moment I returned from my initial project in 2003, in the capacity of a participant. To say that it took me a year to realise my hope of leading a project back to Yuksam, West Sikkim is no understatement. When the offer came to lead this project, it was one that I could not refuse ...

Our group of twenty-four participants took full ownership of the project ... it was a heartening sight to see the drive, commitment and passion of this group of individuals thrown into the big unknown. (ID 60)

This team leader took pains to organize his project and, when it materialized, he had to navigate participating youth through the experience with his team-handling skills. On the day of their arrival at the project country, problem solving and flexibility was reflected when this leader had to decide to change plans due to a workers' strike. In the same report, one of the team members remarked on the efficacy of their team leader:

'On the night we arrived, we were told ... that the next day would herald an area-wide workers' strike ... There would be chaos and unpredictable danger if we were to travel during the strike ...So, under the instructions of [team leader], we stealthily snuck off to the airport in the wee hours ... But I was supportive of going off early ... I was relieved in the knowledge that everything we did, we did for the safety and well-being of the group and the project itself. (ID 60)

Resilience and positive developmental outcomes after the service learning expedition were further reflected in the post-survey of the 'resilient' team leader:

I have no regrets whatsoever leading this group... We left for Sikkim as two leaders with 24 eager participants going into the big unknown. We came back with 24 individuals ready to dip their hands into service-learning activities locally. This is, in itself, sufficient reward for me and showed that all the hassle of the administration I had to go through for this trip was worth every single effort. The lessons in life that they taught me, through their simple and basic acts, have helped me develop into a holistic individual both psychologically and emotionally.

## Discussion

Although all youth in this study were participating in community service learning through the same program, there appears to be variation in the quality of the youth's learning experiences, depending upon age, educational level, and the service learner's own personal characteristics. Several results were consistent with findings from the resilience and positive development research literature (Finn & Rock, 1997; Jew et al., 1999; Letzring, Block, & Funder, 2005).

Inspection of the mean profile for resilient youth showed more positive outcomes on the CASQ scales in two aspects: interpersonal and problem-solving skills. Resilient youth used problem-focused coping strategies more than non-resilient youth. These findings reflect the argument in resilience literature that the capacity for problem-solving behaviour is a powerful means of adaptation (Block & Kremen, 1996; Chan, 2000; Jew et al., 1999; Letzring et al., 2005; Lim, 2002). Resilient youth in this study also seemed to possess higher self-esteem and self-efficacy than non-resilient youth. These characteristic differences mirror those of resilient individuals found in the resilience literature (Finn & Rock, 1997; Lim, 2002; Luthar, 1991). This could be explained by the fact that high self-esteem may offer significant benefits, since enhanced mood and greater capacity contribute to more positive engagement in adaptive learning and, subsequently, the development of resilience.

In terms of personality as measured by ego-resiliency and ego-undercontrol, findings show that, consistent with Block's own findings, resilient youth scored higher on ego-resiliency, (Block & Kremen, 1996; Letzring, Block, & Funder, 2005). ego-resiliency represents abstractions that are intended to encompass the observable phenomena of motivational control and resourceful adaptation. These qualities are relatively enduring, structural aspects of personality (Block & Kremen, 1996; Letzring et al., 2005). Ego-undercontrol, however, was negatively correlated with coping abilities, self-esteem, and efficacy and mastery of goal orientation.

While many of the resilience factor scores discriminated between resilient and non-resilient YEP participants, some of the resilience measures did not show any direct association with resilience in these youth. Specifically, there were no significant differences in social support and ego-undercontrol.

In sum, results of this study are in line with the view of McMillan and Reed (1994), who contend that resilient individuals possess personality traits such as self-efficacy, goal orientation, personal responsibility, optimism, internal expectations, and coping ability or adaptability. Results also suggest, however, that resilience is a capacity anyone can develop, reflecting Masten et al.'s (1990) apt definition of resilience as 'the process of, capacity for, or the outcome of successful adaptation despite challenging or threatening circumstances' (p. 425). Findings may suggest that, given an opportunity such as the YEP experience, one may be likely to develop or increase resilience.

### Limitations and Recommendations for Future Research

These results should be considered in light of the study's limitations. The sample was confined to 347 participants, although the initial sample in the pre-survey was 428 respondents. Although a response rate of 81.07% was still acceptable, a larger overall sample size would have been preferred. Furthermore, the study was limited by the relatively brief period during which data were collected. Further research is needed to understand the long-term effects of service learning as a context for developing resilience in youth. In addition, cross-cultural understanding of the nature of the process requires lengthier studies than this. Follow-up with these participants would enhance insight into the nature of the resilience process.

Further investigations using more varied measures to characterize constructs related to resilience could focus on specific aspects of positive development that contribute to attitude change and competence in youth. Moely et al. (2002) contend that specific youth characteristics – and how they interact with community service learning – are important to consider in future investigations of positive developmental outcomes in youth.

### Conclusion

This preliminary study seems to confirm that adaptive coping, together with positive affective personality traits and attitudes, are critical factors that contribute to positive development of youth attitudes and competence. Findings show that there are significant relationships between resilience measures, civic attitudes, and competence. This study also found that resilient youth use more problemfocused coping strategies and possess higher self-esteem and self-efficacy. Ego-resiliency mean scores are also higher for the resilient group than for non-resilient youth, and resilient youth scored significantly higher in political awareness, leadership skills, and interpersonal and problem-solving skills.

Furthermore, results from this study suggest that resilient participants who have higher levels of coping abilities, self-esteem, self-efficacy, and mastery goal orientations and who possess ego-resiliency personality characteristics are likely to experience higher levels of civic awareness and competency as a result of the overseas community service learning experience. On the other hand, non-resilient participants who are not able to cope with demanding or challenging situations, who have lower self-esteem, self-efficacy, and mastery goal orientations, and who possess ego-undercontrol personality characteristics may have lower competency outcomes and may be less likely to become involved in civic engagement.

Nevertheless, the findings demonstrate that overall, given an opportunity such as the overseas community service learning experience, participants may be able to develop a sense of civic responsibility, competence skills, and positive sense of self. Therefore, through meaningful participation in programs like YEP, youths may be given the opportunity to develop their capacities and strengths, specifically with regard to future civic participation and interpersonal, problemsolving, and leadership competencies, as well as to develop confidence and belief in future possibilities.

It is likely that youth development programs such as YEP foster resilience and promote asset building among youth. A synthesis of research identifies opportunities for meaningful participation, high expectations, and caring and support as critical factors in building resilience in youth (Luthar et al., 2000; Masten et al., 1999; Ungar, 2005). Resilience and positive youth development are not considered to be static personal qualities, but rather changing levels of readiness, disposition, or capacity. Organizations need to assess the level of support needed by youth and facilitate the provision of optimal conditions, with poised guidance, as some life challenges are necessary stepping stones for wellness and thriving (Lerner et al., 2005). Results from this study suggest that properly and responsibly designed overseas service learning provides youth with rich opportunities for positive development through hands-on experiences and immersion in a community different from their own.

## REFERENCES

Batchelder, T.H., & Root, S. (1994). Effects of an undergraduate program to integrate academic learning and service: Cognitive, prosocial cognitive, and identity outcomes. *Journal of Adolescence*, *17*(4), 341–55.

Block, J., & Kremen, A.M. (1996). IQ and ego-resiliency: Conceptual and empirical connections and separateness. *Journal of Personality and Social Psychology*, *70*(2), 349–61.

Bringle, R.G., & Duffy, D.K. (1998). *With service in mind: Concepts and models for service-learning in psychology*. Washington, DC: American Association for Higher Education.

Bronfenbrenner, U. (1979). *The ecology of human development: Experiments by nature and design*. Cambridge, MA: Harvard University Press.

Bronfenbrenner, U. (1993). *The ecology of cognitive development: Research models and fugitive findings*. Hillsdale, NJ: Lawrence Erlbaum.

Chan, D.W. (2000). Dimensionality of hardiness and its role in the stress-distress relationships among Chinese adolescents in Hong Kong. *Journal of Youth and Adolescence*, *29*(2), 147–61.

Chong, E. (2000). *The impact of teacher behaviour on the classroom engagement of normal stream students*. Unpublished master's thesis, Nanyang Technological University, Singapore.

Constantine, N.A., & Benard, B. (2001). California healthy kids survey resilience assessment module: Technical report. *Center for Research on Adolescent Health and Development*. Berkeley, CA: Public Health Institute. Available online at http://crahd.phi.org/projects/HKRAtech.PDF.

Egeland, B., Carlson, E., & Scroufe, L. (1993). Resilience as process. *American Journal of Orthopsychiatry*, *64*(4), 545–53.

Eyler, J., Root, S., & Giles, D.E. (1998). Service learning and the development of expert citizens: Service learning and cognitive science. In R.G. Bringle & D.K. Duffy (Eds.), *With service in mind: Concepts and models for service-learning in psychology* (pp. 85–100). Washington, DC: American Association for Higher Education.

Ferrari, J.R., & Chapman, J.G. (1999). *Educating students to make a difference: Community-based service learning*. New York: Haworth.

Finn, J.D., & Rock, D.A. (1997). Academic success among students at risk for school failure. *Journal of Applied Psychology*, *82*(2), 221–34.

Fredrickson, B.L. (2001). The role of positive emotions in positive psychology: The broaden-and-build theory of positive emotions. *American Psychologist*, *56*(3), 218–26.

Frydenberg, E., & Lewis, R. (1993). *Adolescent Coping Scale: Administrator's manual*. Victoria: Australian Council for Educational Research.

Garmezy, N. (1990). A closing note: Reflections on the future. In J. Rolf, A. Master, D. Cicchetti, K. Nuechterlein, & S. Weintraub (Eds.), *Risks and protective factors in the development of psychopathology* (pp. 527–534). New York: Cambridge University Press.

Garmezy, N., Masten, A.S., & Tellegen, A. (1984). Studies of stress resistant children: A building block for developmental psychopathology. *Child Development*, *55*(1), 97–111.

Giles, D. E., & Eyler, J. (1994). The impact of a college community service laboratory on students' personal, social, and cognitive outcome. *Journal of Adolescence*, *17*, 327–39.

Hauser, S.T. (1999). Understanding resilient outcomes: Adolescent lives across time and generations. *Journal of Research on Adolescence*, *9*(1), 1–24.

Hill, F., Grange, L., & Newmark, R. (2003). The use of qualitative and quantitative methodologies in a special educational needs study. *International Journal of Special Education*, *18*(2), 62–72.

Holahan, C.J., Holahan, C.K., Moos, R.H., & Cronkite, R.C. (1999). Resource loss, resource gain, and depressive symptoms: 10-year model. *Journal of Personality and Social Psychology*, *77*(3), 620–9.

Huan, S.L. (1998). *The relationship between different parenting techniques and the social adjustment of adolescents*. Unpublished master's thesis, National University of Singapore, Singapore.

Ikeda, E.K. (1999). *How does service enhance learning? Toward an understanding of the process*. Doctoral diss., University of California, Los Angeles.

Jacoby, B. (1996). Service-learning in today's higher education. In B. Jacoby (Ed.), *Service-learning in higher education: Concepts and practices* (pp. 3–25). San Francisco: Jossey-Bass.

Jew, C.L., Green, K.E., & Kroger, J. (1999). Development and validation of a measure of resiliency. *Measurement and Evaluation in Counseling and Development*, *32*(2), 75–89.

Khoo, H.N. (2002). *Coping behaviour of secondary school students in Singapore*. Unpublished doctoral dissertation, Nanyang Technological University, Singapore.

Kobasa, S.C. (1979). Stressful life events, personality, and health: An enquiry into hardiness. *Journal of Personality and Social Psychology*, *37*(1), 1–11.

Larson, R.W. (2000). Toward a psychology of positive youth development. *American Psychologist, 55*(1), 170–83.

Lerner, R.M. (2003). Developmental assets and asset-building communities: A view of the issues. In R.M. Lerner & P.L. Benson (Eds.), *Developmental assets and asset-building communities* (pp. 3–18). New York: Kluwer Academic.

Lerner, R.M., Almerigi, J.B., Theokas, C., & Lerner, J.V. (2005). Positive youth development: A view of issues. *Journal of Early Adolescence, 25*(1), 10–16.

Letzring, T.D., Block, J., & Funder, D.C. (2005). Ego-control and ego-resiliency: Generalization of self-report scales based on personality descriptions from acquaintances, clinicians, and the self. *Journal of Research in Personality, 39*(4), 395–422.

Lim, T. M. (2002). *Coping with school: Personality of at-risk students.* Unpublished Master Degree Dissertation, Nanyang Technological University, Singapore.

Lund, R.M. (1998). *Service learning educational experiences: How they influence academic achievement and attitude about motivation for schooling, academic self-concept-performance based, academic self-concept-referenced based, students' sense of control over performance, and students' instructional mastery of schoolwork among Avon Lake City School Student.* Doctoral Dissertation, Cleveland State University, Cleveland, OH.

Luthar, S.L. (1991). Vulnerability and resilience: A study of high-risk adolescents. *Child Development, 62*(3), 600–16.

Luthar, S. L., & Cichetti, D. (2000). The construct of resilience: Implications for interventions and social policies. *Development and Psychopathology, 12*(4), 857–85.

Luthar, S.L., Cichetti, D., & Becker, B. (2000). The construct of resilience: A critical evaluation and guidelines for future work. *Child Development, 71*(3), 543–62.

Maluccio, A.N. (2002). Resilience: A many splendoured construct? *American Journal of Orthopsychiatry, 72*(4), 425–44.

Markus, G.B., Howard, J.P.F., & King, D.C. (1993). Integrating community service and classroom instruction enhances learning: Results from an experiment. *Educational Evaluation and Policy Analysis, 15*(4), 410–19.

Marzano, R.J. (1998). *A theory-based meta-analysis of research on instruction.* Aurora, CO: Midcontinent Research for Education and Learning.

Masten, A.S. (2001). Ordinary magic: Resilience processes in development. *American Psychologist, 56*(3), 227–38.

Masten, A.S., Best, K.M., & Garmezy, N. (1990). Resilience and development: Contributions from the study of children who overcome adversity. *Development and Psychopathology, 2*(3), 425–44.

Masten, A.S., & Coatsworth, J.D. (1998). The development of competence in favorable and unfavourable environments: Lessons from research on successful children. *American Psychologist, 53*(2), 205–20.

Masten, A.S., Hubbard, J.J., Gest, A.T., Garmezy, N., & Ramirez, M. (1999). Competence in the context of adversity: Pathways to resilience and maladaptation from childhood to late adolescence. *Development and Psychopathology, 11*(1), 143–69.

Masten, A.S., & Powell, J.L. (2003). A resilience framework for research, policy, and practice. In S.S. Luthar (Ed.), *Resilience and vulnerability: Adaptation in the context of childhood adversities* (pp. 1–25). Cambridge: Cambridge University Press.

Mau, R., & Seng, S.H. (1997, 22–25 September). Developing resiliency in children and adolescents. Paper presented at proceedings of the 9th Asian Workshop on Child and Adolescent Development. Universiti Brunei Darussalam, Gadong.

McMillan, J.H., & Reed, D.F. (1994). At-risk students and resiliency: Factors contributing to academic success. *Clearing House, 67*(3), 137–40.

Midgley, C., Maehr, M.L., Hruda, L.Z., Anderman, E., Anderman, L., Freeman, K.E., et al. (2000). *Manual for the patterns of adaptive learning scales.* Ann Arbor, MI: University of Michigan.

Ministry of Education, Singapore (2004). Desired outcomes of education. Available online at http://www.moe.gov.sg/corporate/desired_outcomes.htm.

Moely, B.E., Mercer, S.H., Ilustre, V., Miron, D., & McFarland, M. (2002). Psychometric properties and correlates of the civic attitudes and skills questionnaire (CASQ): A measure of students' attitudes related to service-learning. *Michigan Journal of Community Service Learning, 9,* 1–11.

Mullins, M.M. (2003). *The impact of service learning on perceptions of self-efficacy.* Doctoral dissertation, University of Dayton, Dayton, OH.

Reeb, R.N., Sammon, J.A., & Isackson, N.L. (1999). Clinical application of the service-learning model in psychology: Evidence of educational and clinical benefits. In J.R. Ferrari & J.G. Chapman (Eds.), *Educating students to make a difference: Community-based service learning* (pp. 65–82). New York: Haworth.

Roeser, R.W., Midgley, C., & Urdan, T.C. (1996). Perceptions of the school psychological environment and early adolescents' psychological and behavioral functioning in school: The mediating role of goals and belonging. *Journal of Educational Psychology, 88*(3), 408–22.

Rosenberg, M. (1965). *Society and the adolescent self-image.* Princeton, NJ: Princeton University Press.

Roth, J.L., & Brooks-Gunn, J. (2003). What exactly is a youth development program? Answers from research and practice. *Applied Developmental Science, 7*(2), 94–111.

Rutter, M. (1985). Resilience in the face of adversity: Protective factors and resistance to psychiatric disorder. *British Journal of Psychiatry, 147*(3), 598–611.

Rutter, M. (1987). Psychosocial resilience and protective mechanisms. *American Journal of Orthopsychiatry, 57*(3), 316–31.

Seligman, M. (2002). *Authentic happiness.* New York: Free Press.

Singapore International Foundation. (2002). *SIF/Youth Expedition Project* (YEP). Available online at http://www.sif.org.sg.

Ungar, M. (2005). *Handbook for working with children and youth: Pathway to resilience across cultures and contexts.* Thousand Oaks, CA: Sage.

Ungar, M., & Liebenberg, L. (2005). The International Resilience Project: A mixed-methods approach to the study of resilience across culture. In M. Ungar (Ed.), *Handbook for working with children and youth: Pathway to resilience across cultures and contexts* (pp. 211–26). Thousand Oaks, CA: Sage.

Walsh, F. (2003). Family resilience: A framework for clinical practice. *Family Process, 42*(1), 1–18.

Wang, M.C., & Gordon, E.W. (1994). *Educational resilience in inner-city America: Challenges and prospects.* Hillsdale, NJ: Lawrence Erlbaum.

Werner, E., & Smith, R. (1982). *Vulnerable but invincible: A study of resilient children.* New York: McGraw-Hill.

Werner, E., & Smith, R. (1992). *Overcoming the odds: High risk children from birth to adulthood.* London: Cornell University Press.

WestEd. (2002). *California healthy kids survey. Resilience & Youth Development Module.* Spring 2002 report, California USD. Available online at http://www.wested.org/hks.

Wyman, P.A., Cowen, E., Work, W.C., & Kerley, J.H. (1993). The role of children's future expectations in self-system functioning and adjustment to life stresses: A prospective study of urban at-risk children. *Development and Psychopathology, 59*(4), 649–61.

# 11 Australian Approaches to Understanding and Building Resilience in At-Risk Populations

LISBETH T. PIKE, LYNNE COHEN, AND JULIE ANN POOLEY

There is little doubt that the earlier an intervention occurs in the life of the child, the more successful it is likely to be. One of the most effective ways of increasing resilience in all children is to implement intervention programs within the school context. However, many educational authorities have yet to recognize that early intervention is preferable to remedial programs, and ultimately beneficial to both the individual and the wider community.

Schools play an important role in the development of a child's competence, self-efficacy, self-determination, cognitive development, and behaviour patterns. Schools do, however, have a difficult task in addressing the diversity of needs associated with their students. When the programs that are implemented are targeted at all students, these interventions become all-encompassing, connecting students with each other as well as the broader school community. Therefore, embedding programs within a school setting fosters the intellectual, academic, and behavioural development of children not only at the individual level but also at the wider, collective level. In this way all students are provided with the opportunity of participating in and being exposed to a range of programs. Students are able to utilize the positive elements of the environment and incorporate these into their daily lives and processes, which ultimately increases their capacity to integrate successfully into the wider community (Pooley, Pike, Drew, & Breen, 2002). In this milieu, students are encouraged to develop a sense of belonging, linkages, and bonding with others within the educational setting. Schools may therefore be regarded as an important change agent in the lives of children (Pooley, Breen, Pike, Drew, & Cohen, in press).

This chapter describes the Western Australian implementation of TALK, an intervention program aimed at increasing resilience within a school community. The chapter begins by providing the reader with some context in terms of current Australian government policies at both the national and state level that are targeted at promoting resilience in children. This is followed by a description of the TALK program, its aims, implementation, outcomes, and evaluation findings. The chapter concludes with a discussion of implications for mental health professionals working in an educational context.

## Context

Western Australia is one of six states and two territories in Australia. It is the largest state geographically, covering a vast area, with a population of almost two million people. Most of the population (1.5 million) are concentrated on the coastal fringe areas within two hundred kilometres of the state capital, Perth. The state is resource rich with a long history of mining (especially for gold and iron ore) and has a large primary production sector. It is not surprising, therefore, to find that it has a very mobile population. As a result, families are often isolated from extended family members in the eastern states or indeed from each other. Typically, mothers and children reside in the southwest coastal areas while fathers or partners work away from home in interior or the northern areas of the state. It is suspected that these work patterns contribute to Western Australia's having the highest per capita divorce rate in the country (Australian Bureau of Statistics, 2003).

### Current Government Policies Impacting on Resilience

Australian and international evidence confirms that the early years of a child's life are critical to his or her future development (Wyman, Cross, & Barry, 2004). It is at this time that a child's brain is rapidly developing and the foundations for learning, behaviour, and health over the life course are set. The path to poor outcomes often begins in early childhood with a range of associated risk factors, including poor attachment, inadequate social skills, parenting styles, family factors, school difficulties, welfare dependency, and poor physical and mental health (Nelson & Prilleltensky, 2005). Community factors include those such as socio-economic disadvantage and lack of support services (Nelson & Prilleltensky, 2005).

These risk factors, however, can be offset by protective factors such as quality prenatal care, maternal health and nutrition, parental communication, positive attention from both parents, family harmony, and participation in broader social networks (Olds et al., 1998). In line with such findings, the Australian government at both the federal and state levels has funded and implemented a series of initiatives designed to promote the health and well-being of its citizens.

*Federal Level*

The Stronger Families and Communities Strategy is an Australian government initiative providing families, their children, and communities with the opportunity to build a better future. The program was first announced in April 2000 with funding of AUD$490 million committed for the period 2004–2009, and is aimed at empowering communities to develop local solutions to local problems. Funds are intended to set the stage for positive development of children in the earliest stages of life and in their multiple roles as youth, students, workers, and future parents. The government has prioritized early childhood initiatives and undertaken an extensive consultation process to develop a national agenda for early childhood intervention. Among these is Communities for Children *(C4C)*, a program that focuses on well-targeted early intervention approaches that bring about positive outcomes for young children and their families, providing a good grounding for future development. These interventions include a *community parks project*, aimed at promoting richer social networks among families with young children with an emphasis on breaking down cultural barriers. Regular activities are held in community parks especially for children under the age of five, to provide them with a broader range of social and developmental experiences. Another program establishes *play groups* in partnership with local schools. The play groups provide a learning environment and promote healthy play for children and their caregivers. Play group staff also work with families to identify and address the developmental needs of children.

A second federal strategy, the National Investment for the Early Years (NIFTeY), is the result of a meeting of academics, practitioners, and government officials in 1999. Their main focus has been the development, implementation, and evaluation of strategies in the first three years of childhood to advance the health, development, and well-being of all children in Australia. NIFTeY is a national initiative that operates in all states and territories through the establishment of local boards. Its overall goal is to increase knowledge in the community and provide support for parents and their young children.

Reconnect is a Commonwealth-funded service that provides a range of community-based early intervention programs aimed at family reconciliation and support for young people aged twelve to eighteen years who are homeless or at risk of becoming homeless. The aim of the program is to engage the young people with family, work, education, training, and the community.

With the growing global incidence of mental illness, particularly depression, there is also awareness at the federal level of the need for the provision of initiatives, such as MindMatters, to address mental health. MindMatters targets students at secondary schools, acting as a support resource, promoting positive mental health, and preventing suicide by means of a holistic approach (Mullett, Evans, & Weist, 2004). The major goals of the program are to improve the social and emotional health and well-being of young people through producing a resource kit that is distributed to all secondary schools. Examples of the booklets available include *A Guide for School-Based Responses to Preventing Self-Harm and Suicide*, and *Enhancing Resilience through Communication, Changes and Challenges*, and *Stress and Coping*. Each book contains activities and worksheets that teachers may use when addressing these topics.

Similarly, the Australian Network for Promotion, Prevention, and Early Intervention for Mental Health (Auseinetter), funded under the national mental health strategy by the Commonwealth Department of Health and Aging, is a print and electronic (www.auseinet.com) informational resource for professionals working in the mental health area.

*State Level*

Programs and innovative strategies are not only the domain of the federal government. The state government of Western Australia plays a significant role in offering wide-ranging programs, particularly in collaboration or partnership with different organizations. In this regard, the state government has consulted widely with communities and NIFTeY to develop a vision for children. This shared vision suggests that all children:

• be nurtured and treated according to their best interests, with access to quality education, health care, welfare, housing, and social justice;

- be valued, respected, and appreciated for their diversity, including that of location, culture, abilities, and aspirations;
- be free from the detrimental effects of abuse, trauma, and stress;
- live satisfying, enjoyable, fulfilling, and creative lives, with opportunities to achieve in the fields of their choosing; and
- be consulted and participate in decision making on important issues that affect them, from the time they demonstrate the ability to understand.

(*NIFTeY Vision for Children in Western Australia*, 2003).

With this vision guiding project development, a number of initiatives have been developed. For example, the Making the Difference Health and Wellbeing Program and the Robust Sense of Self Worth Program are provided by the West Australia Department of Education and Training (DETWA). Each project is designed to promote the development of resilience in young people from kindergarten to year 12, the final year of formal schooling. This is done by recognizing 'the ability of an individual to successfully recover from or adapt to adversity and to develop social and emotional competence despite exposure to life's problems' as a prerequisite to successful academic achievement (*NIFTeY Vision* 2003). To this end DETWA has implemented policy at state and district levels that recognizes the importance of fostering resilience through adopting preventive strategies and embedding a holistic strategy to the development of positive health and well-being outcomes for students within the curriculum framework. DETWA has also been proactive in developing a series of videos and CD-ROMs on resilience, including *Deal With It*. This multimedia package aims to increase coping skills of teenagers especially with regard to issues related to stress and mental health.

The Ministerial Council for Suicide Prevention has also been established at the state level and is responsible for developing and coordinating suicide prevention initiatives across Western Australia. Whilst the council's aim is to reduce the incidence of suicide and the prevalence of self-harming behaviours amongst people of all ages in Western Australia, it maintains a focus on youth (Ministerial Council for Suicide Prevention, 2004). Two of the council's main objectives are to (1) reduce the impact of suicide and suicidal behaviours on individuals, families, and communities and (2) enhance the capacity of individuals, families, and communities to reduce the prevalence of risk factors for suicide.

Finally, in accordance with evidence of the importance of early intervention, the Early Years Strategy is part of the state government's Children First agenda, which aims to engage communities to work collaboratively with government and non-government agencies to assist in the positive development of young children. The program is inclusive of all young children, particularly indigenous children and others from culturally diverse backgrounds. New services build on the strengths and resources of children, parents, families, and communities through the use of evidence-based practices and ongoing evaluation to ensure that effective strategies are implemented.

Given this wide-ranging set of policies and initiatives at both the federal and state levels, it is clear that Australia is taking a systemic approach to enhancing resilience by building social and community capacity with a focus on health and well-being, and by recognizing the role of early intervention and prevention initiatives. It is against this background that we worked in collaboration with local education district officers to implement the TALK program for at-risk children in one particular school district where children's behavioural and social problems were deemed by school personnel to be most acute. This program, an exemplar of early intervention to promote resilience, is the focus of the remainder of this chapter.

**The TALK Program**

The TALK program is a language enrichment and social skills enhancement program that originated in the United States. The program was based on the Rap Groups model that began in Oakland, California (Cherry Goodier, personal communication, 7 June 2000). The original goals of this program included:

- creating a safe environment for the children where they will have the opportunity to express their ideas without fear of prejudice;
- allowing children to experience a sympathetic adult who will listen to their ideas and value their opinions;
- improvement of communication skills of students;
- improvement of oral communication that focuses on a student's ability to communicate fluently and accurately by listening, speaking, and engaging in familiar topics such as hobbies, the environment, entertainment, sport, and friendships;
- provision of the opportunity for modelling appropriate communi-

cation patterns between adults and children and among the children themselves;
- the capacity to enhance the self-esteem, coping strategies, and problem-solving skills of children by creating a climate of trust and caring between young people and adults;
- provision of opportunities to increase the sense of belonging of children by involving their school and community in their lives, and where students can facilitate the development of new friendships; and
- inclusion of the program within a whole-school approach to develop a caring school community.

## Western Australian Implementation

The TALK program was an initiative between a local Education District Office and a university located in the same district. Organization and implementation of the program were undertaken by the authors (academic psychologists) in conjunction with graduate psychology students who also served as group leaders.

The program was implemented in a primary school of a recently established suburb of the north metropolitan area of Perth. The community is a low socio-economic status area characterized by many single-parent and blended families, low levels of disposable income, high levels of unemployment, low levels of completion of high school, and lack of community resources such as public transport (Australian Bureau of Statistics, 2003; Hart, Brinkman, & Blackmore, 2003). Primary school–aged children in this community have been identified as being at risk in aspects of their development as a result of impoverished home backgrounds or lack of parental involvement. Earlier administration of the Early Development Index (Hart et al., 2003), for example, identified this locality as having a significant number of children whose psychosocial development is at risk. The EDI is a teacher-completed checklist that measures five developmental domains: social competence, emotional maturity, language and cognitive skills, physical health and well-being, and communication skills and general knowledge. As the instrument's authors note, 'The EDI reflects the influence of experiences of the first five years of life. The results of the behavioural checklist are combined to develop an index for a suburb' (Hart et al., 2003, p. 6). Based on these findings, the local Education District Office, Edith Cowan University, and the principal of a local primary school decided to implement the TALK program in this community in the hope of improving children's functioning. Specifically, TALK was implemented in order to address problems of poor verbal interaction skills and a lack of emotional expression skills.

Principles underpinning the program implementation were that (1) young children need exposure to good models of adult conversation and verbal skills if they are to engage with fellow students and school staff in a constructive way; (2) children who are ill-equipped to express themselves through verbal interactions may resort to physical violence, disruptive behaviours, or delinquent acts that are not conducive to the development of a sense of belonging to the school; and (3) fostering a sense of belonging to promote a sense of community within the school will enhance the well-being of both the children and their teachers.

Prior to initiation of the TALK program, senior primary school personnel expressed increasing concern regarding the growing number of children engaged in antisocial behaviours and vandalism in and out of the classroom. Many of the children had been identified as at risk by virtue of the school's designation as a *priority school*, a term used to indicate schools operating in educational districts characterized as poor or disadvantaged. The primary school staff believed that later behavioural problems were related to the need for remediation in the oral language skills of the children across the whole school population. Teachers also believed that many of the inappropriate externalizing and acting out behaviours demonstrated by children in the classrooms and school yard were attributable to the inability of these children to verbally express themselves adequately.

## Risk and Resilience

The goals of TALK fit well within a resilience paradigm. There are many definitions of resilience in the literature that examine the contributions of diverse and complex factors to positive outcomes for children and young people growing up under the kinds of adversity confronting children in this Perth suburb. Ungar (2005), for example, explains that resilience 'generally refers to an individual's ability to bounce back from adverse experiences, to avoid long-term negative effects or otherwise to overcome developmental threats' (p. xi). Resilience is also often referred to as invulnerability and stress resistance (Garmezy, 1985) and may be conceived as those qualities possessed by children that result in positive outcomes despite adversity (Kaplan, 1999). The achievement of positive outcomes in the face of adversity is ameliorated by protective factors. Kumpfer and Hopkins (1993) suggest that resilience comprises seven personal factors: optimism, empathy, insight, intellectual competence, self-esteem, direction or mission, and determination and perseverance. For our purposes here, we have conceptualized resilience as comprising several components including a sense of belonging (SoB), self-esteem, social and emotional development, and coping with factors related to depression. Implementation of the TALK program was hypothesized to effect SoB most, with additional influence expected for these other factors.

## Sense of Belonging

Derived from Maslow's (1968) hierarchy of needs, SoB is a construct identified as a psychological need present in most individuals. The construct has been developed and refined in terms of its application and measurement, especially in the educational domain (Goodenow, 1993). Comparisons have been drawn between SoB and related concepts of sense of community and social capital (Pooley, Cohen, & Pike, 2005) and attachment (Hagerty, 2002; Ron, 2004) in areas such as education and health.

In the educational context SoB has been defined as 'the extent to which students feel personally accepted, respected, included, and supported in the school social environment' (Goodenow, 1993, p. 35). An ongoing program of research into SoB in children and adolescents has demonstrated the importance of conceptualizing the construct developmentally, linking it with the emergence of the concept of 'community self' in both educational and community contexts (see Pooley, Breen, et al., in press; Pooley, Pike, et al., 2002; Rowland, Cohen, Pooley, Pike, & Breen, 2005; Stumpers, Breen, Pooley, Cohen, & Pike, 2005).

Previous research has also identified the importance of SoB as a key ingredient for measuring children's educational resilience (Wang, Haertel, & Walberg, 1997). SoB is necessary for students for a number of reasons. First, children's feelings of belonging within their schools, families, and communities, are correlated with good mental health outcomes (Routt, 1996). Second, students spend a substantial portion of their time at school and participate in school-related activities, making their school experience highly influential in their lives (Battistich, Solomon, Watson, & Schaps, 1997; Edwards, 1995). Third, peer relationships become more important with age (Cauce, 1986), with intimacy between peers increasing markedly from middle childhood to adolescence (Berndt, 1982). Finally, common school stressors, such as personal safety (Weldy, 1995), can be minimized by a caring and responsive school environment to which a child feels attached (Schumaker, 1998).

Studies have shown that a sense of belonging in educational settings is associated with numerous positive effects. These include a positive orientation towards school and learning, liking school, respect for teachers, educational aspirations, self-esteem, a cooperative learning style, an ability to make friends, higher attendance and retention rates, greater classroom and extracurricular participation, and academic success (Battistich et al., 1997; Edwards, 1995; Royal & Rossi, 1997; Schmuck & Schmuck, 1992; Zeichner, 1980). A sense of belonging, then, is a key aspect of academic motivation (Weiner, 1990). Thus, we may conclude that a child's experience of membership is an integral aspect of a classroom and school, as learning occurs in a social context (Schmuck & Schmuck, 1992). Research such that of Beck and Malley (1998) supports this notion, finding that most children who fail at school do so because they feel isolated.

However, schools alone may not be to blame. Traditional forms of belonging have diminished as a result of family breakdown, increases in parental working hours, increasing rates of single parenthood (with the result being greater stress on the parent), and an increasingly mobile society (Beck & Malley, 1998). Feelings of not belonging in school may be linked to overall experiences of alienation both at home and within the child's school community, leading to decreased functioning and threats to the child's well-being (Edwards, 1995).

An examination of SoB provides insight into the mechanisms by which aspects of risk and resilience act as inhibiting and enabling factors in children's development. We have used SoB as suggested by Albert (1991) to provide a link between the educational literature and the risk and resilience literature. SoB can also be conceptualized as the link between the individual and the collective, as well as an indicator of a child's well-being in the academic setting. Promoting SoB is, therefore, one of the most important goals of the TALK project.

## Implementation

TALK aimed first to build a relationship between primary school students and adult facilitators. The program created an environment in which students felt secure and confident about sharing their feelings and concerns. It then aimed to enhance verbal interaction skills and emotional expression. It was anticipated that developing a 'sense of belonging' to the school community through TALK would reduce students' inappropriate externalizing and acting out behaviours within the school environment. The program was initiated with the consent of parents; however, there was no parental involvement in the implementation of the program.

As in the original U.S. model, primary school students were offered the opportunity to meet in small groups with an adult leader to talk about any topic of interest to their specific age group. The groups ran for eight weeks and involved twenty-five graduate psychology students (five males and twenty females) who met on a weekly basis for a period of thirty minutes. There were 145 primary school students involved in these small group discussions: sixty-seven students were in year two (average age eight) and seventy-eight students from year seven (average age twelve).

Prior to implementation of the program, all graduate psychology student group leaders underwent comprehensive training over a period of six hours. As all these students had already completed an undergraduate psychology degree, training content focused on an orientation to working with primary school–aged groups. Topics such as the leader's responsibility, developing and enhancing observation and listening skills, methods of opening group discussion, problems and opportunities that may arise with the target population, and how to end a group were all addressed. Group leaders were also informed that children might reveal information that would need to be referred to the school psychologist for further discussion.

The program was co-facilitated by the children's classroom teachers, who were available to assist with any group management issues as well as generally to support the university students if required. The format of the weekly group meetings was informal so that the primary school students regarded the group as fun and a special time to share with their peers. Although the group was never intended to be therapeutic, it soon became a place where troubled children experienced a safe listening environment.

*How TALK Has Evolved*

TALK has now been embedded in the school program for six years. We have followed the same group of students from age seven (primary year two) through to age twelve (primary year seven) when they are in their final year of primary school. The program started with seventy-four participants. This school has a high transient population, and thirty-five students have been with the program since its inception. We have gained insights into the most effective ways to implement the program in terms of organization, training of group leaders, and the usefulness of different research measures.

Successful implementation requires a high level of organization, necessitating a program manager. This development provides opportunities for postgraduate community psychology students through the articulation of practicum placements. Issues of organization have also extended to the composition of the group. Initially, group structure and size were determined randomly by the primary school. Currently, group size is kept to a maximum of five primary school students, with careful attention paid to the composition of each group in terms of gender and other characteristics. This decision has been taken based on our experience and knowledge of the school and children and in consultation with the teachers at the primary school. Our experience indicates that both mixed and gender-specific groups are equally effective. However, there needs to be careful consideration of individual behavioural characteristics.

Although teachers have always been supportive and involved with TALK, we have had to carefully define their role within the program. Teachers have a duty of care towards their students and are legally required to be present at all times. Simultaneously, however, they need to be cognizant of being minimally intrusive, particularly during group activities.

Initially, we began by being very prescriptive about group activities. In pursuit of standardization of program delivery we required each group leader to implement the same activity. Experience has now shown that activities need to be flexibly tailored to the appropriate age and interests of the children. To this end we have now developed a training program and accompanying manual that is continually updated. This manual is for use by the university students and program manager. It is structured to contain basic information about the program as well as provide the opportunity for the university students to document and outline their proposed program on a weekly basis. In this way, the manual is flexible in that it allows for personal input each week. None of the activities are prescribed, and university students are free to design their own. We also modify and alter the types of measures required in order to capture data gauging the efficacy of the program. We have learnt over the duration of the program that certain aspects of the children, such as resilience, were not being captured by the original measurements. In a longitudinal research project, the alteration of measures complicates the comparison of results across time periods. This has been an issue in that some of the results are not comparable each year. However, some of the instruments have remained constant throughout the research (the measurement of sense of belonging and depression, for example), and this has allowed us to compare these results each year. Over the course of six years we have gathered a significant amount of empirical data as to the efficacy of TALK.

### TALK Outcomes and Evaluation

We have evaluated the program every year since its implementation. Evaluation has employed both quantitative and qualitative methods. Quantitative evaluation has used pre- and post-program administration of measures. These include Harter's Self Perception Profile (SPPC) (Harter, 1985) and Goodenow's Psychological Sense of School Membership Scale (PSSM) (Goodenow, 1993). In an effort to more effectively measure the impact of the program, we have refined our evaluations to also include measures of depression using the Child Depression Inventory (CDI) (Kovacs, 1992) and resilience using the Resilience Scale for Adolescents (READ) (O. Hjemdal, personal communication, 25 February 2005). In addition, qualitative data have been collected annually. Due to the challenges encountered by changing measurements each year, and the transient nature of the cohort, it has been difficult to consistently analyse the data with accuracy. The main forms of analysis have been utilizing *t-tests* and correlations and analysing the qualitative information.

*Outcomes*

Our results have been mixed with measures demonstrating significant changes in performance by students over the years since TALK's inception. For example, the use of Goodenow's Psychological Sense of

School Membership Scale over a five-year period has shown a statistically significant increase in scores: from a mean score of 31.5 (SD = 2.91) in 2001 to 65.8 (SD = 13.92) in 2005 (p < .001), with a maximum possible score of 90 (p < .001). Scores on the CDI, by contrast, were not significant, indicating no change in children's level of depression during this time.

Conversely, some measures have not been used consistently during the past six years. The resilience measure (READ), for example, was not introduced until 2005 due to unavailability of an appropriate measure. Therefore, no comparisons can be made at this stage. An initial analysis indicates that the READ correlates significantly with the PSSM (r = .072, p < .01). This relationship does, however, require further investigation. Nonetheless, we have noted that school membership (as measured here by the PSSM) has been associated with increased performance and self-esteem and decreased depression. We speculate that given these trends, resilience will be positively correlated with school membership. SPPC (Harter's Self Perception Profile) scores have not shown significant differences.

As the program operates only during the school term (eight weeks), it is unlikely that we would see any significant changes in competence during its operation. This is not an intensive intervention in which one would expect to see an effect immediately and on follow-up. We are cognizant that the measure of self-esteem we have used is not ideal. However, ease of administration and availability of the instrument make it a viable option to consider, as well as its being the most widely used measure of self-esteem in the literature.

This increase in the children's PSSM scores presents us with a conundrum. We would expect an increase in sense of belonging over time: the longer children attend the school, the greater their attachment. However, out of all of the children participating in the program only thirty-five children (less than 50%) have been in the TALK program since its inception. This would suggest that the effect of an increase in PSSM scores is a combination of the context of the school and of the TALK program. The school would seem to be operating at a level where the children feel safe, and where their needs are to some extent being met.

*Qualitative Findings*

Qualitative data were collected from three separate participant groups: children, teachers, and graduate psychology student group leaders.

Data from all three sources are consistently positive and supportive of the program. The comments provided by the children can be grouped into various themes, including:

- *Sense of belonging*
  'I like coming to school ... because that's where my friends are.'
  'The school is terrific ... we have fun here and the teachers are really nice.'
  'The new principal is a great guy, he knows all of us.'

- *Self-esteem*
  'If I do good work, [the teacher] always tells me how hard I'm trying.'
  'I like being in the small groups because we all get a chance to talk.'

- *Connection with group leaders*
  'I am happier talking with the group leader than the teacher.'
  'My leader never favours any of us, she treats us all the same.'
  'I wish my dad was more like [the group leader].'

- *Empowerment*
  'I always look forward to Thursdays when we have our small groups.'
  'I like the way we each take turns ... it makes me feel important.'

Comments by the teachers were equally supportive of the program and its outcomes. They viewed TALK as having had a positive impact on the children's behaviour in the classroom and on the school playground:

- *Sense of belonging*
  'The program has helped to create a sense of attachment to the school.'
  'The students view the school from a different perspective.'
  'They look forward to the program each week and it has become part of the curriculum ... they [students] get very upset if the groups are cancelled.'

- *Self-esteem*
  'The students feel important and have developed a confidence which I haven't seen before.'
  'The groups have helped [the students] to respect each other and value the opinions of others.'

- *Connection with group leaders*
  'It has been valuable for the students to have someone not connected to the school with whom they could talk.'
  'I see that the group leaders have become role models for the children ... they are always saying, for example, that they were told not to interrupt when someone is talking.'

- *Empowerment*
  'The program has built language skills and communication skills for many of the children.'
  'The children have learnt to take responsibility for many things since the TALK program started.'

Finally, the group leaders consistently comment on how much they have enjoyed the practical experience applying theoretical constructs to work with at-risk children:

- *Sense of belonging*
  'The kids learn to love what they are doing and that this opportunity has been provided by the school.'
  'Sometimes it was not so easy to get the kids to be part of the group ... the school definitely helps in fostering a sense of connectedness with the kids.'

- *Self-esteem*
  'The TALK program provides an opportunity for the students to learn and grow.' 'From the first time we met the children, till now, they have developed such confidence in the group ... it was just marvellous to watch.'

- *Connection with group leaders*
  'The best for me was when one student came up to me and said, "Thank you for making this such fun and for being here," for me that has made it all worthwhile.'

- *Empowerment*
  'The children learn how to participate in a group discussion.'
  'There is so much of value in this program, that it really can't be measured by a bunch of questionnaires. The students learn social skills in a safe, secure environment; they have the opportunity to practice social skills and talking without fear of being ridiculed or shouted at; they learn how to listen to the opinions of others ... where else do you have such a marvellous opportunity?'

- *Personal reflection*
  'I love getting my hands "dirty," it's a great professional experience.'
  'I think the school needs more of the program. It provides a different perspective for the teachers and assists them to manage some of the problems in their classrooms. '
  'My one disappointment is that the program is so short. We need to find a way to run it all year.'
  'We need to add another dimension to the program that involves teaching the parents communication skills, and how best to interact [with] or talk to their children.'

## Summary

As demonstrated above, TALK shows promise of being a low-cost effective school-based intervention for at-risk children. It provides children with an opportunity to develop some important communication skills that may be generalized to other aspects of their behaviour. The program has provided an opportunity for teachers to rethink their role and relationship with their students while providing graduate psychology students with some valuable training opportunities.

There are, however, important considerations for those that work in the area of mental health in an educational context with regard to the implementation of programs designed to address issues of risk and resilience. The implementation of TALK was initially meant to assist the school with students who were at risk. It was a reactive intervention. Over the years, however, the program has become embedded in the primary school curriculum. It is now seen as a prevention program that attempts to enhance positive outcomes such as SoB that are associated with resilience. While the ultimate aim is to operate from a preventive framework, sometimes it is important to start with a reactive intervention, as many programs begin with an intervention capacity.

While results to date have been far from conclusive, accounts by participants (children, teachers, and graduate students) captured through our qualitative data seem to support continuation of the program. However, more rigorous and comprehensive research will be needed to understand the positive reactions to the program that have yet to be demonstrated conclusively through quantitative data using standardized instruments. This highlights another of the key considerations: the appropriate selection of psychometric measures at the initial implementation of the program. For us, it has become apparent that there needs to be a capacity to evaluate and revise the utility of measures for assessing behavioural change as the program develops and evolves. This suggests that intervention projects need to be more action research based, as action research more readily supports the approach required for implementing and evaluating this type of intervention in a real-life setting. This clearly has implications for aspects of program design and measurement of outcomes. This in turn has implications for attracting funding, as many funding bodies require evidence-based outcomes that don't often include the capacity for action research. Mental health professionals working in this type of setting need to be aware of the challenges in terms of balancing these competing needs for flexibility in program implementation and evaluation and production of rigorous evidence-based outcomes.

We can only speculate that the intrinsic qualities of the TALK program create conditions that facilitate children in joining with adults and finding a sense of attachment to school. As McMillan and Chavis (1986) assert, 'a healthy community system is one that can resist social, psychological, and physiological problems, in addition to enabling individuals and their collectivity to grow to their maximum potential' (p. 338). The TALK program may benefit children by creating such a system of interaction between children and adults at school and beyond. We believe our findings, though tentative, point to support for the importance of community as a protective factor (Puddifoot, 1996). An intervention such as the TALK program provides children with the opportunity to participate in small groups and to feel empowered while they develop a connection and attachment to their group and the school. Our next step needs to account for behavioural as well as psychological outcomes. Anecdotally, teachers report evidence of a decline in behavioural problems and difficulties that would be expected given related research (Ma, 2003).

TALK and other initiatives by both state and federal governments have the potential to create caring communities that foster a sense of belonging for children (Schaps & Solomon, 1997; Wehlage, 1989). This initiative suggests that to maximize the benefits of community interventions, programs based at the school level should involve informal support for children that can compensate for difficult family and personal situations (see also Luthar & Zelazo, 2003).

## REFERENCES

Albert, L. (1991). *Cooperative discipline.* Circle Pines,MN: American Guidance Service.

Australian Bureau of Statistics. (2003). *Population, Australian states and territories 2003.* Canberra: Australian Government Publishing Service.

Battistich, V., Solomon, D., Watson, M., & Schaps, E. (1997). Caring school communities. *Educational Psychologist, 32*(3), 137–51.

Beck, M., & Malley, J. (1998). Research into practice: A pedagogy of belonging. *Reclaiming Children and Youth, 7*(3), 133–37.

Berndt, T.J. (1982). The features and effects of friendship in early adolescence. *Child Development, 53,* 1447–60.

Cauce, A.M. (1986). Social networks and social competence: Exploring the effects of early adolescent friendships. *American Journal of Community Psychology, 14*(6), 607–28.

Edwards, D. (1995). The school counselor's role in helping teachers and students belong. *Elementary School Guidance and Counseling, 29*(3), 191–97.

Garmezy, N.Z. (1985). Stress-resistant children: The search for protective factors. In J.E. Stevenson (Ed.), *Recent research in developmental psychopathology* (pp. 213–33). New York: Pergamon.

Goodenow, C. (1993). Classroom belonging among early adolescent students: Relationships to motivation and achievement. *Journal of Early Adolescence, 13*(1), 21–43.

Hagerty, B. (2002). Childhood antecedents of adult sense of belonging. *Psychosocial and Personality Development, 58*(7), 793–801.

Hart, B., Brinkman, S., & Blackmore, S. (2003). *How well are we raising our children in the North Metropolitan Area?: Early Development Index.* Report prepared for Population Health Program, North Metropolitan Health Service, Perth, Western Australia. Western Australia: Government of Western Australian Printing Office.

Harter, S. (1985). Competence as a dimension of self-evaluation: Towards a comprehensive model of self-worth. In R.L. Leahy (Ed.), *The development of self* (pp. 55–121). Orlando, FL: Academic Press.

Kaplan, H.B. (1999). Toward an understanding of resilience: A critical review of definitions and models. In M. Glantz & J. Johnson (Eds.), *Resilience and development: Positive life adaptations* (pp. 17–83). New York: Kluwer Academic.

Kovacs, M. (1992). *The Children's Depression Inventory*. New York: Multi–Health Systems, Inc.

Kumpfer, K.L., & Hopkins, R. (1993). Prevention: Current research and trends. *Recent Advances in Addictive Disorders, 16,* 11–20.

LaGrange, R.D. (2004). Building strengths in inner city African-American children: The task and promise of schools. In C.S. Clauss-Ehlers & M.D. Weist (Eds.), *Community planning to foster resilience in children* (pp. 83–97). New York: Kluwer.

Luthar, S.S., & Zelazo, L.B. (2003). Research on resilience: An integrative review. In S. Luthar (Ed.), *Resilience and vulnerability: Adaptation in the context of childhood adversities* (pp. 510–50). Cambridge: Cambridge University Press.

Ma, X. (2003). Sense of belonging to school: Can schools make a difference? *Journal of Educational Research, 96,* 340–49.

Maslow, A. (1968). *Towards a psychology of being*. Princeton, NJ: Van Nostrand.

McMillan, D.W., & Chavis, D.M. (1986). Sense of community: A definition and theory. *Journal of Community Psychology, 14,* 6–23.

Ministerial Council for Suicide Prevention. (2004). *Suicide prevention gatekeeper training manual*. Telethon Institute for Child health Research. Perth, Western Australia: Author.

Mullett, F., Evans, S W., & Weist, M.D. (2004). A whole school approach to mental health promotion: The Australian MindMatters Program. In C.S. Clauss-Ehlers & M.D. Weist (Eds.), *Community planning to foster resilience in children* (pp. 297–310). New York: Kluwer.

Nelson, G., & Prilleltensky, I. (Eds). (2005). *Community psychology: In pursuit of liberation and well-being*. New York: Palgrave Macmillan.

*NIFTeY Vision for Children in Western Australia*. (2003). National Investment for the early Years. Retrieved 10 April 2006 from www.niftey.cyh.com.

Olds, D., Henderson, C.R., Cole, R., Eckenrode, J., Kitzman, H., Luckey, D., et al. (1998). Long-term effects of nurse home visitation on children's criminal and antisocial behaviour: Fifteen-year follow-up of a randomized controlled trial. *Journal of the American Medical Association, 280,* 1238–44.

Pooley, J.A., Cohen, L., & Pike, L.T. (2005). Can sense of community inform social capital? *Social Science Journal, 42*(1), 71–9.

Pooley, J.A., Pike, L.T., Drew, N.M., & Breen, L. (2002). Inferring Australian children's sense of community: A critical exploration. *Community, Work and Family, 5*(1), 5–22.

Pooley, J.A., Breen, L., Pike, L.T., Drew, N.M., & Cohen, L. (in press). Critiquing the school community: A qualitative study of children's conceptualizations of their school. *International Journal of Qualitative Studies in Education.*

Puddifoot, J.E. (1996). Some initial considerations in the measurement of community identity. *Journal of Community Psychology, 24*(4), 327–36.

Ron, Y. (2004). No man is an island: The relationship between attachment styles, sense of belonging, depression and anxiety among homeless adults. *The Sciences and Engineering, 65*(5B), 2648.

Routt, M.L. (1996). Early experiences that foster connectedness. *Dimensions of Early Childhood, 24*(4), 17–21.

Rowland, A., Cohen, L., Pooley, J.A., Pike, L.T., & Breen, L. (2005). *Peer social networks after the transition to secondary school: Adolescents' perspectives.* Manuscript submitted to Merrill Palmer Quarterly for publication.

Royal, M.A., & Rossi, R.J. (1997). Schools as communities. *Office of Educational Research and Improvement.* Retrieved 1 May 2000 from http://web.ovid.unilinc.edu.au.

Schaps, E., & Solomon, D. (1997). Schools and classrooms as caring communities. *Educational Leadership, 48,* 38–42.

Schmuck, R.A., & Schmuck, P.A. (1992). *Group processes in the classroom* (6th ed.). Dubuque, IA: Wm C Brown.

Schumaker, D. (1998). The transition to middle school. *Office of Educational Research and Improvement.* Retrieved 1 May 2000 from http://web.ovid.unilinc.edu.au.

Stumpers, S., Breen, L., Pooley, J.A., Cohen, L., & Pike, L.T. (2005). A critical exploration of the school context for young adolescents completing primary education. *Community, Work and Family, 8*(3), 251–70.

Ungar, M. (Ed.) (2005). *Handbook for working with children and youth: Pathways to resilience across cultures and contexts.* Thousand Oaks, CA: Sage.

Wang, M.C., Haertel, G.D., & Walberg, H.J. (1997). Fostering educational resilience in inner city schools. In H. Walberg, O. Reyes, & R. Weissberg (Eds.), *Children and youth: Interdisciplinary perspectives* (pp. 119–40). Thousand Oaks, CA: Sage.

Wehlage, G.G. (1989). Dropping out: Can schools be expected to prevent it? In L. Weis, E. Farrar, & H. Petrie (Eds.), *Dropouts from school* (pp. 1–22). Albany: State University of New York Press.

Weiner, B. (1990). The history of motivation research in education. *Journal of Educational Psychology, 82*(4), 616–22

Weldy, G.R. (1995). Critical transitions. *Schools in the Middle, 4*(3), 4–7.

Wyman, P.A., Cross, W., & Barry, J. (2004). Applying research on resilience to enhance school-based prevention. In C. Clauss-Ehler & M. Weist (Eds.), *Community planning to foster resilience in children* (pp. 13–26). New York: Plenum.

Zeichner, K.M. (1980). The development of an instrument to measure group membership in elementary school classrooms. *Journal of Experimental Education, 48*, 237–44.

# PART THREE

## Cultural Relevance

# 12 Synchronicity or Serendipity? Aboriginal Wisdom and Childhood Resilience

JEAN LAFRANCE, RALPH BODOR, AND BETTY BASTIEN

This chapter describes what has been learned thus far in the search for new ways of providing child welfare services that are more in keeping with both traditional aboriginal world views and modern theories of youth resilience. The framework for this dialogue will, therefore, take place within traditional aboriginal knowledge and resilience theory. This is in keeping with advice from Sahtouris (1992), who argues that 'the most promising survival path for humans is to merge existing technology with the knowledge, wisdom, and ecologically sound practice of indigenous and traditional peoples' (p. 1).

Our goal in this chapter is to recognize that indigenous people have for millennia had a very different cosmology and epistemology that, in spite of a recent history of colonization and oppression, continues to permeate their total being. Many communities have endeavoured to develop programs and practices that are more consistent with the aboriginal world view. There have, however, been significant challenges to these efforts, not the least of which is a fundamental lack of understanding and respect on the part of funding sources and policy makers who wield the power to constrain efforts. The historical and current factors that contribute to this situation will be described, as well as contemporary thinking in aboriginal communities in Canada as they chart their own course in the development of child welfare services that better meet their needs. Community recommendations for change are outlined and compared to broad categories of protective factors that contribute to resilience. It is suggested that this preliminary examination is promising as a means of reconciling aboriginal and Western knowledge for the purpose of creating more relevant and creative programs for all communities.

## Resilience

One of the most easily understood descriptions of resilience is the 'capacity to be bent without breaking and the capacity, once bent, to spring back' (Vaillant, 1993, p. 284). A resilient person is usually seen as someone who lives a successful life as defined by such factors as steady employment, a stable marriage, and overall well-being in spite of having been exposed to high levels of emotional, mental, or physical distress (Rutter, 2001). Resilience is the result of interaction between a variety of risk and protective factors. Risk factors such as poverty, parental alcoholism, and early childhood neglect can increase the likelihood of negative outcomes, while protective factors such as a positive relationship with an adult, church involvement, or positive school experiences can help to counteract risk factors.

Gilligan (2003) believes that

> resilience in children and young people grows out of a strong sense of belonging, out of good self esteem, and out of a sense of self efficacy or being able to achieve things and make a difference. Fundamentally these qualities grow out of supportive relationships with parents, relatives, teachers or other adults (or sometimes peers) who offer in-depth commitment, encouragement, and support. (p. 3)

He warns against looking for a 'magic bullet' with which to inoculate children against social adversity and social inequality, focusing instead on supporting and complementing the efforts of parents, schools, and neighbourhoods. Such support moves beyond the narrow confines of child protection to working with the 'natural allies' of the children where they live, collaborating with the natural supports and resources that they have around them.

It is suggested that aboriginal children and their communities have been subjected to far more risk factors than the general population in Canada, as have many indigenous people in all parts of the world. One of the more significant set of risk factors has been a result of the planned genocide of aboriginal people in Canada.

## Cultural Genocide

The term 'genocide' is commonly linked to the mass killings of Jews and other minorities during the Holocaust. However, while some narrow definitions of the term relate to the physical annihilation of a group, other definitions are much broader (Churchill, 1998). The term was first coined by Lemkin in 1944, during the Second World War, to encompass a range of acts meant to persecute and destroy a particular group. Lemkin described genocide in this way:

> [It] does not necessarily mean the immediate destruction of a nation, except when accomplished by mass killings of all members of a nation. It is intended rather to signify a coordinated plan of different actions aiming at the destruction of essential foundations of the life of national groups, with the aim of annihilating the groups themselves [even if all individuals within the dissolved group physically survive]. (p. 79)

In line with this, Lemkin discussed different types of genocide. One such type was related to wars and physical extermination, while another type involved the destruction of a culture without the physical extinction of the group. A third type of genocide combined the annihilation of some of the people and the assimilation of others (Churchill, 1998).

Genocide that does not involve physical extermination has also been called *cultural genocide*. Tinker (1993) explains cultural genocide as the destruction of a culture's integrity as well as the 'values that defines a people and give them life', destroying 'a sense of holistic and communal integrity ... limiting a people's freedom to practice their culture and to live out their lives in culturally appropriate patterns ... eroding both their self-esteem and the interrelationships that bind them together as a community ... by attacking or belittling every aspect of [their] culture' (p. 6). Cultural genocide is, thus, the systematic destruction of a culture, including the weakening of the will of the people to live (Davis & Zannis, 1973).

The history of aboriginal people in Canada, much like in other parts of the Americas, has traditionally been conceptualized as colonization and assimilation resulting from the settlement of Europeans. However, it has also been suggested that 'Canada's treatment of Aboriginal peoples in general, and its creation and operation of Residential Schools in particular, was and continues to be nothing short of genocide' (Chrisjohn, Young, & Marion, 1994, p. 41). Neu and Therrien (2003) add that genocide 'is an excellent starting point for thinking about the consequences of government initiatives directed at indigenous people' (p. 16).

Davis and Zannis (1973) discuss the link between colonialism and genocide, and propose that 'genocide is the means by which colonialism creates, sustains, and extends its control to enrich itself' (p. 30). Colonialism is the deliberate and systematic application of power and implementation of activities designed to make a group of people – be it a racial, political, or cultural entity – forcefully dependent. Since native people do not voluntarily surrender their independence, they must be overwhelmed and controlled by brutal force to secure their dependency (Davis & Zannis, 1973). Thus, genocide is the method or process through which colonization occurs, as 'colonization cannot take place without systematically liquidating all characteristics of the native society' (Davis & Zannis, 1973, p. 32). Neu and Therrien (2003) refer to this type of genocide (i.e., that which is undertaken or allowed as part of achieving goals of colonization or developing territory belonging to Indigenous people) as genocide in the course of colonization. In Canada, the assimilation or genocide of aboriginal people 'by forcing them into colonial institutional structures and norms has been the most persistent objective of Canada's long-term Indian policy' (Boldt, 1993, p. 169). However, it is important to note that genocide is not new or exclusive to the aboriginal peoples in Canada or the Americas. Genocide still exists today and is expected to continue to be part of colonization and 'conflict resolution' policies and practices around the world and in the future (Churchill, 1998, 1999).

## Cultural Genocide in Canada

The intent to commit genocide could not have been described more bluntly than it was by the then deputy superintendent general of Indian Affairs, Duncan Campbell Scott, in 1920. A poet and essayist as well as government official, Scott encapsulated the prevailing attitude of his day, during a House of Commons discussion on proposed changes to the Indian Act: 'Our object is to continue until there is not a single Indian in Canada that has not been absorbed into the body politic, and there is no Indian question, and no Indian department. That is the whole object of this bill' (Aboriginal Justice Implementation Commission, p. 6). According to Scott and government policy of the time, it was imperative to do away with Indian culture. Many shared the view that it was with the young that substantial change would come, as adults were irredeemable and therefore a hindrance to the process of 'civilizing.' This intent seems to clearly fit within the definition of genocide put forth by Lemkin (1944).

The strategy for achieving this objective was the creation of the residential school system as a primary instrument of assimilation. Removal of aboriginal children from the influence of their families and communities was the instrument used to destroy the culture and identity of the First Nations people. This instrument was pursued in spite of earlier objections by Frank Oliver, superintendent general of Indian Affairs, as early as 1908, after the foundations of the residential school system had been laid:

> I hope you will excuse me for so speaking but some of the most important commandments laid upon the human by the divine are love and respect by children for parents. It seems strange that in the name of religion, a system of education should have been instituted, the foundation principle of which, not only ignored but contradicted this command. (Royal Commission on Aboriginal People [RCAP], 1994, p. 2)

Despite this caution, the residential school system was implemented. The Canadian government soon realized that it was recreating a model already recognized by child care professionals as damaging to children. Furthermore, this model failed to meet the prevailing standards of the day in almost every respect, and often fell short of the most basic humanitarian expectations, including those of the Declaration of Human Rights of 1948. In spite of the evidence that children were not well served and were rendered ill-prepared for life in contemporary society as well as in communities of origin, the model was expanded. The creation of a 'total institution' to destroy a people was a deliberate and planned effort by its architects, crippling many communities in the process. The removal of aboriginal children from parents to be raised in residential schools deprived those children of a cultural legacy, as well as the benefits of a tightly knit community of extended family and relatives who shared the task of child rearing by providing nurturing and security.

In addition to the trauma of being removed from their families and communities, children suffered numerous abuses in residential schools, including physical, sexual, psychological, and emotional abuse (e.g., verbal abuse and forbidding aboriginal languages and spiritual practices), as well as unsuitable living conditions (e.g., inadequate nutrition) (RCAP, as cited in Chrisjohn et al., 1994). The Aboriginal Healing Foundation (1999) has identified the following outcomes for aboriginal people as a result of this program:

> Low self-esteem; dysfunctional families and interpersonal relationships; parenting issues such as emotional coldness and rigidity; widespread depression; widespread rage and anger; chronic physical illness related to spiritual and emotional states; unresolved grief and loss; fear of personal growth, transformation, and healing; unconscious internalization of residential school behaviours such as false politeness, not speaking out, passive compliance; patterns of paternalistic authority linked to passive dependency; patterns of misuse of power to control others, and community social patterns that foster whispering in the dark, but refusing to support and stand with those who speak out or challenge the status quo; the breakdown of the social glue that holds families and communities together, such as trust, common ground, shared purpose and direction, a vibrant ceremonial and civic life, cooperative networks and associations working for the common good, etc.; disunity and conflict between individuals, families, and factions within the community; spiritual confusion; involving alienation from one's own spiritual life and growth process, as well as conflicts and confusion over religion; internalized sense of inferiority or aversion in relation to whites and especially whites in power; toxic communication – backbiting, gossip, criticism, put downs, personal attacks, sarcasm, secrets, etc.; becoming oppressors and abusers of others as a result of what was done to one in residential schools; cultural identity issues – the loss of language and cultural foundations has led to denial (by some) of the validity of one's own cultural identity (assimilation), a resulting cultural confusion and dislocation; destruction of social support networks (the cultural safety net) that individuals and families in trouble could rely upon; disconnection from the natural world (i.e. the sea, the forest, the earth, living things) as an important dimension of daily life and hence spiritual dislocation; acceptance of powerlessness within community life. (p. 1)

Among the most detrimental effects of residential schools reported in the literature are a sense of alienation, loss of identity and self-esteem, lack of parenting skills, family breakdown, intergenerational trauma and violence, and loss of language, culture, spirituality, and pride (Ing,

1991; RCAP, 1994; Spicer, 1998; Stout & Kipling, 2003; Wesley-Esquimaux & Smolewski, 2004).

By the early 1940s Canada had begun to press provincial authorities to provide alternate care for aboriginal children in need of protection. Two decades later, during the early 1960s, the provinces assumed this role, on the condition that the federal government reimbursed them for such care. Tragically, neither level of government ensured that community and familial supports required to keep families together were available. This contributed to the so-called 60s scoop (the forced adoption of particularly large numbers of aboriginal and Métis children in Canada during the 1960s and after) and the admission of thousands of children to white institutions and foster homes, often well outside of the children's communities and, in some cases, outside of Canada.

## From Residential Schools to Child Welfare

Residential schools were replaced by ... child welfare ... in a second attempt to ensure that the next generation of Indian children was different from their parents. (Armitage, 1993, p. 131)

Provincial child welfare agencies began to establish a presence on First Nations by the early 1960s in the Canadian West. Systemic factors involved in the genocide of aboriginal people by means of the residential school system were perpetuated by the child welfare system during the 60s scoop that, in effect, continued until the early 1980s.

By the mid-twentieth century, residential schools had become a *de facto* child welfare system, without any of the legal or policy safeguards of mandated child welfare systems. By that time, some children were being placed in residential schools because of the inability of parents to care for them and concerns about abuse and neglect (Milloy, 1999). As Milloy points out, however:

Beyond social factors (alcoholism, illegitimacy, excessive procreation), neglectful 'home circumstances' were often economic, the product not of some flaw in the character of Aboriginal parents but of the marginalization of Aboriginal communities ... it was more likely to be unemployment, a general lack of opportunity and access to resources, marking the poverty of families, that undercut the material quality of care that parents afforded their children. (p. 213)

By 1966, up to 75% of children in residential schools were 'from homes which by reasons of overcrowding and parental neglect or indifference [were] considered unfit for school children' (Milloy, 1999, p. 214). During the 1960s and 1970s, the federal government made legislative arrangements with provincial governments to assume 'protection' of aboriginal children. Thus, child welfare took over the protective function of residential schools, and played an important role in the closing of residential schools (Milloy, 1999). In fact, some children were directly transferred from residential schools to the child welfare system (Milloy, 1999).

By the end of the 1960s, aboriginal children represented 30–40% of all children in the child welfare system in Canada, and even higher numbers in the prairie provinces (e.g., 50% in Alberta) (Bennett & Blackstock, 2002). These children were often placed in non-aboriginal foster or adoptive homes, continuing the process of Aboriginal assimilation into Canadian mainstream society (Blackstock, Trocmé, & Bennett, 2004; Hudson, 1997; Sinclair, 2004).

Although the child welfare system purported to be acting in the best interests of the child, this second mass removal of children from their homes and communities paralleled the residential school experience and perpetuated the genocide of aboriginal people. The impact on aboriginal children, families, and communities perpetuated the loss of culture, connection, identity, and relationships; the development of a new generation of aboriginal people without parenting skills; the further disempowerment of aboriginal people; and the continuation of problems such as alcoholism, poverty, and violence (Native Child and Family Services of Toronto, Stevenato and Associates, & Budgell, 1999).

A number of other studies have examined the long-term impacts of the child welfare system on aboriginal children (e.g., Armitage, 1993; Baden, 2002; Bennett & Blackstock, 2002; McRoy, Zurcher, Lauderdale, & Anderson, 1982; Native Child and Family Services of Toronto et al., 1999; Richard, 2004; Spicer, 1998). These studies have found that some children raised in non-aboriginal homes experienced racism as well as physical, emotional, and sexual abuse by foster or adoptive parents (Bennett & Blackstock, 2002; Timpson,1995). In addition, many children experienced identity issues as they tried to understand their own racial and cultural identity in a non-aboriginal environment (Bennett & Blackstock, 2002; Richard, 2004). Exacerbating identity issues, several adoption agencies that placed aboriginal children into homes did not keep records that would later assist children in finding their biological families (Bennett & Blackstock, 2002). Further studies have suggested a range of negative long-term outcomes for aboriginal children raised in the child welfare system, such as poverty, unemployment, incarceration, alcohol and drug addiction, family violence, and an increased risk of having their own children placed in care (e.g. Bennett & Blackstock, 2002; Spicer, 1998).

## Delegated Child Welfare Authority in First Nations

By the early 1980s a greater understanding generated a sense of alarm at the growing numbers of children that were cared for by white caregivers. This gave rise to a system whereby provincial authorities delegated First Nations communities to deliver a range of child protection services to their children and families. The legislation was intended to establish self-determination in the development and delivery of child services in First Nations communities and in some instances to off-reserve members.

The most common model has beento establish a tripartite agreement between the federal government, the provincial government, and the local band council. The role of the federal government is to fund the programs in fulfilment of their fiduciary obligations, while the province is to delegate mandated authority and ensure that the intent of legislation is met by delegated First Nations child welfare agencies.

Many of the current problems contributing to the ever-growing numbers of aboriginal children in care flow from the manner in which these responsibilities are carried out. The *Wen: De: We are coming to the light of day* (First Nation Child & Family Caring Society of Canada, 2005) report reveals that funding continues to be a significant problem. Most resources are allocated to the removal of children from their families and, often, communities, with precious little designated for primary and secondary prevention services that would keep families intact. Although the funding formula is slowly changing, the situation does call for a total revamping if current reality is to change (First Nation Child & Family Caring Society of Canada, 2005). First, increased funding is necessary, as inadequate resources have placed First Nations child and family service agencies in an untenable situation. Second, substantial policy and program changes for the delivery of programs by both the federal and provincial governments are required, as aboriginal people fight for increased self-determination and to create programs that are congruent with their cultural traditions.

In addition, coordination of federal, provincial, and tribal jurisdictions seems fraught with problems. The *Wen: De* report states that of the twelve agencies surveyed, there were a combined 393 jurisdictional disputes over a one-year period requiring an average of 54.25 person hours to resolve each incident. Of these disputes, 36% arose between federal government departments while 27% were between provincial departments and 14% were between federal and provincial departments. Only 23% involved tribal jurisdictions.

Ultimately, Canada's historical pattern of inadequate federal funding accompanied by a lack of accountability for quality of service is inexorably leading to predictable outcomes: family breakdown, loss of children to the community, and the creation of yet another lost generation of aboriginal people, perpetuating the cycle begun in the 1800s.

## Intergenerational Impacts on Aboriginal People

> Residential schools have had a devastatingly negative impact on the lives of individuals. (Chrisjohn et al., 1994, p. 61)

The devastating individual and cultural impact of residential schools on aboriginal people is well documented. The abuse and neglect suffered not only affected these children's future, but also the lives of their descendants, whose families have been characterized by further abuse and neglect. As the Royal Commission on Aboriginal Peoples (1994) concluded, 'these effects have carried over to several generations and may well be the basis for the dysfunction we see in individuals, families, and entire Native communities' (p. 83).

The trauma that aboriginal people experienced through their history of genocide and that has been passed on from generation to generation continues to affect lives and perpetuate many of the problems manifested in aboriginal communities (Milloy, 1999; Wesley-Esquimaux & Smolewski, 2004). According to the Aboriginal Healing Foundation (1999):

When trauma is ignored and there is no support for dealing with it, the trauma will be passed from one generation to the next. What we learn to see as 'normal' when we are children, we pass on to our own children. Children who learn that ... sexual abuse is normal, and who have never dealt with the feelings that come from this, may inflict physical and sexual abuse on their own children. This is the legacy of physical and sexual abuse in residential schools. (p. A5)

Residential schools and welfare placements have also impeded the transference of positive parenting skills from one generation to the next, which has led to troubled family relationships and difficulties raising children (Milloy, 1999; York, 1990). Milloy adds that 'In residential schools, [children] learned that adults often exert power and control through abuse. The lessons learned in childhood are often repeated in adulthood with the result that many survivors of the residential school system often inflict abuse on their own children' (p. 299), resulting in intergenerational cycles of abuse.

Other well-documented impacts linked to this history include suicide, post-traumatic stress disorder, alcohol and drug abuse, gambling, somatic disorders, domestic violence, crime, and child abuse (Bennett & Blackstock, 2002; Berry & Brink, 2004; Stout & Kipling, 2003; Wesley-Esquimaux & Smolewski, 2004).

Aboriginal communities continue to deal with many of these and other problems today. Indeed, the number of children in care is only one of a range of issues facing aboriginal children, families, and communities today. For example, in Canada aboriginal youth are more likely to live in single-parent homes, drop out of school, be homeless, abuse alcohol and drugs (including solvents), commit suicide, and live in poverty than non-aboriginal youth (Indian and Northern Affairs Canada, 2004; Richard, 2004; Statistics Canada, 2004; Trocmé, Knoke, & Blackstock, 2004). Similarly, aboriginal people in general are disproportionately affected by a range of social, economic, and health issues such as poverty, unemployment, crime, violence, alcohol and drug abuse, HIV/AIDS, diabetes, sexually transmitted infections, tuberculosis, and suicide (Health Canada, 2000; Lee, 2000). Suicide, for example, is the leading cause of death for youth and adults up to forty-four years old, and urban aboriginals are more than twice as likely to live in poverty as non-aboriginal people (Health Canada, 2000; Lee, 2000). Indian and Northern Affairs Canada further reported that 16% of homes on reserves were in need of major repairs, and 5% were unsafe or uninhabitable (Health Canada, 2000). Likewise, a study by the Department of Indian and Northern Affairs (1996, as cited in Bennett & Blackstock, 2002) concluded that aboriginal people living on reserves would rank eightieth in the world if measured by the United Nations Human Development Index. By contrast, as a country, Canada ranks first in the world. It seems clear that the risk factors identified in childhood resilience theory are far more prevalent within aboriginal communities than they are for the general population.

## Aboriginals in Canada: A Resilient People

It is remarkable that, in spite of the destructive impacts of policy aimed at First Nations communities, aboriginal people have survived and maintained their culture and traditions to the extent that they have. The traditional resilience of aboriginal people was acknowledged early on when the Indian and Eskimo Residential School Commission prepared policy recommendations on the education of aboriginal children in 1930. The prevailing belief was that aboriginal people had already acknowledged European superiority in dealing with the 'forces of nature,' what today would be referred to as technological superiority:

> So far as the Indian himself is concerned, he has already seen with his own eyes that many of the white man's ways are superior to his own. He has seen, for instance, that the white man's methods and education have given him control over many of the forces of nature and over many of these circumstances of life. (Indian and Eskimo Residential School Commission Report, 1930, p. 2)

In spite of this perception, the commission's debates highlighted two fundamental assumptions about aboriginal people, having far-reaching implications for the shaping of policy about aboriginal education:

> Further as to the question of providing the best system of education for the Indigenous people of this country is one which had to be faced in other parts of the world where superior races invaded and possessed the territories occupied by similar peoples. Careful consideration is demanded in connection with two other important factors which have a direct bearing on the subject. The first is as to whether the Indians' exist-

ing need is to be taken as the foundation upon which our education is to be built and by which it would, in effect, be limited. Two, are we to assume that the white man's education is the most perfect yet devised by the ingenuity of man and impose that education upon them without necessarily considering whether, in fact, it is the best, the form best suited to their capacity or their needs. Both methods have been employed in dealing with various primitive peoples in other parts of the world and as might be expected, with various results.

The policy decision focused on two clear but contradictory alternatives. One alternative recognized the strength and history of aboriginal people and proposed

> grafting onto the deeply rooted stock of what already exists. The Indians successfully occupied this continent for 12,000 or possibly, 20,000 years. They ... have displayed unsurpassed human qualities of loyalty to unseen powers and adaptability to the practical; have a living past capable of energizing their present[,] and any system of education which destroys all their faith in their own institutions and traditions will create in them, a sense of permanent inferiority and an unfortunate belief that everything which is peculiarly your own is not only worthless but an obstacle to progress.

The second alternative rejected this notion and contended that the only hope for progress among Indigenous people lay in 'the complete application to their condition of the white man's experience, knowledge, and skill.' It was only in this way that they could benefit from 'the education needed to advance them to higher levels of civilization and to enable them to use to their own advantage, the natural resources which surround them' (ibid.). The latter was to prevail despite the recognition that the traditional qualities of aboriginal people were worth preserving. These included:

> The quality of loyalty to family and friends which is capable of expansion into loyalty to a wider circle.
> The deep love of children from which can be developed the strong desire to help the children of the race to be well-born.
> The generosity and hospitality which are outstanding characteristics of the Indian races which may be developed as some of the finer elements of social living.

The traditional quality of courage and admiration of brave leadership and which can be used to spur the young Indian on in the face of discouragement and the hard grind of monotonous routine.

The engrafted dignity and serenity of the leaders of the race and which should be preserved as a help in restoring to the hectic world in which we live, the poise and calm of which we have been robbed by our numerous mechanical inventions.

In spite of these fine qualities, history is clear about which view had the most influence on policy decisions, contributing to conduct of what can only be seen as a concerted effort to destroy a people. Meanwhile, aboriginal leaders continued to work towards increased self-determination and recognition as the original people of Canada. By the early 1990s Canada had begun to acknowledge the desperate situation of many aboriginal people and created the Royal Commission on Aboriginal People that consulted widely on how to address the problems that aboriginal people were confronting. Although many of the recommendations have not been accepted, a movement towards healing and reconciliation has been funded, supporting a new era of healing and reconciliation.

## Towards Healing and Reconciliation

It is clear that most aboriginal communities have placed much of their hope for changing the situation described thus far in a return to traditional values. As a speaker at the Royal Commission on Aboriginal Peoples (1994) said:

Those communities who have had the most success in dealing with the psychological legacy of colonialism are those that have found a way to operate within their cultural context and drawing on ... the spiritual and other strengths that are present in their culture. (p. 48)

In recent years, aboriginal people have resolved to overcome the pain and loss that were the legacy of colonization through healing, reconciliation, and self-determination (Aboriginal Healing Foundation, 1999; Berry & Brink, 2004). A major part of healing and reconciliation is the building on of the strengths and resilience of aboriginal people and the reclaiming of aboriginal culture, identity, and pride (Aboriginal Healing Foundation, 1999; Berry & Brink, 2004). Indeed, aboriginal people are mobilizing to recover from the trauma and oppression of residential schools and genocide, revitalizing their language, customs, spirituality, traditions, values, and beliefs (York, 1990). York concludes that today, 'evidence of a cultural revival can be seen across Canada ... [It] is just one step toward regaining what has been lost' (pp. 264, 269).

## Aboriginal World View

From a broader perspective, the healing of aboriginal people may be facilitated through cultural approaches based on an aboriginal world view. The colonization of aboriginal people introduced an Anglo-European ideology based on values of individualism, power, control, and efficiency (Cajete, 2000). These are radically different from aboriginal world views and philosophy, which are based on an 'organic, holistic concept of the world; spiritual and harmonious relationships to the land and all life forms; communalism; personal duties and responsibilities to the band/tribe; social and economic justice, equality, and sharing; [and] universal and consensual participation in decision making' (Boldt, 1993, p. 183). An aboriginal world view can also be conceptualized as an eco-philosophy that values the interconnectedness of people to the universe and to each other, emphasizing cooperation, creativity, connectedness, balance, ritual, and ceremony (Cajete, 2000). Cajete concludes that aboriginal philosophy or science is 'in every sense an expression of the evolutionary interrelationship of Native people with nature' (p. 58).

Boldt (1993) further emphasizes that in order for aboriginal people to thrive, aboriginal culture must be adapted and developed to be relevant, practical, and successful for the modern world. This adaptation 'speaks to the need to bridge the past and present in such a way as to allow Indians to be part of the twentieth century without betraying the fundamental philosophies and principles of the ancient covenants' (p. 183). Such a bridge demands ongoing planning, collaboration, and cooperation between elders and youth, as elders transmit the philosophies and principles of the culture, and youth help to make these relevant to today's economic, political, and social environment (Boldt, 1993). However, in order for aboriginal people to develop their culture in ways that allow them to thrive in a contemporary world while identifying with their own heritage, they must first break from the culture of dependence created during years of colonization (Boldt, 1993). Breaking this cycle of dependency represents a significant challenge for aboriginal communities in Canada today.

## Resilience and Aboriginal People

Research suggests that there is, possibly, a high level of congruence between aboriginal world views and modern theories of childhood resilience. A number of aboriginal writers have recently focused on aspects of resilience that resonate with the cultural solutions advocated by their elders (Blackstock, Trocmé, & Bennett, 2004; Dion Stout & Kipling, 2003; Hunter & Lewis, 2006; LaBoucane-Benson, 2005).

LaBoucane-Benson (2005) argues that 'for Aboriginal families a resilience framework must consider and reflect their worldview, including a need for balance, fluidity, and the interconnectedness of family members, the community, and the cosmos' (p. 7). She goes on to describe how during the research process for the Royal Commission on Aboriginal People many aboriginal people reiterated that 'families are at the core of the process of renewal in which they are engaged' (Canada, 1996, p. 1). The renewal process of aboriginal families is a continuation of the resilience demonstrated by aboriginal people, and their survival in the face of genocidal policies. In a powerful testament to the resilience of their people, two presenters from the Victorian Aboriginal Child Care Agency propose:

> In order to have a positive future our children need to be resilient. Not only resilient to the past which is imprinted on their genes and the living memory of their parents, grand parents, families, and communities, but also resilient to a colonized environment which denigrates their very sense of identity and being. So many Aboriginal child and family service practitioners seek to build on the one positive fact for today's Aboriginal and Islander communities – we have survived: we have proved resilient. (Hunter & Lewis, 2006)

Similarly, in his description of identity formation and cultural resilience in aboriginal communities Lalonde (2006) states:

> Resilience implies transcendence. While there is perhaps no happy ending to be found in the story told by these data, there is hope. Within a population that suffers the highest rate of suicide in any culturally iden-

tifiable group in the world, and that even after the 60s scoop continues to see a disproportionate number of children taken into care, there is evidence of resilience. The surprising outcomes – the transcendence – is [sic] not found in the single 'hardy' or 'invulnerable' child who manages to rise above adversity, but in the existence of whole communities that demonstrate the power of culture as a protective factor. When communities succeed in promoting their cultural heritage and in securing control of their own collective future – in claiming ownership over their past and future – the positive effects reverberate across many measures of youth health and well-being. (p. 23)

Aboriginal communities are clear about the essential values and philosophy that must guide the development of programs and services. These include shared parenting and community responsibility for children, the importance of language as a source of renewed culture, knowledge of history and tradition as an essential element of identity, the importance of kinship and connection to each other, and a respectful approach to all of life.

Congruent with these aspects of aboriginal culture, resilience theory describes protective factors that include having one person in life who values and respects the child (mentor/elder), a connection to community (history and tradition), a connection to a church (spirituality), healthy peer relationships (identity), development of at least one talent or skill (traditional skills such as drumming and dancing), and contribution to one's community or school (being seen as part of the solution for one's people).

A more systematic application of both aboriginal and resilience perspectives can enrich communication between aboriginal and non-aboriginal practitioners, and improve the quality and relevance of services to aboriginal children and families. Such applications to service development and their potential for successful cross-cultural communication of important concepts between aboriginal and white society will be explored. We will compare and contrast what aboriginal elders and their communities in Alberta have told us is important with what youth resilience theory has been advancing for many years with a view to enhancing protective factors in day-to-day practice. Our hope is that by juxtaposing these words and resilience theory we can begin to develop a common language that resonates with all people in the development of innovative practice models that enhance child and family well-being. The quotations that follow come from elders at a sharing circle at a conference entitled 'Creating

Hope for the Future.' It will be left to the reader to determine to what extent the quotations reflect what we know about resilience as explored elsewhere in this volume. In Table 1 we have gathered the quotations under a number of themes relevant to both health perspectives.

*Kinship and Connection to Each Other – Connection to
a Community*

> I'm thinking about ... just getting back to the way I was raised by my grandparents. It is hard to talk about because they are not here anymore. I want to see my grandkids being there with me like I was with my grandparents, because they were really into the culture and my grandmother actually taught me a lot of things. We used to go berry picking, and making dry meat and stuff like that and that is what I would like to see for myself and other families. I want to see the closeness back the way it was.

*Spirituality and Respect for Nature – Church and Religious
Connections*

> I took up believing and trusting in God because I couldn't trust anything else, that's what I had. And he was always there and he never left me, my creator was there all the time and that's my inspiration. I've learned to forgive and to start trusting, little children, people, and adults, I try to help them in every way I can today.

> This elder chose me as I was standing there beside the fire. I didn't know what was supposed to be done ... I stood there and this elder came and talked to me ... about the creator and about the grandfathers and the grandmothers, relatives that had passed on. He explained to me ... the four principles of life, the four directions ... Then he said 'Jesus was never here, the man in the black robe ... he brought him over in a big ship ... your grandfather and your grandmother never knew who Jesus was.' And that day, that word stuck in my mind and ever since then, I have followed the traditional way of life.

*Sharing and Respect for Each Other – Contributing to the Community
and School*

> I want to be able to see [a] community that's unified, that can discuss things together, and that can work together as opposed to fighting

Table 1: A comparison of key aboriginal world views and resilience concepts

| Aboriginal world view | Resilience concept |
| --- | --- |
| Kinship and connection to each other | Connection to a community |
| Spirituality and respect for nature | Church and religious connections |
| Sharing and respect for each other | Contributing to the community/school |
| Knowledge of history, culture, and language | Sense of identity |
| Development of traditional skills (i.e., drumming, dancing) | Sense of competence |
| Shared parenting and community responsibility for children | Healthy parenting |

against each other. If we could take our negative energy and turn it into positive energy the things we can accomplish are phenomenal ... but we have to believe in ourselves. I would like to see people taking responsibility for themselves ... if we choose a more positive lifestyle and take the responsibility for ourselves and say 'yes we're a part of it and we want to make things happen,' then things can change.

I would like to see people not being afraid of people. There is [so much] fear, they are scared to talk to people. The trust is lacking [and people] are scared to even share their pain. I can remember people would come to the road, say 'hi, what's your name, where are you from, come in have coffee, come in rest up,' even [if you were] just walking a little ways. I would like to see that happen again, just feeling free with no fear of anything. Just saying how you feel or 'Hey! I need to talk to somebody' and if you could just take that time to sit down and have some coffee.

## Knowledge of History, Culture, and Language – Sense of Identity

I went to a couple of culture camps this year and the things that I saw at the culture camp were good. It was almost as if the people acted differently, not like here in everyday life. In the culture camp they were just laughing and having a good time. I don't know if I was the only one guy who saw this, but you know that would be something I would like to see more of.

Every child should have a Blackfoot name and I think it's very important because that places us in the universe and it places us in connection with all our relatives. So it's a powerful strength that we have is to have our names, our Blackfoot names. But it does not have any meaning if you don't know what those connections are or if you don't know how to be in relationship with those connections or with those alliances. An Elder will give a name and so when you give your name, you say, 'This is who I am and this is the elder who gave me my name,' so there's a connection to an elder and this is the story of why they gave you that name and a lot of it is tied to it. This gives us strength as every time you say your name you have all these connections and all these alliances that place you, who you are, where you came from, and where are you going.

## Development of Traditional Skills – Sense of Competence and Skill

I went to Onion Lake a little while ago and you should have seen the young people dance around; just the young people, even the little kids were playing drums. That's what they should teach. People here should teach the young people to play drums and dance; all the dances [such as] round dances.

I encourage some of traditional values [even if] I know we can't go back in time and survive the way they use to a long time ago. The trap line is different and the fur just is not there and the prices are not there either; but then we still have to survive ... The oldtimers would entertain themselves by picking up the drum and just singing; to me that is a lost art, and they would have fun and tell stories and different things. I have sat and listened to some old timers that passed on. They told me different things and it was a good way of life where there was always humour no matter what. To me in any kind of healing humour is a big part of it.

## Shared Parenting and Community Responsibility for Children – Healthy Parenting

I'm granny. Long ago, as far as I know, our people had their way of raising their families. Like we had the grandparents, we had the aunts and uncles and then we had the parents themselves. Our grandparents were there to teach us. They were our teachers. If we wanted to know something we approached our grandparents and they taught us what they knew and our aunts and uncles were the people that told us when we did something wrong. When we did something wrong it wasn't our parents that scolded us or told us what we did was wrong. It was up to the aunts and uncles. They were the ones that disciplined their nephews and nieces and I still see that sometimes today. Sometimes one of my sons when his nephews do wrong, he tells them they did wrong. He doesn't wait for the parents to tell them. He tells them. That's the way it was long ago and the parents were there just to love their kids. You gave love to your kids and your kids loved you in return. The children didn't have to be taken out of homes and when they were orphaned or the parents were sick, the rest of the family was there to just take them in and look after them. There was no such thing as who is going to take care of this child, somebody just said you can come home and live with me. I'll raise you and take care of you and that was it.

## Discussion

The removal of aboriginal children deprived them of a tightly knit community of extended family and relatives who shared the task of child rearing. The separation of children from parents and the loss of parental role models are responsible for many of the childcare problems of aboriginal parents (McKenzie & Hudson, 1985). Aboriginal children who spent many years in residential schools had limited experience as family members (Haig-Brown, 1988). Atteneave (1977) recollects that 'neither they nor their own parents had ever known life in a family from the age they first entered school. The parents had no memories and no patterns to follow in rearing children except for the regimentation of mass sleeping and impersonal schedules' (p. 30). This lack of positive role modelling has taken its toll on the aboriginal family in Canada today.

Since aboriginal people attribute many of their losses to colonialism and the oppressive systems that attempted to take away their history, traditions, language, and identity, it should not be surprising that many would seek a return to health and autonomy in their history, traditional way of life, rediscovery of language, and sense of identity as an aboriginal person. While many aboriginal child welfare agencies are seeking models of practice more consistent with their own world views, there is a dearth of 'new' models that incorporate 'old' ways to respond to our 'new' understanding of the impact of residential school experiences, as well as the 60s scoop, on aboriginal communities and families. The challenge is to learn from a dialogue that not only will create new knowledge, but can be readily applied to real-world situations.

The creation of this vision is not without its challenges. On the one hand, there is a strong and continuing desire among many aboriginal people and their allies to build upon traditional aboriginal strengths and values such as courage, respect for each other and for nature, the oral tradition and the wisdom of the elders, a deep connection with each other and mother earth, and a consistent application of spirituality to all of life. On the other hand, the loss of culture and tradition that has resulted from colonization continues to affect the lives of aboriginal people as well as their healing processes.

As child welfare services have evolved over the past century, the adoption of a bureaucratic and legalistic paradigm seems to have increasingly rigidified practice through the introduction of overly specialized roles, top-down and fiscally driven policies, increasing disconnection from community, overly prescriptive standards, and other trappings of technologically based approaches that create increasing distances between child welfare practitioners and those they serve. Yet these are the models provided to aboriginal service providers. What we propose is to bring together the best of indigenous and Western approaches by strengthening elements of interconnectedness and spirituality within child welfare practice in all of our communities. Our destinies are so intertwined that only by bringing together the full force of our understanding can we reverse the actions of past generations and create new approaches based upon lessons critical to our common future.

Canada is not alone in this plight. A recent forum in Niagara Falls, Canada, demonstrated that indigenous people from around the world are united in a common vision of serving their people in ways that are true to themselves. Although there is a need to create new knowledge to fill existing service gaps, it is also clear that few communities have a clear notion of how to achieve this. Aboriginal communities are, however, clear about the essential values and philosophy that must guide the development of programs and services (see earlier discussion of resilience and aboriginal people).

In this regard, Little Bear (2000) speaks of the collision of 'jagged world views,' aiding our understanding of the differences between aboriginal and Eurocentric worldviews. By contrast with First Nations, Eurocentric philosophies are more linear than holistic, hierarchical and specialized rather than generalized, more materialistic and self-interested than sharing, less concerned about relationships and kindness than competitiveness, more aggressive than respectful, and more focused on external sources of control and authority than on the development of internal controls. The complex historical interaction of these two approaches has left a heritage of jagged world views among Indigenous people who no longer have a clear grasp on either world view. This leads to a jigsaw-puzzle type of consciousness that each person has to piece together alone.

Yet, as demonstrated by community members' commentary, the fundamentals are still very much alive in aboriginal communities. What made a difference in the lives of those who shared their stories resided in their relationships – some as permanent as that of a grandparent, some as transitory as a chance encounter of a young man with an elder. All these stories contained a common thread: the importance of being respected and acknowledged by another person. All reflected a sense of being viewed as a person with inherent dignity and worth. All recounted being left with a major impression of being a person with potential and hope for the future because someone believed in them, whether they were a student who had demonstrated a talent in school or someone whose grandfather showed her how to properly care for her new baby. In short, these stories related fundamentally human experiences that made an important difference in individual lives.

## Community Recommendations

To create the conditions for the realization of an aboriginal world view that fits with what we know about resilience, we will need to structure our services in ways that reflect what we are learning from communities themselves. Many community members have a clear vision of what this will look like. The following summarizes some key notions of community members that flow from their stories and resilience theory. While space does not allow full expression of the diversity and richness of the perspectives that we gleaned from our encounters, we hope that the following will provide a brief overview of some excellent ideas. Some of these ideas have been derived from community gatherings at Sturgeon Lake, Saskatchewan, and the Blood Reserve, Alberta. Others have come from social work students at Blue Quill College (an aboriginal college in northern Alberta), in response to a question about how we might best address the community issues and concerns that had arisen.

*Kinship and Connection to Each Other*

A synopsis of conversations in all three communities underscored the importance of listening to community stories so that members can feel validated, encouraging aboriginal communities to take the initiative amongst themselves in such settings as elder and youth gatherings. It would be important to deal with isolation from family and community by creating settings and community resources where people can meet to reconnect with each other. Where serious conflict exists, it was recommended that mediation services be provided to deal with long-standing hostility and resentment, reuniting the community by sharing common history and helping to reconnect estranged families.

*Spirituality and Respect for Nature*

Blackfoot scientists from the Blood Reserve in Alberta have expressed the following thoughts about spirituality and respect to guide us:

> When we ask the elders for their wisdom or to guide us … they always ask us is for respect. The Blackfoot interpretation of respect and what it means and how we conduct ourselves is very different from … the Western way … it comes from a very spiritual and sacred connection to life and how we maintain that balance in terms of the sacredness of life.

> In English, respect really doesn't speak to spirituality or the sacredness of life so the understanding is very different. Sometimes when the Elders speak to us … there's a disconnect in our understanding of what the Elders are saying and we can carry that lack of understanding in our day-to-day activities or our programming. We may even say, 'well, the Elders said respect,' but we haven't really understood what they meant.

An aboriginal social worker in child welfare from northern Alberta stated:

> My vision is that these teachings should be available to everyone; teachings from our elders about our spirituality. I would like us to return to some of those teachings and have them incorporated in the way we live our lives. We have strengths and we are making a contribution so why

don't we incorporate where those strengths come from? Incorporate that into the way we live our lives and the way we try to help children. Have spirituality available for our children, our families in need. We're sending one of our kids to a sweat for treatment instead of sending the kid to wherever they send psychotics in Edmonton or Grande Prairie. Why can't we try Sweat Ceremonies or Pipe Ceremonies as ways of healing for our children and our families?

## Sharing and Respect for Each Other

Social work students from Blue Quill College proposed the provision of opportunities for safe expression of affection, and open discussion around feelings, emotions, and inadequacies. Students emphasized people's need to heal, to tell their stories, to learn to trust, to find out who they are as individuals. Communities and the individuals living within them also need to learn to relate to one another and to those in other societies. It is very important for people to learn that they are not what the oppressors said or say they are:

- They are not a thing devalued.
- They are valued as individuals and as a people.
- There is a place for them within this world.
- They can contribute.

These students also proposed that:

Healing groups are needed that allow for group healing and the sharing of stories that embrace the reality that they were the victims and they were wronged. It was not their fault.

We need to find traditions, customs and activities that will draw families and communities together. While this can be done in a traditional context, allowing families to partake in new traditions together, it is the time spent together that counts.

## Knowledge of History, Culture, and Language

Social work students at Blue Quill College also offered the following suggestions based upon their experiences:

We need to encourage the resurgence of old traditions and native language, and allow and provide Aboriginal children to have the opportunity to re-connect with their heritage. Knowledge of one's history is one of the keys to begin to get grounded with self. People that have lost their roots are 'lost.' The lost need to see that the Aboriginal people were once a proud nation and can again become a proud nation. It is important to create hope and a belief in ourselves.

Being a survivor of physical and sexual abuse, all I wanted was to be heard, really heard and validated. I wanted someone to listen to my story. It is about sharing of stories that starts the healing. My journey began being heard (not just a statistic) and feeling real and not a number. Picking the strengths, qualities and positive aspects, I later looked at one step at a time. Culture plays an important component for Aboriginal people that teach the men and women role through culture or respect for self and others, gaining back self-esteem. No longer do I feel like I am a victim, but a survivor through sharing, knowledge, respect, humour, tears, and laughter, spirituality, and Creator.

I tend to connect with the residential school experience because these same principles of colonization happened when I was taken from my home and put in a 'white' foster family who happened to be prejudiced against 'Indians,' spoke French, and called me a 'savage.' I was denied my culture, history, language, family, and home. For these reasons, I can say that to help our residential school survivors and maybe even abused foster children, and the next generations of residential school survivor's children, we need to begin to love ourselves and take pride in which we are as First Nations. We need to learn about the history of Aboriginals before, during, and after colonization. These concepts must be learned before we can heal, not only for the residential school survivors but for their families as well; so everyone connects and stays unified as a family unit.

## Development of Traditional Skills

Members of the Sturgeon Lake Cree Nation explained:

We make the Cree language and culture a part of every curriculum available to all students. It was also important that we have cultural camps where youth can learn ancient arts of canoeing, trapping, hunting, fishing, smoking meat and fish, herbal healing, drum making and drumming, and traditional dances.

Members of the Blood Tribe recommended that:

We carry forward the oral tradition and provide opportunities for the elders to convey their knowledge while they are still with us and that the community continue its efforts to live the traditional Kainai [Blood Tribe] way of life.

*Shared Parenting and Community Responsibility for Children*

Members of various communities emphasized the following with regard to community parenting:

We should providing opportunities for parents to address the pain of not being loved or shown love and listen to what they need to heal from this. We could address the loss of affection that has been experienced by establishing programs that educate families on how to reconnect with one another and how to love one another again.

We can allow the community to gather and exchange information, ideas, and struggles around parenting. As a community we need to support one another with all our family systems. We must recognize that parenting is a community commitment and a child is not raised by one person. Child Welfare systems and Aboriginal people need to understand the differences and similarity of parental skills of our respective systems. To discuss the positive or accepted practices within Aboriginal families may enlighten child welfare and re-kindle traditional values that existed before colonization. Mainstream values concerning parenting within Aboriginal families conflict with collective community and spiritual well-being of our people.

We must learn and honour the traditional parental role. We must seek guidance from elders about what the parental role used to be and talk to the community about healing and reclaiming parenthood.

## Summary and Conclusions

It seems clear that many indigenous people seek a return to more traditional ways of life and that they wish to incorporate these in the manner in which services are delivered to them. It also seems clear that a shift is beginning to take place in terms of a heightened sensitivity to the ecology of our planet, partially in response to warnings about issues such as the imminent crisis of global warming by eminent Western scientists who stress the interconnectedness of all aspects of life. This is not a new phenomenon to indigenous people, who have only relatively recently been exposed to the Western scientific and philosophical paradigm that stresses separation and domination. Many of the elders have continued their traditional beliefs in spite of colonization and oppression. Many indigenous communities continue to seek the elders' advice in spite of mounting pressures to adopt solely technological solutions to human problems. There has been increasing recognition of indigenous perspectives on caring for the ecological health of our planet. Aboriginal elders from around the world have been sounding the alarm for some time, and have been joined by hundreds of esteemed scientists in warning us that our callous disregard for Mother Earth must cease if we are not to destroy ourselves.

While not a panacea for all of these ills, it is suggested that resilience theory is also fundamentally based upon the importance of relationship and connection to each other. Would it be possible to bring about enhanced communication and mutual respect between white caregivers and aboriginal communities by creating a common language based on concepts that unite more than divide? One can only imagine: a human services world where spirituality is imbued in day-to-day practice; where kinship and human connection are valued more than instrumental relationships and interactions; where respect for each other takes precedence in our actions rather than rigid practice standards; where each can take pride in his or her unique culture, tradition, and language rather than discarding them within one or two generations; where parenting is assumed to be a community responsibility rather than that of the nuclear family or a struggling single parent.

Perhaps by reflecting on these fundamental issues we can begin to make a difference, one child at a time, one family at a time, one community at a time. Finally, it seems to us that the hopes and aspirations of aboriginal people in our communities are much the same as those of people everywhere: a harmonious connection to each other, families to love and support, a spiritual connection of some kind, the opportunity to contribute and to learn new skills, a sense of self grounded in one's origins.

## REFERENCES

Aboriginal Healing Foundation. (1999). *Aboriginal Healing Foundation program handbook* (2nd ed.). Ottawa: Aboriginal Healing Foundation.

Aboriginal Justice Implementation Commission. (29 June 2001). *Final Report*. Retrieved 20 October 2006 from http://www.ajic.mb.ca/reports/final_toc.html.

Armitage, A. (1993). Family and child welfare in First Nation communities. In B. Wharf (Ed.), *Rethinking child welfare in Canada* (pp. 131–71). Toronto: McClelland & Stewart.

Atteneave, C. (1977). The wasted strengths of Indian families in the destruction of American Indian families. In Unger, S. (Ed.), *The destruction of American Indian families*. New York: Association on American Indian Affairs.

Baden, A.L. (2002). The psychological adjustment of transracial adoptees: An application of the cultural-racial identity model. *Journal of Social Distress and the Homeless, 11*(2), 167–91.

Bennett, M., & Blackstock, C. (2002). *A literature review and annotated bibliography focusing on aspects of aboriginal child welfare in Canada*. Retrieved 18 July 2005 from http://www.cecw-cepb.ca/DocsEng/RevisedLitReview.pdf.

Berry, S., & Brink, J. (2004). *Aboriginal cultures in Alberta: Five hundred generations*. Edmonton: Provincial Museum of Alberta.

Blackstock, C., Trocmé, N., & Bennett, M. (2004). Child welfare response to aboriginal and non-aboriginal children in Canada: A comparative analysis. *Violence against Women, 10*(8), 901–16.

Boldt, M. (1993). *Surviving as Indians: The challenge of self-government*. Toronto: University of Toronto Press.

Cajete, T.P.J. (2000). *Native science: Natural laws of interdependence*. Santa Fe, NM: Clear Light.

Canada. (1996). *Report of the Royal Commission on Aboriginal Peoples*, Vol. 3. Ottawa: Royal Commission on Aboriginal Peoples.

Chrisjohn, R.D., Young, S.L., & Marion, M. (1994). *The circle game: Shadows and substance in the Indian residential school experience in Canada*. Penticton, BC: Theytus.

Churchill, W. (1998). *A little matter of genocide: Holocaust and denial in the Americas 1492 to present*. Winnipeg: Arbeiter Ring.

Churchill, W. (1999). *Struggle for the land: Native North American resistance to genocide, ecocide, and colonization*. Winnipeg: Arbeiter Ring.

Davis, R., & Zannis, M. (1973). *The genocide machine in Canada*. Montreal: Black Rose Books.

Dion Stout, M. & Kipling, G. (2003). *Aboriginal people, resilience and the residential school legacy*. Ottawa: Aboriginal Healing Foundation.

First Nation Child & Family Caring Society of Canada. (2005). *Wen: de: We are coming to the light of day*. Ottawa: Author.

Haig-Brown, C. (1988). *Resistance and renewal*. Vancouver: Tillacum Library.

Health Canada. (2000). *Statistical profile on the health of First Nations in Canada*. Retrieved 19 February 2006 from http://www.hc-sc.gc.ca/fnih-spni/pubs/gen/stats_profil_e.html

Hudson, P. (1997). First Nations child and family services: Breaking the silence. *Canadian Ethnic Studies, 29*(1), 161–73.

Hunter, S., & Lewis, P. (2006). *Embedding culture for a positive future for Koori kids*. Paper presented at conference of Association of Children's Welfare Agencies, Sydney, Australia.

Indian and Eskimo Residential School Commission. (1930). *Report*. RG 10, Vol. 6730, File 169–62, pt. 2.

Indian and Northern Affairs Canada. (1994). Report of the Royal Commission on Aboriginal Peoples (RCAP). Available from http://www.ainc-inac.gc.ca/ch/rcap/sg/ci2_e.pdf.

Indian and Northern Affairs Canada. (2004). *Basic departmental data 2003*. Retrieved 18 July 2005 from http://www.ainc-inac.gc.ca/pr/sts/bdd03/bdd03_e.pdf.

Ing, N.R. (1991). The effects of residential schools on Native child-rearing practices. *Canadian Journal of Native Education, 18*(Supplement), 65–118.

LaBoucane-Benson, P. (2005). *A complex ecological framework of aboriginal family resilience*. Native Counseling Services of Alberta. First Nations – First thoughts. Centre of Canadian studies 30th anniversary conference, University of Edinburgh, 5 May 2005.

Lalonde, C. (2006). Identity formation and cultural resilience in aboriginal communities. In Flynn, R.J., Dudding, P., & Barber, J. (Eds.), *Promoting resilient development in young people receiving care: International perspectives on theory, research, practice & policy* (pp. 52–71). Ottawa: University of Ottawa Press.

Lee, K. (2000). *Urban poverty in Canada: A statistical profile*. Retrieved 19 February 2006 from http://www.ccsd.ca/pubs/2000/up/.

Lemkin, R. (1944). *Axis rule in occupied Europe: Laws of occupation – Analysis of government – Proposals for redress*. Washington, DC: Carnegie Endowment for International Peace, pp. 79–95.

Little Bear, L. (2000), Jagged world views colliding. In M. Battiste (Ed.), *Reclaiming indigenous voice and vision* (pp. 77–85). Vancouver: UBC Press.

McKenzie, B., & Hudson, P. (1985). Aboriginal children, child welfare, and the colonization of aboriginal children. In K.L. Levitt & B. Wharf (Eds.), *The challenge of child welfare* (pp. 125–41). Vancouver: UBC Press.

McRoy, R.G., Zurcher, L.A., Lauderdale, M.L., & Anderson, R.N. (1982). Self-esteem and racial identity in transracial and in racial adoptees. *Social Work, 27*(6), 522–6.

Milloy, J.S. (1999). *A national crime: The Canadian government and the residential school system, 1879–1986*. Winnipeg: University of Manitoba Press.

Native Child and Family Services of Toronto, Stevenato and Associates, & Budgell, J. (1999). *Repatriation of aboriginal families: Issues, models and a work-plan*. Retrieved 24 July 2005, from http://www.nativechild.org/native child2005/rep_rpt.pdf.

Neu, D., & Therrien, R. (2003). *Accounting for genocide: Canada's bureaucratic assault on aboriginal people*. Black Point, NS: Fernwood.

Richard, K. (2004). A commentary against aboriginal to non-aboriginal adoption. *First Peoples Child & Family Review, 1*(1), 101–9.

Rutter, M. (2001). Psychosocial adversity: Risk, resilience. In J. Richman & M. Fraser (Eds.), *The context of youth violence: Resilience, risk and protection* (pp. 13–42). Westport: Prager.

Sahtouris, E. (1992). The survival path: Cooperation between indigenous and industrial humanity. *Proceedings of the United Nations Policy Meeting on Indigenous Peoples*, Santiago, Chile. Available at www.http://www.ratical .com/LifeWeb/Articles/survival.html.

Sinclair, R. (2004). Aboriginal social work education in Canada: Decolonizing pedagogy for the seventh generation. *First Peoples Child & Family Review, 1*(1), 49–61.

Spicer, P. (1998). Drinking, foster care, and the intergenerational continuity of parenting in an urban Indian community. *American Indian Culture and Research Journal, 22*(4), 335–60.

Statistics Canada. (2004). *Aboriginal peoples of Canada*. Retrieved 23 October 2005 from http://www12.statcan.ca/english/census01/products/analytic/ companion/abor/can ada.cfm.

Stout, M.D., & Kipling, G. (2003). *Aboriginal people, resilience and the residential school legacy*. Retrieved 19 July 2005 from http://www.ahf.ca/newsite/ english/pdf/resilience.pdf.

Timpson, J. (1995). Four decades of literature on Native Canadian child welfare: Changing themes. *Child Welfare, 74*(3), 525–47.

Tinker, G. (1993). *Missionary conquest: The gospel and Native American cultural genocide*. Minneapolis, MN: Augsburg Fortress.

Trocmé, N., Knoke, D., & Blackstock, C. (2004). *Pathways to overrepresentation of aboriginal children in the child welfare system in Canada*. Retrieved 19 July 2005 from http://www.cecw-cepb.ca/DocsEng/PathwaysAug2004Trocme Blackstock.pdf.

Vaillant, G. (1993). *The wisdom of the ego*. Cambridge, MA: Harvard University Press.

Wesley-Esquimaux, C.C., & Smolewski, M. (2004). *Historic trauma and aboriginal healing*. Retrieved 19 July 2005 from http://www.ahf.ca/newsite/ english/pdf/historic_trauma.pdf.

York, G. (1990). *The dispossessed: Life and death in Native Canada*. London: Vintage UK.

# 13 Resilience in Japanese Youth

JULIE ANNE LASER

Resilience has been defined as 'patterns of positive adaptation in the context of significant risk or adversity' (Masten & Powell, 2003, p. 4). Current research has concentrated on assessing protective and risk factors that can either promote or deter normal growth and development. A large body of information has been gained regarding protective factors that the individual may possess or factors that are present in the developing person's environment that promote resilience. Simultaneously, risks factors have been assessed that compromise health or social functioning for the developing individual. Research from North America, Europe, Australia, and New Zealand has shown that there is a great deal of similarity between the risk factors from these areas, as well as protective factors important for Western populations (Butler, 1997; Farrington, 1995; Garmezy, 1985, 1993; Gore & Eckenrode, 1996; Kumpfer, 1999; Luthar, Cicchetti, & Becker, 2000; McMillan & Reed, 1994; Rutter, 1989; Sameroff, 2000; Ungar, 2004; Werner & Smith, 1992, 1998, 2001; Yule, 1992). However, little has been learned about resilience or protective or risk factors from a non-Western perspective.

The Japanese are perceived as a very resilient people given how they were able to reshape their nation into a world power after being decimated at the close of the Second World War. Many researchers have investigated the educational systems, business practices, advanced

The author would like to thank the Yasuda Foundation of Tokyo, Japan, for funding this research. The author also acknowledges the important contributions of the Japanese team: Dr Tom Luster, Toko Oshio, Dr Yasuo Tanaka, Shinichi Ninomiya, Hidemi Shinbo, Narumi Tsukui, Dr Murohashi Harumitsu, Dr Satoshi Miura, Dr Norihiro Ito, Teruko Ikehata, Reiko Morimura, Dr Akio Ishimoto, Yoshimi Akino, Dr Kazuo Suzuki, and Aoi Tamura.

technology, and mechanized industrialization that give Japan its advanced status. Within Japanese culture, there is high regard for individuals who persevere through difficult experiences with dignity. However, there has been no systematic investigation of individual and environmental protective factors that have undergirded such a seemingly resilient people. In fact, the words 'resilience,' 'protective factor,' and 'risk factor' did not exist in the Japanese language at the start of this study. Therefore, the purpose of this study was to investigate whether the protective factors that have been posited by researchers in North America, Europe, Australia, and New Zealand as positive influences on adolescent developmental outcomes in the face of risk, also act as protective factors in Japan. Likewise, risks that have been identified through research as particularly deleterious to Western populations were assessed to determine if they have similarly negative impacts on Japanese adolescent development. In addition, risks that have been viewed as a concern to Japanese youth workers and youth scholars in Japan were measured. In particular, this study examined the relationship between both protective factors and risk factors and six outcome variables: internalizing behavior, delinquency, drug use, alcohol use, tobacco use, and sexual behaviour.

## Methods

### Sample Selection

The sample for this study was selected from the Sapporo area, on the northern island of Hokkaido, Japan. Sapporo is the fifth-largest city in Japan, with a population of approximately 1.79 million. To obtain a diverse and fairly representative sample of post-secondary students in the Sapporo area, a range of vocational schools, colleges, and universities that differed in terms of size and prestige were targeted for inclusion in the study. Post-secondary institutions were the selected venue due to the high level of participation (74.1%) of Japanese youth in post-secondary education (Japan Information Network, 2004). Nine different post-secondary institutions participated in this study, including three vocational colleges (23.9% of the total respondents), two two-year colleges (41.8%), and four four-year universities (34.3%). Even though we were able to obtain high levels of completed surveys from vocational students, their institutions were often very small. Therefore, parity between the different types of institutions was not obtained. In all, 802 students participated in the study. Surveys were completed during class sessions and, with few exceptions, all students in the classrooms filled out the surveys.

*Participants*

Of the 802 respondents, 42.5% were female and 57.5% were male. There were a greater number of male respondents due to the fact that there were fewer females enrolled in the schools that had the largest numbers of respondents. The age of those surveyed was from eighteen to twenty-two years. However, most respondents (90.6%) were between eighteen and twenty years of age.

Slightly more than half (54.3%) of the respondents lived with their families. Less than 10% lived in dormitories, with the remainder living in apartments (35.7%) or with another family (.4%).

Nearly half (49.3%) of the respondents saw their mothers daily; however, only 1.5% saw their fathers daily. The educational attainment of over half of the mothers of the respondents (52.3%) was a high-school diploma, and the other mothers had some level of post-secondary training (28%). Among the fathers of the respondents, 41.5% had a high-school diploma and the rest had some post-secondary education (7%) or had completed a college degree (36.1%). Most respondents (92.4%) had at least one sibling.

*Measures*

Three instruments were used in the investigation: (1) the Laser Ecological Protective Factors for Young Adults, (2) the Life Events Survey for Japanese Youth, and (3) a demographic information questionnaire. The instruments were designed to assess a range of outcomes and contextual factors.

The Laser Ecological Protective Factors for Young Adults (LEPFYA) was designed to assess potential protective factors and has 151 items with responses provided on a five-point Likert scale. Questions regarding individual, family, and extra-familial protective factors are based on a careful review of the literature on protective factors that have been linked to positive individual outcomes for at-risk youth in North America, Europe, New Zealand, and Australia (Butler, 1997; Farrington, 1995; Garmezy, 1985, 1993; Gore & Eckenrode, 1996; Kumpfer, 1999; Luthar et al., 2000; McMillan & Reed, 1994; Rutter,

1989; Sameroff, 2000; Werner & Smith, 1992, 1998, 2001; Yule, 1992). The LEPFYA instrument was developed for this study in collaboration with Japanese researchers who reviewed and modified the wording of each item to ensure cultural relevance and understandability among Japanese youth. Back-translation was used to ensure proper translation. Both translators in this process were bilingual, had studied in both Japanese and American universities, and were familiar with the nuances of psychological language in both cultures.

The LEPFYA was used to assess the following internal protective factors: autonomy, self-efficacy, the creation of a personal myth, optimism, sense of humor, easy temperament, physical attractiveness, moral development, mental flexibility, emotional intelligence, spirituality, and perceptions of social support. Environmental variables assessed include: strength of partner relationship, size of social network, strength of supportive friends, sense of community, perceived collective efficacy, social capital, sense of school belonging, relationship with a school mentor, sense of family belonging, strong parental marriage, parents who impart positive values to their offspring, familial economic stability, strength of paternal relationship, and strength of maternal relationship.

The Life Events Survey for Japanese Youth (LESJY) measures potential risk factors through 114 items with responses given on a five-point Likert scale. The LESJY combines items from Stephen Small's Teen Assessment Project (TAP) Survey (Small & Luster, 1994) with items found in the 1997 National Longitudinal Survey of Youth Center for Human Resource Research, 2002) and items created by the investigator based on the risk literature in North America, Europe, New Zealand, and Australia (Butler, 1997; Farrington, 1995; Garmezy, 1985, 1993; Gore & Eckenrode, 1996; Kumpfer, 1999; Luthar et al., 2000; McMillan & Reed, 1994; Rutter, 1989; Sameroff, 2000; Werner & Smith, 1992, 1998, 2001; Yule, 1992). Also included in the LESJY are items that are of particular concern in Japan. Investigators from both Japan and the United States compiled the LESJY instrument.

A demographic information questionnaire was used to gather basic demographic information from respondents regarding age, sex, family structure, and academic background of respondents' parents. Both Japanese and American investigators also developed this questionnaire.

*Data Analysis*

Multiple regression analyses were used to analyse data. Regression equations for every outcome were run using the full sample and then run again by gender. Doing this made it possible to see if similar results were obtained for each gender or if results varied as a function of gender.

**Protective Factor Variables Assessed**

Twenty-six protective variables were assessed, including both individual and environmental factors. Individual protective factors are personal strengths in the social, emotional, cognitive, physical, or moral domains that promote positive developmental outcomes. Environmental protective factors are the aspects of people and the environments in which they spend time that are believed to promote positive development. Because youth reside in many environments, protective factors in the peer microsystem, neighborhood microsystem, school microsystem, and family microsystem were assessed.

**Risk Factor Variables Assessed**

Twenty-five risk factor variables were assessed that included both individual and environmental risk factors. Risk factors are aspects of either the individual or environment associated with problem outcomes in individuals. Examples of risk factors measured in this study include history of physical illness, history of physical abuse, history of sexual abuse, confusion over sexual orientation, alcohol use, living in an unsafe neighbourhood, being bullied at school, parental depression, witnessing domestic violence, personality differences with parents, parents who lack social support, parents who use alcohol, parents who are not aware of youth's activities, parents who are not available to the youth, parental favoritism of a sibling, frequent changes of residence, and living in a home that is overcrowded. Media influences that may be associated with problem outcomes in individuals were also assessed. In Japan, problematic media influences identified by Japanese youth workers and youth scholars were involvement in hip-hop culture and viewing sex and violence on television.

*Japanese Risk Factor Variables*

We also measured some constructs that have not been studied previously in Japan but have been discussed in the popular Japanese press as potential risk factors for their youth. These risk factors include involvement in *enjo kousai* (translated as school-girl prostitution, but school boys are also found to be involved), having a mother who is involved in *telekura* (telephone sex), having a father who frequents *fuzoku* (brothels), feelings of being undervalued due to gender, and gambling. These Japanese risk factors are often sensationalized in local media as societal evils that erode the healthy development of youth; however, there is virtually no scientific understanding of these social problems.

*Outcome Variables Assessed*

The study examined the relationship between protective and risk factors as well as six outcome variables: internalizing behaviour, delinquency, drug use, alcohol use, tobacco use, and sexual behaviour. Internalizing behaviour involves feelings of sadness, loneliness, suicidal ideation, and self-dislike. These problems may not be apparent to anyone other than the individual who experiences them, in contrast to externalizing problems. Delinquency outcomes include involvement with street gangs or *yakuza*, larceny, youth centre placement or police involvement, substance abuse, and risky sexual behaviour. Drug, alcohol, and tobacco use was assessed in terms of the frequency with which each substance is consumed. Risky sexual activity combines the number of sexual partners, age of first oral sex, and age of first sexual intercourse.

**Results**

Regression analysis identified protective and risk factors significant for each particular outcome (p = .05). Findings are presented in Table 1. Factors relevant to the full sample were designated with an *S*; to the female subsample, an *F*; and to the male subsample, an *M*.

*Risk and Protective Factors Relevant to the Total Sample*

Although there are many aspects of Japanese culture that are unique, there were many risk and protective factors that were similar to those

Table 1: Protective and risk factors that relate to outcomes

| Predictor | Internalizing behaviour | Delinquency | Drug use | Alcohol use | Tobacco use | Sexual activity | Intercourse age |
|---|---|---|---|---|---|---|---|
| **Internal/development factors** | | | | | | | |
| *Protective factors* | | | | | | | |
| Sense of autonomy | | | | | | -F M | -F |
| Self-efficacy | S F | | | | | | -F |
| Creation of a personal myth | | | | | | -F | -F |
| Optimism | | | | | | | |
| Sense of humor | | | -S -M | S | S M | F | F |
| Easy temperament | -S -F | | | | | | |
| Physical attractiveness | S M | | | | | | |
| Increased moral development | | | -S -M | | | | |
| Mental flexibility | | | | | | -S -M | |
| Emotional intelligence | -S -M | | | | -S -M | | |
| Sense of spirituality | | | | | | | |
| Perceived social support | | | | | | | |
| *Risk factors* | | | | | | | |
| History of physical illness | S F M | | S | | | | |
| Feel undervalued due to gender | | | | | -F | | |
| History of physical abuse | S M | | | | | | |
| History of sexual abuse | | | | | | S F M | S F M |
| *Enjo kousai* (Schoolgirl prostitution) | F | | S F M | | | | |
| Confusion over sexual orientation | S F M | | S | | | -S -M | -S -M |
| Alcohol Use | -S | S M | | | M | S F M | S F M |

Table 1 (continued)

| Predictor | Internalizing behaviour | Delinquency | Drug use | Alcohol use | Tobacco use | Sexual activity | Intercourse age |
|---|---|---|---|---|---|---|---|
| **Peer microsystem** | | | | | | | |
| *Protective factors* | | | | | | | |
| Strength of partner relationship | | | | | | S F M | S F M |
| Size of social network | | | | S F M | | | S F M |
| Strength of supportive friends | -M | | | | -F | | |
| **Neighbourhood microsystem** | | | | | | | |
| *Protective factors* | | | | | | | |
| Sense of community | | | | | | | |
| Perceived collective efficacy | | | | | | | |
| **Social Capital** | | | | | | | |
| *Risk factors* | | | | | | | |
| Believes neighbourhood not safe | | S F M | S F M | S F M | S F M | S F M | S F |
| **School microsystem** | | | | | | | |
| *Protective factors* | | | | | | | |
| Sense of school belonging | | | | | | | |
| Relationship with school mentor | | | | -F | | | |
| *Risk factors* | | | | | | | |
| Bullied | S F M | | | | | | |
| **Family Microsystem** | | | | | | | |
| *Protective factors* | | | | | | | |
| Sense of family belonging | | | | | | | |
| Strong parental marriage | | | | | | | |
| Positive parental values imparted | -F | | | -S -F-M | | | |
| Familial economic stability | | | | | -S | | |
| Strength of paternal relationship | | | | | | | |
| Strength of maternal relationship | | -S -M | | | | | |

Table 1  (continued)

| Predictor | Internalizing behaviour | Delinquency | Drug use | Alcohol use | Tobacco use | Sexual activity | Intercourse age |
|---|---|---|---|---|---|---|---|
| **Family Microsystem**  (continued) | | | | | | | |
| *Risk factors* | | | | | | | |
| Parental depression | S F M | | | | | | |
| Domestic violence witnessed | S M | S F M | | | | | |
| Personality differences with parents | | | | | | | |
| Parents lack social support | | S | | | | | |
| Parents use alcohol | | -S -M | | | | | |
| Parents not aware of respondent's activities | S F M | | | | | | |
| Parents not around respondent | | | | | F | | |
| Parental favoritism of sibling | S F | | | | | S F M | S M |
| Believe mom is involved in *telekura* (telephone sex) | F | S F M | S F M | | | | |
| Believe dad visits *fuzoku* (brothel) | | S M | S F | -S -F | | | |
| Parent gambles | | | | | | S F | S F |
| Frequency of moving | S F | M | | | -F | | |
| Home overcrowded | S M | | | | | | |
| **Media influences** | | | | | | | |
| Involved in Hip Hop culture | M | M | | | | | |
| View violence/sex on TV | M | S F M | | | S F | S F | S F |

*Note:* Beta values are p ≤ .05 to be assigned a letter.

of Western youth. Of the twenty-six Western protective factor variables investigated, fourteen were found to be predictive in the Japanese sample in at least one regression equation. Internal or development protective factors included autonomy, self-efficacy, creation of a personal myth, having a sense of humor, easy temperament, moral development, and emotional intelligence. The peer microsystem protective factors partner relationship, social network, and supportive friends were predictive of at least one outcome. No neighbourhood microsystem protective factor variables were significant predictors of the identified outcomes. The sole school microsystem protective factor variable that was predictive of healthy outcomes was a relationship with a school mentor. Finally, family microsystem protective variables included having parents who imparted values, family economic stability, and having a strong maternal relationship.

Regarding the twenty-five risk factor variables, all were significant in at least one regression equation with the exception of personality differences with parents. These findings highlight the similarity of harmful risks facing both Western and Japanese youth. Additionally, the risk factors identified in Japanese press, that is, involvement in *enjo kousai*, having a mother who is involved in *telekura*, having a father who visits *fuzoku*, feelings of being undervalued due to gender, and parental gambling, were all found to have a harmful effect on participating youth.

*Risk and Protective Factors Relevant to Gender*

Splitting the sample by gender was an important step in better illuminating the influence of the protective and risk factors. Size of social network, strength of partner relationship, and parents who imparted positive values appear to be important protective factors for both sexes for the same outcomes. The remaining eleven predictive protective factors varied by gender.

Relationships would have been masked if they had not been evaluated by gender. This underscores the relevance of protective factors to specific genders with regard to specific outcomes, rather than identifying protective factors as relevant to both sexes for particular outcomes. This insight could be used to create prevention programs that target gender-specific interventions. For example, the protective factor of sense of autonomy differed drastically for females and males. For females, the absence of a sense of autonomy was related to increased sexual activity. Conversely, for males, a strong sense of autonomy increased sexual activity. Therefore, for a frontline worker wishing to affect rates of adolescent sexual activity, offering support and education to foster a greater sense of autonomy in female youth may be an effective strategy to reduce rates of sexual activity. However, offering the same support and education to foster a greater sense of autonomy in male youth may have the opposite outcome.

There are some protective factors that when absent for a particular gender actually became risk factors. For example, for males, the lack of emotional intelligence and moral development were deleterious. However, the absence of these protective factors for females did not prove to be problematic. Therefore, creating programs that foster greater development of emotional intelligence and moral development may be particularly salient for male youth but may not be relevant for female youth. Similarly, for males the absence of a strong maternal relationship was important for delinquency. Thus, creating programs that build strong relationship between mothers and sons may provide a reduction in male delinquent behaviour.

On the other hand, for females the absence of a school mentor proved problematic, but not so for males. Hence, from an intervention perspective where funding will not stretch to providing mentors for all students, it may be most advantageous to supply mentors to female students. Likewise, lack of a personal myth was related to increased sexual behaviour in young women only. A personal myth serves as a lens by which the individual sees the world and her place in the world. The creation of a personal myth provides the individual with a goal to strive for and a future that holds better possibilities. The establishment of programs that support the exploration and conception of a personal myth for females may be particularly important in reducing rates of sexual activity.

Risk factors had a substantial overlap for females and males regarding outcomes. Variables relevant to both groups included having a history of physical illness, a history of sexual abuse, involvement in *enjo kousa*, confusion over sexual orientation, alcohol use, living in a neighbourhood that was not safe, being bullied, having a parent who was depressed, having a parent who was not aware of the youth's activities, having a parent who was not around, having a mother that was involved in *telekura*, and increased viewing of violence or sex on television.

However, the majority of risk factors (thirteen out of twenty-five) were predictive by gender for particular outcomes. This has important implications for understanding how particular outcomes are connected to specific risks. This finding reflects recently published research by the National Center on Addiction and Substance Abuse at Columbia University (Califano, 2003) that posits that the risks that were predictive of females' drug use were different from the risks associated with males' drug use. In the Japanese study, parental gambling, for example, was linked to increased female drug use but not male drug use. Additionally, having a history of physical abuse increased internalizing behavior in males but not females. Conversely, the risk factor of involvement in *enjo kousai* increased internalizing behaviours in females but not males. This research helps to support the creation of prevention and intervention programs that focus on the reduction of risks by gender — not only general risk factors for youth. For the outreach worker, familiarity with both general risk factors and risk factors that are particularly deleterious for each gender could greatly improve client assessment and intervention.

### Unique Constellations of Risk and Protective Factors

Interestingly, there was no particular protective or risk factor that proved to be a significant predictor for every outcome. Rather, certain risk or protective factors were associated with specific outcomes. Unfortunately for the interventionist, this means that there is no single 'magic' protective factor that could be augmented or one risk factor that could be reduced to improve client functioning. This being said, however, one risk variable (living in a neighbourhood that was not safe) was predictive in all the equations except for the internalizing behaviour outcome. This underscores the importance of the environment in which youth function and the impact that environment has on youths' externalizing behaviour.

### Conclusion

This study highlights the relevance not only of culture in understanding protective and risk factors associated with youth outcomes, but of gender as well. Findings show that no particular protective or risk factor variable is predictive for all outcomes, and the combination of protective factor variables and risk factor variables is distinct for each outcome by gender. These connections between individual protective and risk factors are reflective of the review of resilience literature done by Luthar et al. (2000). The authors concluded that resilience is often limited to a particular domain rather than across all areas of an individual's life, preventing a 'one size fits all' approach to interventions and the grouping of variables for outcomes. For the interventionist, depending on the outcome she or he is wishing to address, there may be particular risk and protective factors that need to be assessed and either augmented or reduced; however, a particular focus on a specific outcome may improve functioning regarding that outcome but not necessarily across all outcomes for the individual.

## REFERENCES

Butler, K. (1997). The anatomy of resilience. *Networker, 2*, 22–31.

Califano, J. (2003). *The formative years: Pathways to substance abuse among girls and young women ages 8–22.* National Center on Addiction and Substance Abuse (CASA). New York: Columbia University.

Center for Human Resource Research. (2002). *NLSY97 user's guide.* Columbus: Ohio State University.

Farrington, D. (1995). The development of offending and antisocial behaviour from childhood: Key findings from the Cambridge Study in delinquent development. *Journal of Child Psychology and Psychiatry, 360*(6), 929–64.

Garmezy, N. (1985). *Stress-resistant children: The search for protective factors.* Elmsford, NY: Pergamon.

Garmezy, N. (1993). Children in poverty: Resilience despite risk. *Psychiatry, 56*, 127–36.

Gore, S., & Eckenrode, J. (1996). Context and process in research on risk and resilience. In R. Haggerty, L. Sherrod, N. Garmezy, & M. Rutter (Eds.), *Stress, risk, and resilience in children and adolescents* (pp. 19–63). Cambridge: Cambridge University Press.

Japan Information Network. (2004). *Rate of advancement to post-secondary education.* Retrieved 4 September 2006 from (http://www.webjpn.org/stat-ndex.html).

Kumpfer, K. (1999). Factors and processes contributing to resilience: The resilience framework. In M. Glantz & J. Johnson (Eds.), *Resilience and development: Positive life adaptations* (pp. 179–224). New York: Kluwer.

Luthar, S., Cicchetti, D., & Becker, B. (2000). The construct of resilience: A critical evaluation and guideline for future work. *Child Development, 71,* 543–62.

Masten, A., & Powell, J. (2003). A resilience framework for research, policy, and practice. In S.S. Luthar (Ed.), *Resilience and vulnerability: Adaptation in the context of childhood adversities* (pp. 1–25). New York: Cambridge University Press.

McMillan, J., & Reed, D. (1994). At-risk students and resiliency: Factors contributing to academic success. *The Clearing House, 67* (3), 137–40.

Rutter, M. (1989). Pathways from childhood to adult life. *Journal of Child Psychology and Psychiatry, 30*(1), 23–51.

Sameroff, A. (2000). Ecological perspectives on developmental risk. In J. Osofsky & H. Fitgerald (Eds.), *WAIMH handbook of infant mental health* (Vol. 4, pp. 1–33). New York: John Wiley & Sons.

Small, S., & Luster, T. (1994). Adolescent sexual activity: An ecological, risk-factor approach. *Journal of Marriage and Family, 56,* 181–92.

Ungar, M. (2004). *Nurturing hidden resilience.* Toronto: University of Toronto Press.

Werner, E., & Smith, R. (1992). *Overcoming the odds: High risk children from birth to adulthood.* Ithaca, NY: Cornell University Press.

Werner, E., & Smith, R. (1998). *Vulnerable but invincible.* New York: Adams, Bannister and Cox.

Werner, E., & Smith, R. (2001). *Journeys from childhood to midlife.* Ithaca, NY: Cornell University Press.

Yule, W. (1992). Resilience and vulnerability in child survivors of disasters. In B. Tizard & V. Varma (Eds.), *Vulnerability and resilience in human development* (pp. 182–97). London: Jessica Kingsley.

# 14 Chinese Approaches to Understanding and Building Resilience in At-Risk Young People: The Case of Hong Kong

FRANCIS WING-LIN LEE AND KENNEDY KWONG-HUNG NG

Resilience, commonly defined as the innate ability of human beings to overcome adversity, has attracted increasing attention during recent decades. Literally, resilience means the ability of a spring to return to its original shape after being stressed (Bernard, 1991; Flach, 1997; F.W.L.Lee, 2005). This concept is applied to people who are believed to have a similar ability to recover after facing adversity in their own lives (Glantz & Johnson, 1999; Werner & Smith, 1992). A resilient person is one who shows characteristics such as social competence (the ability to seek appropriate help from peers and adults), problem-solving skills, confidence, autonomy to plan and act independently, a sense of purpose, and belief in the future. Resilience results from long-term, systematic change that is reflective of the communities in which young people live and work (Wolin & Wolin, 1993).

Different cultures have different beliefs in the ability of their people to counter adversities. As Lau and Yeung (1996) observe, 'Developmental researchers who have worked in different cultures have also become convinced that human functioning cannot be separated from the cultural and immediate context in which children develop' (p. 29). Highly influenced by Confucianism (Chue, 2000; Creel, 2003; Lu, 1997), Chinese people have their own interpretation of this innate ability of human beings. This chapter will thus begin with an introduction to the Chinese understanding of resilience, followed by an examination of how resilience is fostered and enhanced among the at-risk youth population of Hong Kong, over 90% of whom are Chinese. Specifically, we will discuss the Understanding the Adolescent Project, a government-subsidized program for promoting resilience of at-risk young people. We will look at its implementation, plans for future development, and main limitations. Finally, we will offer recommendations on how to further enhance resilience in Chinese youth in general.

## Conceptions of Resilience in Chinese Culture

As children develop and grow, their belief systems are gradually established. Pepitone (1994) explains beliefs as 'concepts about the nature, the causes, and the consequences of things, persons, events and processes' that are socially constructed parts 'of a culture and have guided the socialization of those who share that culture' (p. 140). Shek (2004) reminds us that it is 'important to ask how cultural beliefs about adversity are related to resilience' (p. 64). According to Lau and Yeung (1996, p. 32), 'Chinese perspectives on child development are more like philosophies than theories of nature.'

In Chinese, resilience is translated as *Kwong yee lik*, meaning 'the ability to resist adversity.' It is believed that everyone has the ability to face adversity in their lives and to self-heal. This belief is best illustrated by Chinese proverbs that indicate strength in people. The Confucian proverb *Yee chin chau chuen*, for example, means 'to strive for survival under adversity.' Similarly, *Yee chin zee chang* means people have the ability of 'self-strengthening in adversity' in order to counteract unfavourable situations.

One has to understand that beliefs revealed by these proverbs are deeply embedded in the value system of the Chinese and penetrate deeply into the ways Chinese people face personal challenges, especially those who experience chronic and acute stressors throughout their lives. In constructing the Chinese Beliefs about Adversity Scale (CBAS), for example, Shek (2004, p. 70) has suggested that expressions such as *Chi de ku zhong ku, fang wei ren shang ren* (Hardship increases stature), *You zhi zhe shi jing cheng* (When there is a will there is a way), *Chi yao you heng xin, tie zhu mo cheng zhen* (If you work hard enough, you can turn an iron rod into a needle), and *Ren ding sheng tian* (Man is the master of his own fate) demonstrate the capacity for resilience in Chinese culture.

## The Need to Build Resilience among Young People in Hong Kong

Hong Kong is a Special Administration Region of the People's Republic of China (PRC). Previously a British colony, it had its sovereignty returned to the PRC in July 1997. Hong Kong has a population of close to seven million people of which more than 30% are below twenty-four years of age (Information Services Department, 2004). Since the change of sovereignty, young people in Hong Kong have experienced several challenges, including political uncertainty, economic hardship, interpersonal problems, and cultural challenges (Choi et al. 2003; Shek, 1995). These psychosocial stressors have increased the vulnerability of young people to mental health problems. Shek (1996) has reported that between 8.1% and 23.7% of adolescents in Hong Kong demonstrate psychological or psychiatric morbidity. A more recent study has revealed that the younger generation of Hong Kong has encountered serious mental and psychological health problems related to personal, familial, and social factors (CHEI IP, 2002). Au and Tang (2003) have pointed out that mental health problems faced by Hong Kong adolescents include substance abuse, eating disorders, Triad (gang) membership, unplanned pregnancies, suicide or suicidal ideation, depression, violent tendencies, retreat and alienation, low self-image, and poor school performance and truancy. These studies indicate that a considerable number of adolescents in Hong Kong are at risk physically, psychologically, and socially. Read with a focus on health rather than illness, these findings indicate the need to enhance resilience among young people in Hong Kong.

### Building of Resilience in At-Risk Young People in Practice: Understanding the Adolescent Project

In spite of cultural beliefs relating to the innate resilience of the Chinese community, there is little emphasis on promoting such ability within individuals. Consequently, when the concepts of resilience are put into practical terms, Western theories have to be borrowed to implement health-related theories. Although Chinese culture has, as noted, emphasized the innate abilities of individuals to overcome adversity, borrowing Western ideas of resilience has shifted the focus to a more ecological perspective on successful human development. To enhance the resilience of people, one must help develop both the internal and external resources available to individuals (Henderson, Bernard, & Sharp-Light, 2000; Krovetz, 1998). Internal resources include competency (C), belonging (B), and optimism (O); external resources include participation (P), expectation (E), and support (S). Such an approach is in line with the Confucian proverbs of *Yee chin chau chuen*, meaning 'to strive for survival under adversity,' and *Yee chin zee chang*, meaning 'self-strengthening in adversity,' reflecting the need to develop ones' internal resources so as to counteract unfavourable situations. Furthermore, building a harmonious relationship with the surroundings (environment) has always been a main teaching of Confucianism (Lu, 1997).

According to Hepworth, Rooney, and Larsen (1997), human existence presents 'a broad array of problems of living' where 'no single approach or practice model is sufficiently comprehensive to adequately address them all' (p. 16). A variety of interventions and practice models are therefore required based on the principles of equifinality (i.e., different intervention models providing different pathways to the same destination) and multifinality (interventions having the same starting point but arriving at different outcomes) (Hepworth et al., 1997). The Understanding the Adolescent Project (UAP) could be regarded as one entry point for practicing systemic intervention with youth at risk, incorporating ecological systems theory and life model theory.

Ecological systems theory is a 'unifying framework' for integrating different intervention theories (Hepworth et al., 1997). It is developed from 'a biological theory which proposes that all organisms are systems, composed of sub-systems and are in turn part of super-systems' (Payne, 1991, p. 135). The characteristics of systems theory include:

1 Non-summativity: the whole is more than the sum of its parts
2 Boundary work: systems are organized by boundaries
3 Reciprocity: changes in one subsystem will effect changes in others
4 Input: feeding energy into the system for maintenance
5 Entropy: system dismissing unless energy is input
6 Equilibrium: system maintaining its stability by output (Payne, 1991).

The life model theory of Germain and Gitterman (1980) suggests that individuals are continuously adapting to and interacting with their environment. They change and are changed by their environment in order to maintain equilibrium via the process of 'reciprocal adaptation.' Individuals try their utmost to maintain a good fit with their environment by giving input to their context physically or psychologically or both, and attempting to divert stress arising from the system itself. Stress may result from life transitions, environmental pressures, and interpersonal process. Individuals cannot function efficiently, however, in social contexts where resources for maintaining adaptation and influencing the environment are scarce. From this perspective, the ultimate goal of UAP is to help vulnerable at-risk youth to adapt and influence the environment through enabling, teaching, facilitating, mediating, advocating, and organizing (Payne, 1991).

Interventions for at-risk youth should therefore provide a continuum of interventions that affect behaviour 'within an individual ... between the individual and the environment or within the individual and the environment, or within the environment' (Parsons, Hernandez, & Jorgensen, 1988, pp. 417–18). The UAP is designed to address issues facing youth at risk as they adapt to their environment. Often, these youth do not have satisfactory connections with systems such as families, schools, and communities. Connecting youth with such systems and exploring resources within interactions and transitions in the community can result in personal and interpersonal empowerment. Building a culture of resilience in families, schools, and related communities is the main goal of the UAP.

Building on this systemic view of people and their environments, program elements of the UAP include boundary work that promotes the interface and exchanges between individuals and their environment (DuBois & Miley, 2005). That said, youth at risk need helpers who work collaboratively and employ 'multi-level systems intervention' (Parsons et al., 1988).

*From Theory to Practice*

In July 1994, the Working Group on Services for Youth at Risk of the Social Welfare Department (SWD) of the Hong Kong government commissioned a joint project team comprising Breakthrough Ltd., a nongovernmental organization, and the Faculty of Medicine, Chinese University of Hong Kong, to carry out the UAP. The goal of the project was to develop 'a comprehensive screening tool for early identification of development needs of young people [in secondary schools] for early intervention with appropriate primary preventive programs so as to prevent the emergence of behavioural problems' (Lau, 2003, p. 94). The UAP employed the concept of resilience enhancement in its intervention with identified adolescents, borrowing theoretical and operational concepts from the West and combining them with Chinese under-standings of adolescent development. The UAP was conducted in Shatin region (a satellite town in the New Territories region of Hong Kong), from July 1994 to the end of 2000, with five million Hong Kong dollars in financial support from the Lotteries Fund. The project was launched in three phases: UAP1, UAP2, and UAP3.

*Brief Review of the Implementation of UAP in Hong Kong*

During UAP1 (July 1994–January 1997), a screening questionnaire for identifying at-risk adolescents was developed, the 'Hong Kong Students Information Form' (HKSIF). The instrument comprised a student version (S) and a teacher version (T).

UAP2 (February 1997–June 1999) involved validating the HKSIF and developing primary preventative programs based on the concept of resilience. The project was then started in twelve secondary schools as part of a pilot implementation and evaluation of the programs (including workshop and small-group activities).

UAP3 (July 1999–December 2000) involved refinement of the programs developed in UAP2 for future territory-wide implementation. A relatively small-scale project was also started in July 1999, to develop the conceptual framework of resilience in order to prepare for large-scale implementation.

During 2001 and 2002, 150 secondary schools in Hong Kong implemented the UAP program. Each school was subsidized with one hundred thousand Hong Kong dollars for their participation in the project. While the UAP in secondary schools ended in 2005 owing to the depletion of funds, the Education and Manpower Bureau (EMB) (a policy branch in the government) started full implementation of UAP in all primary schools during 2004–2005, subsidizing each school with sixty-six thousand Hong Kong dollars.

An evaluation report of the UAP was compiled during 2001–2002. The report demonstrated that various stakeholders participating in the UAP, such as students, parents, teachers, and social workers, found the project useful in enhancing different aspects of student resilience (Lau, 2003). Specifically, prominent and sustainable improvement of students' 'anger management, resolution of conflicts, communication and relationship with teachers, classroom performance, communication skill and social relationship' (Lau, 2003, p. 47) was demonstrated.

*Structural Components of the UAP*

### GOALS AND NEEDS
The UAP served as a tailor-made primary prevention program for fostering resilience in youth and preventing them from developing at-risk behavior (Lau, 2003). The goal of the UAP was to facilitate resilience in youth with regard to three operational components: competence (C), optimism (O), and belonging (B).

### FORM OF BENEFIT
The UAP was used to train youth to deal with adverse life circumstances. Specifically, it aimed to 'protect them from developing psychiatric problems despite growing up in adverse social circumstances' (Lau, 2003, p. 7). The conceptual framework of UAP also worked on improving the school, family, and mental health situations of young people by enhancing the resilient culture of school and family (Lau, 2003). Both individual and community components of resilience enhancement were designed to obtain long-term benefits for participants, and their families and schools.

### ELIGIBILITY
The UAP recruited at-risk secondary-one (grade 7, aged thirteen to fourteen years) students as participants. According to the SWD user's manual, secondary schools could apply to join the project on a voluntary basis. Participating schools would receive funding upon the approval of their application. The respective school social workers would work with school teachers to determine the final list of participating students, who would then complete the HKSIF-S form for screening.

### LEVEL OF ADMINISTRATION OF UAP
The Youth Section of SWD and the Regional Strategic and Planning Group were responsible for coordinating and assisting secondary schools in implementing UAP (SWD, 2004). School social workers became team leaders and coordinators for the UAPs in their schools, responsible for forming task forces of the projects by recruiting class, counselling, and disciplinary teachers in schools. They also had to perform administrative work and were responsible for the coordination between the schools and SWD, including finding agents to deter-

mine the contents of the project, as well as executing and monitoring progress of the project.

## Implementing the UAP

Using Dolfoff and Feldstein's (2003) schema for examining social welfare programs, factors necessary for the successful implementation of the UAP include adequacy, financing, coherence, and latent consequences.

### Adequacy

Adequacy consists of horizontal adequacy and vertical adequacy. Horizontal adequacy refers to the coverage of the target population, whereas vertical adequacy is defined as in-depth sufficient coverage of the recipient of the target population (Dolfoff & Feldstein, 2003).

Horizontal adequacy was achieved by implementing the UAP in all secondary schools within Hong Kong. This endeavour was facilitated by non-government organizations (NGOs) and funding from SWD starting in 2001 (Lau, 2003). As previously mentioned, funding was allocated if the school's application was approved, and at-risk youth were identified by means of the screening tools (HKSIF-S & T). Although all schools could potentially receive funding, SWD provided only enough funding to serve approximately twenty to thirty students at each school, limiting the number of at-risk students being supported. Funding allocation may, therefore, not always have been sufficient to cover all the at-risk students identified. As such, there is a need to modify the UAP's funding mechanism so as to incorporate all youth in need, enhancing horizontal adequacy. The project should be universal and preventive in principles rather than selective and remedial.

Vertical adequacy of UAP was achieved through implementation of a series of activities aimed at fostering youth resilience. These activities included an opening ceremony, a day camp, a three-day two-night camp, some community services, a parent-child camp, sessions for sharing and review, a final review session, and a closing ceremony (Lau, 2003). Although these activities formed the actual program activities of the UAP, from the experience of the workers the hardware, software, and humanware (therapeutic use of workers' selves) were vital to achieving vertical adequacy of UAP.

Hardware refers to equipment, facilities, venues, and staff for technical support. The basic framework of UAP activities was closely related to group work and adventure-based counselling (ABC), requiring adventure equipment, training facilities, and outdoor facilities or campsites. Together with this, well-trained staff with adequate knowledge and skills for running the programs were required.

Workshops, day camps, and training camps to improve participants' sense of competence, belongingness, and optimism were designed by means of the UAP-enhanced software support. Development of the UAP's user's manuals and train-the-trainer program was essential for successful implementation of related components of various initiatives. These manuals guided workers through implementation of the programs in accordance with the project's conceptual framework, introducing the background, conceptual framework, and implementation mechanism. Manuals also contained program session plans for various proposed activities. Manuals were complemented with train-the-trainer programs, including training camps and workshops, for social workers and teachers involved, organized by the SWD. Actual training was carried out through a government–community agency partnership with Breakthrough Ltd.

The user's manuals were important to social workers and teachers, as they helped to clarify and guide implementation as well as evaluate different aspects of the UAP. However, professionals assigned with carrying out the program elements reported that the manuals were too brief and not detailed enough to help them to conduct the programs. A step-by-step user's guide incorporating more practical skills with various program options that assists smoother implementation of the program by practitioners should be developed. Despite this shortcoming, Lau (2003) argues that UAP's train-the-trainer program was crucial for helping workers to understand the project's conceptual framework, objectives, and practical skills and to transform the concepts into practice, enhancing enthusiasm and commitment of workers to carry out the intervention.

Humanware is 'the therapeutic use of self through the integrating of personal-self, professional-self, and technical-self of the workers' (Edwards & Bess, 1998, p. 89). The proper use of self by a social worker can enhance the therapeutic relationship with clients, thus further enhancing the therapeutic process. As Satir (1987) states, 'use of the self by the therapist is an integral part of the therapeutic process and it should be used consciously for treatment purposes' (p. 24).

Similarly, Coady and Wolgien (1996) comment that 'the most important factor [a worker brings] into therapy is [him or herself]' (p. 337). The UAP is therefore highly dependent on workers' involvement. As we learned, nurturing humanware is critical to the success of any youth-at-risk programs. Preparing humanware takes time, and should therefore be included in the strategic planning for training and developing workers for youth-at-risk intervention programs such as the UAP.

## Long-Term Strategic Financing

To ensure the success of primary prevention programs, which should be developmental in nature, there is a need for both strategic planning and long-term commitment. Therefore, strategic financing coupled with a solid youth developmental policy is needed for programs such as UAP if they are to be sustainable. The funding of the UAP was one hundred thousand Hong Kong dollars per year for the fiscal year 2001–2004, after which it was reduced to forty thousand Hong Kong dollars for 2004–2005. To ensure smoother, long-term implementation of the project, long-term financial commitment on the part of the government is required. Unfortunately, even with the advocacy of concerned bodies, no improvement has been seen.

## Coherence between Government Departments

Different UAPs in primary and secondary schools were conducted by different departments of the government. SWD was responsible for secondary school UAPs, while EMB took care of the primary school UAPs. Experience gleaned from the project gave rise to various questions regarding the disconnection between service providers in the delivery of UAP. The effectiveness of two or more different government departments handling the same project, even when different 'client communities' are being served, is questionable. Under such conditions, the challenge of transferring learning between the two different departments persisted, along with the risk of resource overlap and waste. There was also the challenge of reconciling different strategies for youth at risk as evidenced by the service perspectives of EMB and SWD. Although these strategies are of great importance to the success of the UAP, effective program administration would encourage the exchange of acquired wisdom. This is more easily facilitated if concurrent projects are organized and carried out by one department.

*Latent Consequences*

The UAP reinforced the current phenomenon of low-paid, short-term contract work or part-time jobs in the social services sector of Hong Kong. Worse still, there is no long-term planning for youth-at-risk services from the SWD, meaning that NGOs can only offer short-term jobs on a contract or a part-time basis. As a result, the UAP had both a high staff turnover rate and incorporated many inexperienced social workers in frontline work, ultimately affecting the quality and fidelity of programs offered to youth. Owing to the limited financial resources for various NGOs under the existing lump sum grant system in Hong Kong, successful bidding of the UAP was, however, a good way of obtaining money for the NGOs.

*Recommendations for Implementing UAP*

### EMPLOYING A STRENGTH PERSPECTIVE

UAP aims to empower youths by building their strengths and concept of self. Traditional Chinese beliefs stress human strengths when facing adversities, making this facet relevant to youth in Hong Kong. Such emphasis is seen in expressions such as *You zhi zhe shi jing cheng* (When there is a will there is a way) and *Chi yao you heng xin, tie zhu mo cheng zhen* (If you work hard enough, you can turn an iron rod into a needle) (Shek, 2004). In line with these beliefs, social workers responsible for implementing UAP should adopt a strength perspective and look at the UAP participants 'in the light of their capacities, talents, competencies, possibilities, visions, values, and hopes' (Saleebey, 1996, p. 297). Workers are encouraged to respect participants' uniqueness and have more appreciation for their positive attributes and capabilities.

### ADOPTING A HOLISTIC APPROACH

Incorporating a holistic approach, mirroring resilience theory as well as the Confucian emphasis on whole-person development (Lu, 1997), the programming of UAP requires social workers to be sensitive to participants' behaviour, emotion, cognition, and sense of inner selves. Workers attempt to help individuals to change positively by observing their needs and using the constructed experiences of participants as teachable moments. The goal is to allow participants opportunities to experience 'challenge by choice,' through making their own decisions (Schoel, Prouty, & Radcliffe, 1988).

### USING ADVENTURE-BASED COUNSELLING

The employment of ABC in UAP is prevalent and should be continued. The main goal of ABC is to improve the self-concept of participants (Schoel et al., 1988) by helping them become aware of their own strengths and weaknesses, developing a sense of competence and belongingness, and developing an optimistic view of problem solving. UAP workers design problem-solving programs suitable for participants, allowing them a sense of peak experience, personal breakthroughs, and a feeling of success or satisfaction upon completion of programs. A goal of ABC is to help participants transfer their learning to their everyday lives through experience. From an ABC perspective, adventure activities for UAP should be well-designed with proper sequencing (briefing, leading, and debriefing), where the meaning and relevance of the activities to participants' everyday lives can be explored (Schoel et al., 1988). During adventurous activities, for example, participants are faced with personal challenges by struggling within the 'groan zone' (an area of struggle within a person) (Luckner & Nadler, 1997). During this time, there will be moments in which participants need group support and trust before they are able to face challenges set before them by group facilitators. However, facilitators should take care during this time regarding the level of challenge participants face. Activities should be paced to match participants' needs and competencies.

### FORMING PARENT-TEACHER SELF-HELP COMMUNITIES

Workshops and activities for teachers and parents involved in UAP require some structural improvements. For these components to be more effective, integrated work between teachers and parents needs to be established, incorporating long-term cooperation. As the UAP terminates at the end of the school year, there is a need for working teams (teachers, school workers, and parents) to form parent-teacher self-help communities to ensure continuous care of young people through vacation periods. This arrangement would help participants of UAP to maintain enhanced resilience over time. Such parent-teacher associations may organize many therapeutic programs for participating youth. If the skills and talents of parents are incorporated into the development of programs for students, both parents and students could be empowered. A community care model of nurturing social networks and volunteer services within the communities aimed at marginalized groups, such as children in poverty, may assist in achieving these outcomes. This model promotes two central tenets of Chinese culture: self-help and care by community members on a volunteer basis. Depending on the level of professional participation, a community care model may take on three forms: permanent professional participation, professional initiation and support for a period of time, and no or little professional participation (Popple, 1995).

There is also a need for parents, teachers, school social workers, and school principals involved in UAP to form long-term self-help groups employing the community care approach to incorporate young people and their parents via meaningful participation. The parent-teacher self-help communities should place emphasis on nurturing personal efficacy, enhancing personal competence, developing personal consciousness, establishing personal strengths, and applying personal power (Miley, 1999). The parent-teacher community is the best environment for individuals to learn, re-learn, or un-learn their socializing techniques. For group members who may not have good socializing skills, the group is a good forum for them to observe and practise new skills. Making use of imitative behaviour and interpersonal learning, group members learn functional interaction skills within their community. This learning can also promote understanding emotion, cognition, and behaviour within the group stemming from dynamics that may originate from participating youths' own families and life experience. In this way, the parent-teacher community provides youth an arena for healing, personal growth, and enhanced social functioning through a supporting network (Yalom & Leszcz, 2005).

## Conclusion: Building Resilience in Young People

In order to help build resilience of young people – especially those who are regarded as at risk – it is important to help them develop their strengths as well as to consider the elements of the broader systems with which they interact. One method to develop their potential is to actively engage them in decision making and work roles (F.W.L. Lee,

2005). Cultivation of a supportive environment is also important to enhance resilience. Programs like UAP tackle both aspects of individuals, developing their internal and external resources (Henderson et al., 2000). Specifically, UAP was designed to develop young people's internal resources. It also sought to provide opportunities to develop external resources, so that youth are able to receive appropriate support and guidance when needed.

Our experience has shown that to promote resilience of young people by means of activities associated with the UAP, several principles should be observed (A.T.S. Lee, 2003; F.W.L. Lee, 2005). These principles include program, process, people, and partnerships.

The best design of programs or activities would promote the development of internal and external resources associated with survival. Programs should, therefore, offer opportunities for youth themselves to engage in the decision-making process to ensure that their needs are met in ways relevant to them.

Programs should focus on encouraging young people to reflect on the process of activities, rather than solely emphasizing outcomes. Specifically, participants should be encouraged to reflect on what they have learned throughout the activities. With adventure-based counselling, for example, the debriefing processes following participation in the related activities are the main emphasis of exercises in which reflections on experiences are stressed.

Belief in the strengths of young people and commitment to lead them to engage in the programs are essential if workers are to be effective leaders. The leaders should also be competent to assist participants through the programs and activities as well as guide their personal reflections.

Finally, genuine and open communication between leaders and participants is an essential and effective means of contributing to increased resilience of participants. The leaders and the participants are equal partners, sharing the same context, programs, and activities. This partnership experience provides a meaningful basis for leaders to guide participants' reflections, which are essential in UAP.

Although the operation of the UAP draws its theoretical framework from Western theories, traditional Chinese beliefs have put much emphasis on innate human abilities to face and overcome adversities. Such a cultural approach is well matched with aspects of Western resilience theories. Accordingly, with a genuine will to enhance the resilience of at-risk youth, it is believed that an appropriate integration of traditional Chinese beliefs and Western theories on resilience is possible. Furthermore, if appropriate attention is paid to program limitations outlined in this chapter, positive development of at-risk youth in Hong Kong can be promoted through such programs.

## REFERENCES

Au, R.C.K., & Tang, A.C.W. (2003). Concepts, studies and intervention models of resilience. In P.Y.W. Choi, R.C.K. Au, A.C.W. Tang, L.S.M. Sum, J.S.Y. Tang, J.F.M. Choi, & A.T.S. Lee (Eds.), Making of 'young unfallen man': Handbook for families and schools to build up resilience of young people (pp. 34–57). Hong Kong: Breakthrough Ltd. (in Chinese)

Bernard, B. (1991). Fostering resiliency in kids: Protective factors in the family, school, and community. Minneapolis, MN: National Resilience Resource Center, University of MInnesota.

CHEHP (Centre for Health Education and Health Promotion). (2002). Health crisis of our new generation: Surveillance on youth health risk behaviors. Hong Kong: Centre for Health Education and Health Promotion, Chinese University of Hong Kong.

Choi, P.Y.W., Au, R.C.K., Tang, A.C.W., Sum, L.S.M., Tang, J.S.Y., Choi, J.F.M., & Lee, A.T.S. (Eds.) (2003). Making of 'young unfallen man': Handbook for families and schools to build up resilience of young people. Hong Kong: Breakthrough Ltd. (in Chinese)

Chue, H.T. (Ed.). (2000). Confucionism in Chinese culture. Selangor Darul Shsan, Malaysia: Pelanduk.

Creel, H.G. (2003). Confucius and the Chinese way (X. Wang, Trans.). Taipei: Wei bo wen hua guo ji chu ban you xian gong si. (in Chinese)

Coady, N.F., & Wolgien, C.S. (1996). Good therapists' view of how they are helpful. Clinical Social Work Journal, 24(3), 333–52.

Dolfoff, R., & Feldstein, D. (2003). Understanding social welfare (6th ed.). New York: Allyn & Bacon.

DuBois, B., & Miley, K.K. (2005). Social work: An empowering profession (5th ed.). Boston: Allyn & Bacon.

Edwards, J.K., & Bess, J.M. (1998). Developing effectiveness in the therapeutic use of self. Clinical Social Work Journal, 26(1), 89–105.

Flach, F. (1997). Resilience: How to bounce back when the going gets tough! New York: Hatherleigh.

Germain, C.B., & Gitterman, A. (1980). The life model of social work practice. New York: Columbia University Press.

Glantz, M.D., & Johnson, J.L. (Eds.). (1999). *Resilience and development: Positive life adaptations*. New York: Kluwer Academic/Plenum.

Henderson, N., Bernard, B., & Sharp-Light, N. (Eds.). (2000). *Mentoring for resiliency.*Berkeley, CA: Resiliency in Action, Inc.

Hepworth, D.H., Rooney, R.H., & Larsen, J.A. (1997). *Direct social work practice: Theory and skills* (5th ed.). Pacific Grove: Brooks/Cole.

Information Services Department, HKSAR. (2004). *Hong Kong 2003*. Hong Kong: Government Printer

Krovetz, M.L. (1998). *Fostering resiliency: Expecting all students to use their minds and hearts well*. Thousand Oaks, CA: Corwin.

Lau, J. (2003). *Report on evaluation of the nderstanding the Adolescent Project (UAP) in secondary schools 2001/02*. Hong Kong: Centre for Clinical Trials and Epidemiological Research, School of Public Health, Chinese University of Hong Kong.

Lau, S., & Yeung, P.P.W. (1996). Understanding Chinese child development: The role of culture in socialization. In S. Lau (Ed.), *Growing up the Chinese way: Chinese child and adolescent development* (pp. 29–44). Hong Kong: Chinese University Press.

Lee, A.T.S. (2003). *Notes on lecture on resilient youth work.* Unpublished manuscript, Hong Kong University, Hong Kong.

Lee, F.W.L. (2005). *Understanding and working with young people.* (Asian ed.). Singapore: McGraw-Hill.

Lu, G. (1997). *Confucianism and essences of Chinese and Western cultures: Revelations and integration.* Taipei: Yang zhi wen hua shi ye gu fen you xian gong si. (in Chinese)

Luckner, J.L., & Nadler, R.S. (1997). *Processing the experience: Strategies to enhance and generalize learning* (2nd ed.). Dubuque, IA: Kendall/Hunt.

Miley, K. (1999). Empowering processes for social work practice. In W. Shera & L. M. Wells (Eds.), *Empowerment practice in social work* (pp. 2–12). Toronto: Canadian Scholars Press.

Parsons, R.J., Hernandez, S.H., & Jorgensen, J.D. (1988). Integrated practice: A framework for problem solving. *Social Work*, September/October, 417–21.

Payne, M. (1991). *Modern social work theory: A critical introduction*. London: Macmillan.

Pepitone, A. (1994). Beliefs and cultural social psychology. In L.L. Adler & U.P. Gielen (Eds.), *Cross-cultural topics in psychology* (pp. 139–52). Westport, CT: Praeger.

Popple, K. (1995). *Analysing community work: Its theory and practice*. Buckingham, UK: Oxford University Press.

Saleebey, D. (1996). The strengths perspective in social work practice: Extensions and cautions. *Social Work, 41*(3), 296–305.

Satir, V. (1987). The therapist story. In M. Baldwin & V. Satir (Eds.), *The use of self in therapy* (pp. 7–25). New York: Haworth.

Schoel, J., Prouty, D., & Radcliffe, P. (1988). *Islands of healing: A guide to adventure based counselling*. Hamilton, U.S.A.: Project Adventure.

Shek, D.T.L. (1995). Adolescent mental health in different Chinese societies. *International Journal of Adolescent Medicine and Health, 8*, 117–55.

Shek, D.T.L. (1996). Mental health of Chinese adolescents: A critical review. In S. Lau (Ed.), *Growing up the Chinese way* (pp. 169–99). Hong Kong: Chinese University Press.

Shek, D.T.L. (2004). Chinese cultural beliefs about adversity: Its relationship to psychological well-being, school adjustment and problem behaviour in Hong Kong adolescents with and without economic disadvantage. *Childhood, 11*(1), 63–80.

Social Welfare Department. (2004). *Understanding the Adolescent Project: User's manual*. Hong Kong: Youth Section, SWD.

Werner, E., & Smith, R. (1992). *Overcoming the odds: High-risk children from birth to adulthood*. Ithaca, NY: Cornell University Press.

Wolin, S.J., & Wolin, S. (1993). *The resilient self: How survivors of troubled families rise above adversity*. New York: Villard Books.

Yalom, I.D., & Leszcz, M. (2005). *The theory and practice of group psychotherapy* (5th ed). New York: Basic Books.

# PART FOUR

---

# Government Policy and Service Provision

# 15 Raising Youth Voices in Community and Policy Decision Making

JACKIE SANDERS AND ROBYN MUNFORD

In this chapter we explore the intersection of the individual and service-policy components in public decision-making processes regarding physical resources that are accessible to young people. Our discussion is located within the strengths and positive youth development paradigms as they relate to resilient outcomes in youth. These theoretical frameworks provide us with a means of centring the voices of young people (Mauthner & Doucett, 1998; Sanders, 2004), critically analysing the experiences young people have as they go about the business of their daily lives. They give us ways of understanding the challenges many young people face in finding safe, nurturing, growth-oriented spaces. Most importantly to us, as practitioners and researchers, these paradigms provide us ways of finding solutions that create alternative spaces for young people. It is in these spaces that young people are able to become participating citizens with much to contribute to the quality of our communities.

Our chapter begins with a brief overview of strengths and positive youth development theories. This discussion provides a foundation upon which we can consider the case example used to structure the remainder of the chapter. The example is drawn from recent research examining factors that most and least contributed to young people's well-being. This research provided us with numerous opportunities to build detailed and rich understandings of the ways in which young people's lives unfold and the matters that make the most difference to positive outcomes. We present some of these observations during our discussion. We conclude with a set of key lessons learned from our involvement in this research in terms of shaping resilience possibilities for young people. In our conclusion we draw together key strands from the chapter and revisit four important principles that strengths-based theory and positive youth development para-digms have for undertaking work that enhances the resilience of young people.

## Understanding Resilience through Strengths Theories and Positive Youth Development Lenses

Resilience literature has examined a diverse range of factors able to differentiate children from high-risk settings who will do well from those who will not. This literature has also identified those factors in the lives of high-risk young people and their *whanau*, or families, that could be harnessed to create sustainable change (Barton, 2005). While developmental literature has documented a wide range of factors possibly related to the development of resilience in young people, the strengths-based literature has focused on understanding the way in which individual and structural factors work together to create contexts within which people are more or less able to experience well-being (Saleebey, 2002). Researchers have explored family, school, and community – three of the primary systems in young people's worlds – in an effort to identify those aspects that contribute most to the development of resilience. The consensus seems to be that caring, support, high expectations, participation, and involvement in each of these systems all make a difference to successful youth outcomes. One of the most frequently cited findings is that positive relationships have a more profound impact on outcomes than do specific risk factors. In particular, caring and support appear to be the most critical. As Atwool (1997) has argued, resilience is unlikely to develop in a child unless they have a relationship 'with at least one other adult in which they feel worthy and lovable' (p. 159). Morison Dore (1993) has also noted the pivotal importance of significant emotional attachment in the development of resilience. She has also drawn attention to the importance of the experience of being cared for in long-term development to the capacity to care for others. Given these findings, strengths-based theories have begun to exert a strong influence on approaches to youth work and support provided to families (Saleebey, 2002; Scott & O'Neill, 1996; Ungar, 2004).

Strengths-based approaches situate their understanding of the development of human capacity and resilience within a consideration of the complex contextual interactions at micro and macro levels, reflecting the influence of wider theoretical frameworks such as critical social theory. They require that we critically examine the relationship between private and public worlds; that we recognize that what happens in the individual lives of young people will be influenced by wider social forces and responses. For example, responses to poverty and homelessness may individualize social issues that have a significant structural component to them. Similarly, public policies that place curfews on all young people in an area don't account for the diverse lives lived by young people in a locality. Rather, they assume that all young people are a risk to themselves and others and therefore should be treated the same.

Workers have a key role in mediating these private and public worlds, facilitating the hearing and understanding of voices of marginalized young people and finding spaces where these voices can help shape policy and practice. Such work will inevitably include a critical examination of the reasons why young people become excluded and why the marginalized label implies a lack of resilience rather than positive social capacity (Barry, 2005; Ungar, 2004). Workers have an important role to play in challenging dominant discourses and social practices that function to exclude young people from participation. Here, deeper understandings around marginalization and the explanations and perspectives of young people are paramount. A major commitment is to move from a focus on youth as 'deficient citizens' and 'citizens in the making' to a recognition of young people as citizens of today (Burke, 2005) who have a right to be heard and to have their views incorporated into the policies that govern social life (Barry, 2005).

Critical theory also challenges workers to interrogate notions of power, to understand culturally specific origins of knowledge, and to critically explore relationships between clients and workers, including the ways in which matters such as difference and diversity are addressed (Munford & Sanders, 2005; Sanders & Munford, 2005). Highlighting the centrality of relationships identified above, these approaches also challenge workers to examine their own positions and roles in helping relationships (Maidment, 2006; Saleebey, 2006; Sanders & Munford, 2006).

Strengths theories have their modern origins in the disability movement, and particularly in the works of key writers such as Saleebey (2002). These theories arose from critical reflection on processes of support where people did not 'get better.' Rather, the social work needed to focus upon enabling individuals and their families to creatively and positively manage disability throughout the life course was improved. Strengths theories represent a different approach to social work, one that focuses attention on identifying and harnessing all the resources within individuals' and families' networks, maximizing naturally occurring supports and resources already present in their lives (Munford & Sanders, 1999; Scott & O'Neill, 1996). The important contribution strengths-based theories brought to a professional practice that had been saturated with a pathologized, treatment-oriented, medical approach to supporting families was the premise that individuals and communities have inherent capacities for restoration, growth, and change. Given this, change could best be effected by reinforcing this innate competence through the creation of belief in the possibility of development 'rather than centring exclusively upon risk factors and disease processes' (Saleebey, 1997, p. 301).

In practice, strengths-based work involves the following sorts of activities (Munford & Sanders, 1999, p. 13):

- building a relationship (Saleebey, 2006) where the worker enters the client's world on the client's terms, taking time to let this relationship develop through affirmation and support; once trust is established, gentle challenges are used to encourage the client to critically reflect upon things that may need to change;
- the use of active listening strategies in order to identify strengths and successful achievement of tasks, and being sensitive to the 'teachable moment' (Scott & O'Neill, 1996, pp. 87–91);
- a focus on reframing and providing alternative meanings and interpretations to issues and problems; and
- identifying and building on strengths and capacities in order to address current issues and problems.

Strengths-based support functions at a structural level by identifying and addressing the way that systems impact upon the lives of individuals. It also works at an intensely personal level.

The youth development paradigm provides us with a conceptual framework for applying strengths principles to youth work (Lerner, 2004; Lerner, Lerner, & Almerigi, 2005; Roth, 2004; Ungar, 2004). It constitutes a productive way of understanding the many different perspectives that influence how young people come to understand their worlds and the options these perspectives hold for them. In positive youth development work, youth are explicitly located in the centre of the explanatory frame that seeks to understand how the choices they make represent a combination of active agency and contextual structuring. Youth development approaches begin from the perspectives of the young person and disrupt the 'taken for granted' assumptions about the everyday lives of young people. The following principles are significant:

- All young people have strengths and resources; this challenges workers to identify those resources that enable young people to survive and grow, rather than focusing on the risks and 'wrongs' we see in young people's behaviours.
- A focus on strengths does not diminish the importance of identifying 'risks'. However, risks are contingent and context dependent: they may hold solutions or contain resources such as strong relationships with other young people that can be harnessed to good effect, and they may represent the best set of adaptations a young person can make to his or her environment.
- Young people are active agents in the construction of their everyday lives and adults can unwittingly undermine this agency by interpreting behaviour as troublesome and disruptive. The positive youth development approach encourages us to understand the positive as well as negative components of apparently disruptive or troubling behaviour and to understand how young people actively mediate their worlds.
- Successful interventions with young people are built on strong relationships with workers and significant others who are part of their everyday lives. Effective workers are creative, working with the young person to seek out resources and opportunities for supporting change processes relevant and appropriate to that young person's situation.
- Youth development approaches encourage us to think differently about core concepts such as citizenship, inclusion, and exclusion. Fundamental to this understanding is being able to think about what it may be like to 'walk in the shoes' of young people.

The youth development approach helps us to understand that the systems and policies we have established to assist young people may function to dismiss their experience, further marginalize them, increase their vulnerability, and reduce their capacity to be resilient in the process. The costs of accessing and utilizing services may be too high for these young people. They may refuse to seek help because our services make them feel they have failed and have nothing valuable to contribute. As a result of previous experience, they may not trust help offered by adults, and may choose instead the support of friends who have stood by them through difficult times. They may also feel misunderstood, put down, and devalued (Johnson & Paterson, 2005). Furthermore, to access help they may have to disrupt the very networks that have assisted them to survive and grow in difficult and challenging environments.

Marshall (Kidd & Marshall, 2005), a youth peer educator in South Wales, suggests that many of the policies in place for young people have lost a real focus on young people's needs. Workers have become consumed by complying with procedures and paperwork without understanding the impact of policy and service delivery on the lives of young people themselves. Like Ungar (2004), Marshall suggests that young people may view experiences such as exclusion and non-participation in services differently and not necessarily as being negative. This means that they will have different definitions of the problem and alternative strategies for finding solutions.

Strengths theories and the positive youth development paradigm provide valuable frameworks for helping us to think beyond problems to finding solutions. They encourage us to approach our work with clients in a collaborative frame of mind and to be willing to listen and learn. Both of these frameworks broaden our understanding of expertise and knowledge and ensure that we do not lose sight of the fact that in social work practice we are outsiders in others' lives. They suggest to us a compelling need for humility in the work we do and remind us that while we can walk away, the young people we seek to support cannot. This knowledge helps us to focus on expending effort to understand the factors that influence how young people come to understand their worlds and the options they contain, even when we may not understand why they may make particular choices. It focuses our attention on understanding the priorities of other people and on being endlessly creative and willing to work with all of the resources that clients have.

The frameworks created by the positive youth development paradigm and strengths-based theories in social work practice provide a productive set of approaches for understanding the experiences of children. These theories also encourage us to work alongside youth to frame solutions to the challenges they face, finding environments that are safe and that provide scope for them to work on their life projects (Edwards & Alldred, 1999; Giddens, 1991). Drawing on postmodern understandings, these paradigms remind us that there is always more than one story to be told; they allow us to recognize that young people can be both resilient and troubled, troubling, and resourceful. In terms of framing policies for young people, they require that we focus our attention on the individual, relational, and structural components that shape people's lives. Many of the principles from both of these paradigms now form an integral part of key policy documents in New Zealand concerning children and young people (see, for example, Ministry of Social Development 2001, 2002). However, the easy rhetoric that policy documents often contain can distract us from the reality for many young people, and we may fail to notice that they are still not heard and their experiences are not taken account of in practice or policy, with the result that nothing much changes in terms of the daily lived experience of young people.

## Community Resources and Public Spaces: Young Women as Active Shapers of Policy

Our research takes an action-methods approach: seeking to engage with practitioners, young people, and their families in an action-reflection cycle, generating insight within individual practice and learning. These insights can then be generalized into wider practice and from there, hopefully, into policy settings. Through reflection and insight we become better teachers, practitioners, researchers, and people. We have found that detailed examination of specific cases provides a rich means of expanding understanding. We therefore use a case example here, drawn from our community research. Our discussion is also informed by experiences with numerous other young people who have generously shared their experiences and perspectives with us. In exploring this material we examine the wider lessons it holds for working with young people in ways that enhance their resilience.

Our case example comes from a community well-being study conducted between 1999 and 2005. Ethnographic techniques were used to examine the experiences of sixty young people living in a small city (population seventy-five thousand) aged between thirteen and fifteen years. The project focused on the daily life experiences of participants and included significant others, such as parents, to provide contextual information. The young people were, however, the primary focus of the project. Participants were purposively selected from three different sites. We selected these three groups in order to identify similarities and differences between engaged and marginalized young people. Specifically, young people from group 1 were not participating in mainstream education; young people from group 2 were regularly attending a co-educational high school and, educationally speaking, were functioning at their chronological age level; young people from group 3 were attending a single-sex school and participating in an accelerated educational program that operated at between one and two years above their expected academic level. Background work prior to this project had suggested that there were overlaps between these three groups, both socially and in terms of shared life experiences. In trying to understand resilience, it is helpful if we can avoid seeing troubled young people as totally different from their socially mainstream peers. The connections and similarities not only provide us with clues about ways of drawing young people back from dangerous life circumstances, but they remind us that young people share common experiences in society. They are at one and the same time diverse and also share interests, needs, and expectations.

The young people from group 1, who are the primary focus of this chapter, had all been excluded or had removed themselves from schools prior to the study. Some were continuing with their education at home or through support agencies that offered a variety of training programs. Thus, while they had rejected or been rejected by mainstream education and therefore could no longer avail themselves of the social and cultural capital that being part of that system implied (Ungar, 2001), they nonetheless retained a positive orientation to learning that, given many of their experiences in the education system, was in itself a testament to their resilience.

Reflecting on and learning about the ways in which the young women in our study used public spaces, we also learn about the ways in which young people can be either engaged as active partners in the development of policy or excluded from it. From the chance juxtaposition of two public decision-making processes that took place during our research, we gain the opportunity to reflect upon the resilience of troubled young people and their potential to contribute actively and effectively to public policy and decision making. We also learn about the many different ways of seeing such young people and the importance of understanding the complexity and contradiction that is part of their lived experience. From talking to young people we have learned of the disjunction that often exists between the way in which they experience their lives – particularly in the intensity of their relationships with each other – and how, from the outside, adults view these relationships. Adults find it hard to understand the meaning and depth of the relationships and the ways in which young people construct them. Often these relationships appear loose, casual, fragmented, and harmful, but when we take the time to listen, we learn that underlying this is a strong code about how to be with one's friends. These stories tell us not only about the power of the relationships young people create with each other, but of the gaps these relationships fill that have been created by adults giving up on them.

*The Contested Meanings of Public Space*

Across our three sites, there were remarkable differences in the ways in which the young women experienced and used public spaces, particularly in the central city area. For instance, Jena (from group 2), like her peers from the two mainstream school sites, talked of using the centre of the city in active ways. She also spoke in ways that were consistent with dominant views about how a central city area should be used:

> Like, me and friends sometimes we will go into town and just walk around and just try on clothes for fun, you know, you're not really buying anything. It's quite fun cause we wear things that we would never wear, it's real cool and then my friend, she is like crazy about big trucks and that so like we go to the toy stores and try to find little models and then it is cool cause we have got all these little interests and so we will go around the shops in the malls.

The young women from group 1, however, spoke contradictorily about their use of this area. In explaining the ebb and flow of their daily lives, Arapeta and Iris describe their behaviour as very passive:

*What happens when you are up there [in the centre of town]?*
Sit, drink, watch people walk past. [Arapeta]
*So when you are in town, do you just walk around and that?*
We just sit there and watch people. [Iris]

In contrast, Ani, also from group 1, recounted a particular set of events that unfolded in town and showed herself to be more active than Arapeta and Iris:

Me and my mates, we like to go and play in Timezone [a games arcade] but I got banned from there, I can't go back, man that stinks, it was an awesome place.
*What was that for, babe?*
Well, for fighting for one thing, and also I nicked some of the prizes that they had on the counter, and we were in there just totally wasted and I spewed up on the floor. And they called the cops, they said that we were, what did they say, oh I dunno, we were scaring off customers or some shit like that, and that people were, well, didn't want to walk on the footpath when we were there.

It was clear that when the young women from group 1 talked about specific events or times they were anything but passive. However, as we explored the nature of the young women's relationship to this central city place it appeared that it was even more than these two contrasting voices suggested. In addition to being a place where they simply appeared to observe others – and sometimes a place at which they had powerful adventures that contained significant risks – it was also an important emotional space for them. Paradoxically, it was a place where they could be sure of feeling safe and nurtured, and in this way the central city area was a powerful magnet. Shaan describes this other aspect of the centre of town:

We go and sit up there and just talk about our problems together and try and sort something out.

One of the 'problems' that Shaan is referring to is prolonged sexual abuse from her stepfather. She clearly didn't visit the centre of town to chat about relatively trivial concerns with her mates; the problems these young women sought to resolve together were very real and overpowering, and demanded resources that they did not always possess on their own.

From their narratives, we could see that these young women carried a very contradictory set of relationships to the central city space; it was significant in their lives, and it held different, contested meanings. The deeply contested nature of their relationship to this area was not apparent on the surface. To external observers, these young women were considered a nuisance, and their active-voice descriptions of time spent there were the only account that had resonance with townspeople's perspectives. That the young women might have felt like outsiders, as their passivity suggested, or come to the centre of town seeking solace, support, and nurturing did not figure in public accounts and explanations of their behaviour. The complexity and contradiction would similarly have come as a surprise to local decision makers. The difficult and destructive manifestation of their distress simply crowded out any other understanding.

The issue of contradiction or contestation in meaning and experience is a unifying theme in the stories young people tell us. Contradiction appears to be a fundamental concept that structures the ways in which children manage their relationship to their social worlds in general, and to adults in particular. Child and youth studies internationally have noted the need youth have to speak in a variety of voices (Heywood, 2001; Lesko, 2001; Mayall, 2001; Valentine, 1996). When we work with young people, particularly those who are troubled or troubling, we must actively recognize and understand the fundamental nature of the contradictions they need to balance in living their daily lives. This understanding needs to become a major focus of our work: what does it mean for them to do this; how does understanding this allow us to find places to support them, enhance their well being, and to become more resilient?

*Planning for the Redesign of the City Centre*

As we began our fieldwork the city decided to curb the 'nuisance' and 'destruction' these young people wrought in the centre of town. A bylaw was passed banning liquor consumption in the public spaces, and a major redesign of the city centre was embarked upon. Here is what the city says on its website about this space, before and after the redesign:

The city centre is acknowledged as an important space, both in enjoyment by members of the public, and to the progression of the central business district. However after 130 years of development, planting, and re-design, the city centre had become a confusion of paths and spaces. It became a dangerous, undesirable space, which was very rarely used by visitors or permanent residents. In 2002 the City Council embarked on the 'City Heart' project, with the intent of revitalising the town centre. The major objective of the project was to create a safe, secure, inviting, and vibrant city centre. Today it has become a safe and enjoyable public space that is used by a wide range of people.

The language is very instructive and identifies that, in addition to being an emotional space for the young women, the centre of town was emotionally meaningful for the city decision makers. The shared emotional significance, but profoundly different meanings attached to this emotional content, created a fundamental tension between the city and the young women. The city planners named the project the City Heart Project, underscoring the iconic significance of this central town area. However, the resonance of this for these young women was never realized by the city planners.

The city clearly did not consider the young people who used this space daily and nightly to be 'permanent residents,' people with a legitimate claim to occupy the square. In this statement the city articulated its own sense of exclusion from this iconic space. Of course, the city had the power and authority to deal with the sense of exclusion it experienced from this important central meeting place. It decided to recreate this space, to take control back, and in the design brief it was clear that the primary objective was to reduce the probability of unde-sirable behaviours, the obvious active behaviours of the young women participating in our study.

Applying strengths theories to this situation, we could observe that the manner in which problems were defined and came to be under-stood, and whose perspectives dominated in this process of problem definition and solution construction, were critical in terms of shaping the response. The city declared that the square was 'dangerous' and had become an 'undesirable space.' However, as we had learned from our detailed investigations with the young women, clearly there were a number of different perspectives that could be taken in defining this problem. Additionally, as we know from social work theory, the way in which the problem or issue is defined will have a critical influence

Figure 1   Different ways of defining the problem

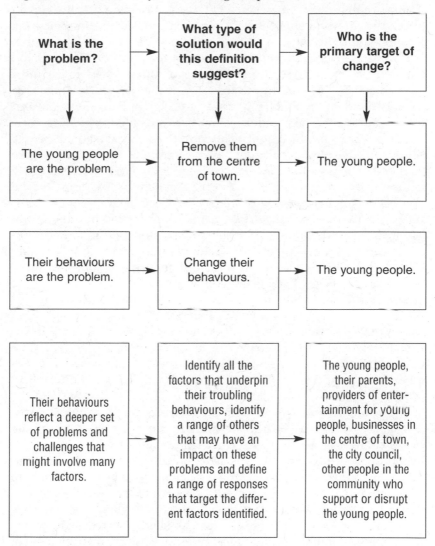

upon the response (see Figure 1). Responses will differ depending on the understanding we have of the problem, and as we can see, only one of the possible definitions of the problem required us to look beyond the young people for a solution.

There is nothing wrong with a city wanting to be safe and wanting inviting central areas. However, what was critical here was the way in which the city went about determining the problem and defining the solution. Typically, when a city embarks upon a process of change it will initiate a public consultation process to run alongside decision making, paying attention to the needs of those likely to be most affected by the decision. In the redesign of the city centre, there was consultation with the public in terms of design options. Retailers and other central city stakeholders were also consulted regarding their needs, but at no time did the city attempt to consult the young people who were the most significant users of this space and who were largely the reason for the redesign. In doing this it substantially ignored the principles expressed in the Agenda for Children and the Youth Development Strategy (Ministry of Social Development, 2001, 2002), the two major policy documents promulgated by our central government for defining appropriate processes to take account of children's and young people's needs in planning and policy-making processes. The city chose to assert its dominance and shut the young people out. It chose to define the young people as the problem and to ignore any contribution they could make to the solution. In this process we can clearly see the gulf that opens up between high-level policy that may well espouse important principles concerning inclusion, involvement, and participation, and local processes that continue to exclude young people and respond to them on the basis of stereotypes or assumptions about the 'type' of people they are (Phillips, 2004).

The young people's presence in the centre of town and their use of this space was seen as illegitimate, and so their potential to contribute to any changes was similarly seen as illegitimate or possibly irrelevant. In the process of occupying this space in disruptive ways, they had disqualified themselves from being residents with a justifiable claim to be drawn into the redesign process. Yet we knew from our interactions with these young women that their violent behaviour was only one dimension of their use of this space. As such, the redesign, which threatened to shut them out, constituted a real threat to their well-being. If the redesign proved successful, where would these young women go? We were worried that they might move to one of the poorly lit inner-city parks and concerned about the risks this might pose for them.

*Planning for a New Community Youth Centre*

Simultaneous with the redesign of the city centre, a youth centre was being reconstructed on the other side of town, the side from which these young women came. A youth community centre had worked for many years out of very limited accommodation. It was desperately in need of new facilities to be able to effectively respond to the increasing numbers of young people who were leaving mainstream education with no school qualifications. An opportunity arose to apply to a large philanthropic trust for funds to build a new facility, complete with a gymnasium, classrooms, meeting areas, and counselling space. We had been involved with the existing youth community centre, and some of the young women had been recruited into our research through this centre that provided an alternative education program for them. We became enthusiastic supporters of the centre's decision to apply for funds for a new building. We helped to write the funding application, canvass local opinion, and gain support for the initiative in the community. This was a valuable learning experience for us and gave great insight into the power of dominant discourses concerning young people – particularly 'troubled youth' – to constrain and shape policy responses.

We were surprised and shocked, however, to realize that what had seemed like such a wonderful idea to us could run into so much resistance from community members and decision makers. One of our tasks in this project was to canvass for support for the initiative from members of the local community and from elsewhere in the city. We were overwhelmed by the level of resistance and hostility to the idea of doing anything positive and constructive for these young people. Residents and decision makers challenged us with the following sorts of responses:

> If they build the gymnasium in that part of town, no-one from anywhere else in the city will use it because those bad kids are there, they will frighten everyone else away and then they will have a nice new building all for themselves, they don't deserve it.

> They will just destroy it, they wont appreciate it like kids in other parts of town would. They already get more than their fair share of local resources for all the trouble they cause.

Why should they get something nice, they just cause trouble?

In order to be one of the successful applicants the project had to demonstrate a wide public appeal. Because the facility was located in a part of town that no one else really wanted to visit and it responded to needs of a group of young people seen as undeserving, this group was immediately at a disadvantage. The young people were not wanted in the middle of town, and they didn't deserve new facilities in their area that might act as a magnet resource and draw them back. They were caught in the crossfire of competing and disabling discourses about young people at the margins, and the public consultation process reinforced for them what they experienced in their daily lives: they were not wanted and they were not deserving of positive attention.

As the community consultation proceeded, it became clear to us and the staff at the centre that the young people needed to become visible in new ways to the community, to be given a voice in the process and to be seen as we saw them: creative, adaptable, responsive, resilient, and strong. While we had started the project attempting, as adults do, to secure resources that young people could then use, we realized that these young people had a critical part to play in the public debate and that with support and encouragement they could become the most powerful advocates for their centre. Having witnessed their exclusion from the redesign of the city centre, we realized that we were also in danger of excluding them from the campaign to secure the new facility. Our motives of course were different, but the process was the same.

Drawing on material that they had shared with us in the research and from confidence-building activities provided by the alternative school, we worked as a large team. Centre staff and researchers helped the young people prepare for active participation in the process. We encouraged them to shape their stories in ways that illustrated the challenges they faced in having nowhere safe to go in the evening, and the impact of school exclusion on their ability to continue to play competitive sport (something the new gymnasium would help resolve). They were also encouraged to practice dealing with challenges and angry responses from people in the community concerning the aggressive and destructive acts that were also a part of their lives. The young women wrote submissions and shaped their experiences into evidence that they presented at public hearings to explain the challenges they faced as vulnerable young people with few resources and little support. They also learned to listen to people from the community tell them about the impact their destructive behaviours had on others. There were several public hearings, some of which required the groups to compete publicly for the funds by proving their case was the most attractive. There were also some very formal hearings concerning consents for the building and change of land use from parks to buildings. The power of these young women's stories and experiences helped shape the process and secure the centre's place as one of the four preferred projects for the city. Finally, once the funds had been granted and approval given, the young women also became involved in the planning for the building and its opening.

These young women's participation in the process of securing the community centre engaged them in new relationships and new types of involvement in their community, as they became drawn into the sometimes very heated public debate about its development. They competently engaged in very formal and quite intimidating public consultation processes to achieve a positive result. Their involvement provided public validation of their experience. In the process of securing the funding and consent for the new community centre, city planners and decision makers heard them speak; they were no longer an inarticulate, faceless mass of threatening youngsters, but individual young people with stories to tell and who had a contribution to make to the development of policy, practice, and community decision making. Furthermore, the young women were given opportunities to actively participate and try out new roles that could open up future possibilities.

Of course, everything hasn't been dramatically changed since then. In spite of the redesign they still create havoc in the centre of the city from time to time, and their lives are far from uncomplicated. If the primary motivation for the redesign of the city centre was to remove these young people from this space, then it has failed. Of course, when a solution is based upon a misunderstanding of the nature of the issues, it is often unsuccessful.

Looking at the community centre initiative, in contrast, we saw the positive, constructive, and incredibly courageous ways in which these young women were able to participate in the public processes required to secure the new centre. These processes were highly contested and hard fought. By participating in these intimidating processes they demonstrated powerfully their hidden resilience, capacity, and competence. Their active engagement in this project illustrated what a powerful resource youth could be at both an individual and a policy level if they were not seen as just a problem. They had never participated in public processes before, but now they competently played a central role in shaping the debate. Decision makers found themselves having to see these young women as more than a problem to be solved or removed. The contradictions in their lives and the complex and demanding roles they had to balance were as much a resource as they were a threat. What was needed was creativity to discover the right ways of harnessing their resilience, and a willingness to really listen to their views about what they needed.

## Lessons for Our Approach to Youth Work

Our experiences working with this group of young women as their haven in the centre of town was redesigned and through the challenge of developing the new community youth centre taught us a number of broader lessons about resilience and work with young people. We learned from observing these young women that very troubled youth have important resources to contribute to social development and the improvement of their opportunities.

Observing these two public processes that had the potential to have significant impacts on the daily lives of young people, we also observed that public policy responses can be enabling or disabling depending on how the problem or issue is defined. The nature of the definition is often dependent on whether or not officials take time to understand how young people have come to the position where their troubling behaviours seem to be the best response they can make to their situation. We learned that what appeared to officials and residents of the city to be chaotic, disorganized, dangerous, and unhealthy behaviour could equally be seen as creative and adaptive responses to the realities of these young people's life circumstances. As Ungar (2004) notes, 'A wide and varied cohort of authors have challenged notions of homogeneity in healthy behaviours. They argue from behind the critical lens of culture, gender, and race that in specific contexts negative and troubling behaviours are, in fact, signs of health' (p. 75).

Understanding these matters means that our support can be targeted more effectively to the core of the problem. We saw, in the two situations of decision making, the difference that involving the young people made. In the first they were defined as the problem and not considered to have anything to offer in its resolution. In the second we saw that with support and encouragement these young women could be powerful and articulate advocates for themselves and other young people. They had resources based on experience, and they knew what might make a difference for people like them. They also had skills of bravery and were able to place themselves in intimidating public encounters with powerful decision makers. In fact, they had learned a lot of valuable skills for interacting with adults while on the streets, and they used these to good effect to manage their interactions in the public hearings. They surprised public officials, who had written them off as having nothing to offer and being nothing but trouble. The research process and community centre project provided opportunities to bring the issues that these marginalized people faced to public notice in ways that invited decision makers into their territory and that provided opportunities for public officials to respond in positive ways.

We learned important lessons too. Early in the process of applying for funds for the new community centre we realized that we had also excluded the young people from the project. We assumed an adult stance, took over the project, began preparing submissions and attending hearings, feeling that this was properly 'adult business' and we wanted to protect the young people from the criticisms of others. We soon learned, however, that while young people sometimes most surely do need our protection, this is not always the case. We must think carefully about our motives and assumptions when we decide to exclude young people from processes and decisions that concern them. In our case, the involvement of young people in the pursuit of funds for the community centre had a major impact upon the project's success. Their presence brought the lived reality of young people to the forefront of the process. This had the effect of moderating the strident and highly critical comments concerning the young people that had been levelled at us when we arranged public meetings on our own. Giving young people a place at the table created a space where they could stand alongside us and argue for their own needs – a much more effective way of establishing a 'deserving case' than when done by a third party.

Finally, reflecting on these two processes highlighted the importance of being able to clearly understand the reality that young people continually balance contradictions in their lives. Understanding the ways in which this works itself out in individuals' lives needs to become a major focus of our work.

## Making Connections

We never achieve perfect understanding when we are working with the dynamic situations presented to us by disturbed or distressed young people and their families. These are complex, often fast-moving situations, involving numbers of different people that require all of our professional and personal resources. What we try to do is to draw widely on the information resources that exist in the numerous locations around young people. We want to carefully and respectfully hear their stories as unique and deeply meaningful, and to recognize that alongside these are many other stories about these situations. We need to make sense of what is before us and to establish sequences of events, causes, and possible effects. Importantly, however, we also need to understand powerful emotions, and identify the connections between the individual, relational, cultural, community, and policy levels. Events at all five of these levels influence the situations we confront on the ground. The example presented here demonstrates resilience as the product of the complex intersections between these five different components as well as being located more or less discreetly within each level. Our example highlights the ways in which individual experience provides the framework within which understanding and meaning is constructed. At the same time a focus on the individual level alone will not provide us with the understanding or resources that we need to support young people to embark on change. Strengths-based, youth-development-oriented work has the potential to provide opportunities to straddle the divide between all four levels of resilience. Understanding that resilience can be nurtured through actions at each of these levels provides us with a working model that can be used, like a checklist, in daily interactions with young people.

Gilligan (2003) reminds us that resilience is not a magical property that is lying around waiting to be picked up; neither is it something we can use like a vaccine to protect ourselves from all risks:

> There is no one-shot magic bullet of resilience which will inoculate children against the effects of social adversity and social inequality. There are no short cuts in policy terms. There is no resilience-based alternative to policy based on justice and serving needs. (p. 3)

As Barton (2005) explains, resilience is a much studied but little understood concept, and the immense research effort that has been directed at identifying and measuring it has generated more heat than light. Thinkers who have been willing to see resilience as extending beyond a set of individual properties that may be acquired if the right combination of preconditions are present, understand it to be something that exists in the spaces between people and that accumulates through positive interactions (see, for example, Gilgun & Abrams, 2005; Gilligan, 2005; Ungar, 2005). Resilience can be created and harnessed through intentional interactions that are informed by principles such as those underpinning the strengths and youth development movements. Knowing this focuses our attention on understanding more about fostering healthful relationships between ourselves as practitioners and those we seek to assist. Working with individuals – youth in particular – can be difficult, as we try through our own efforts to have an impact on the circumstances of others. However, understanding resilience as something that exists between people reminds us to pay attention to working on systems with decision makers who may be quite removed from youth. A relational understanding of resilience also emphasizes an understanding of how past experience and wider context shape possibilities for individual young people. These ideas also remind us that working alongside young people and encouraging them to identify and harness their own expertise is a resilience-enhancing project as well. A full understanding of resilience and work in a strengths mode requires that we work at our chosen level but in relation to the other four.

Finally, we re-visit four key principles that strengths-based workers seeking to enhance the resilience of young people use successfully:

1  Relationships are fundamental to the work done regardless of the level we are focusing on. It is through these that our work is accomplished, and in building relationships with young people we need to listen carefully and ensure that we create a safe environment for our encounters with them.

2 We need to know and understand the circumstances that confront the young people we are supporting. This means that we must take the time required to be around young people, to be in their lives listening to and observing the other people they interact with, the way they react, and the meanings that may lie behind the things they say to us and others. Often decisions and judgments are made about the disposition of young people on the basis of what or how they present. Looking beneath the surface ,we find reasons for this behaviour, and can often learn that if the underlying issues are dealt with the behaviour may disappear and the young person will be more able to function in ways we deem appropriate. Sometimes being there, listening, and trying to understand will bring us into contact with material that will make us uncomfortable; we will hear things we may have preferred not to hear. To be effective, we need to be able to manage difficult information and uncomfortable situations. When we can do this effectively we will more easily find the teachable moment (Scott & O'Neill, 1996) rather than the opportunity to give a lecture. The teachable moment provides the opportunities for long-term sustainable change that grows out of genuine insight.

3 Young people are the authors of their own experience. We need to recognize their agency and capacity, and see the positive adaptations that may lie behind troubling behaviours. Young people have energy, ideas, understanding, and their own capacity. These are invaluable resources that hold the seeds of change. Recognizing young people as competent and as experts also means that we should seek as many opportunities as possible to draw them into public policy-making processes and community projects. We can be confident that they will be direct, and, if the issue is relevant to them, that their contributions will be highly relevant and will likely lead to more sustainable, long-term solutions.

4 Finally, it is important to remember that even when we are successful in supporting a young person to make big changes at the individual level, there may well be wider, unintended consequences. Change in young people can have positive ripple effects. But this is not always the case. There may well be people around the young person who feel that they gain more from her distress and trouble than they will from her harnessing her positive potential. It is important to be attentive to these ripple effects and to develop plans to address them. Early steps towards change will be fragile

and tentative, and a young person who falls back into harmful activities may not necessarily have 'given up' or 'reverted to type'; it may be that others in their network are standing in the way. Hooking into existing networks to identify natural helpers, allies, and resources and activating them can be a very productive way of disabling these other people.

Gilligan (2005) provides salutary observations on the intersections between young people and adults:

> Young people are not passive bystanders in their own development. They are not passive receptacles into which adults pour experiences. They are not wholly dependent. Children are active players in the search for their own destiny ... they can also be seen as resilient authors of experience ... [children and young people see] a crucial difference between being involved and being landed with responsibility for decisions of great enormity. As adults we must listen to and involve children and adolescents, while avoiding any shift of our responsibility for key decisions onto their shoulders. (pp. 8–9)

## REFERENCES

Atwool, N. (1997). Making connections: Attachment and resilience. In N. Taylor & A. Smith (Eds.), *Enhancing children's potential: Minimising risk and maximising resilience* (pp. 155–64). Proceedings of the Children's Issues Centre Second Child and Family Policy Conference, 2–4 July. Otago University: Dunedin.

Barry, M. (2005). Introduction. In M. Barry (Ed.), *Youth policy and social inclusion: Critical debates with young people* (pp. 1–8). London: Routledge.

Barton, W. (2005). Methodological challenges in the study of resilience. In M. Ungar (Ed.), *Handbook for working with children and youth: Pathways to resilience across cultures and contexts* (pp. 135–48). Thousand Oaks, CA: Sage.

Burke, T. (2005). Postscript on citizenship. In M. Barry (Ed.), *Youth policy and social inclusion: Critical debates with young people* (pp. 51–3). London: Routledge.

Edwards, R., & Alldred, P. (1999). Children and young people's views of social research: The case of research on home–school relations. *Childhood*, 6(2), 261–79.

Giddens, A. (1991). *Modernity and self identity: Self and society in the late modern age.* Cambridge, MA: Polity.

Gilgun, J., & Abrams, L. (2005). Gendered adaptations, resilience, and the perpetration of violence. In M. Ungar (Ed.), *Handbook for working with children and youth: Pathways to resilience across cultures and contexts* (pp. 57–70). Thousand Oaks, CA: Sage.

Gilligan, R. (2003, March). *Promoting children's resilience: Some reflections.* Paper presented at the 2003 Launch Event for the Glasgow Centre for the Child and Society, Glasgow, Scotland.

Gilligan, R. (2005). Promoting strengths and resilience in vulnerable children and families: Some reflections on the role of social worker and other professionals. *Childrenz Issues, 9*(2), 15–2.

Heywood, C. (2001). *A history of childhood: Children and childhood in the west from medieval to modern times.* Cambridge, MA: Polity.

Johnson, J., & Paterson, J. (2005). Postscript on homelessness. In M. Barry (Ed.), *Youth policy and social inclusion: Critical debates with young people* (pp. 183–185). London: Routledge.

Kidd, S., & Marshall, K. (2005). Postscript on policy and practice. In M. Barry (Ed.), *Youth policy and social inclusion: Critical debates with young people* (pp. 27–31). London: Routledge.

Lerner, R. (2004). *Liberty: Thriving and civic engagement among America's youth.* Thousand Oaks, CA: Sage.

Lerner, R., Lerner, J., & Almerigi, J.B. (2005). Positive youth development, participation in community youth development programs, and community contributions of fifth-grade adolescents. *Journal of Early Adolescence, 25*(1), 17–71.

Lesko, N. (2001), *Act your age: A cultural construction of adolescence.* New York: Routledge-Falmer.

Maidment, J. (2006). The quiet remedy: A dialogue on reshaping professional relationships. *Families in Society: The Journal of Contemporary Social Services, 87*(1), 115–21.

Mauthner, N., & Doucet, A. (1998). Reflections on a voice-centred relational method: Analysing maternal and domestic voices. In J. Ribbens & R. Edwards (Eds.), *Feminist dilemmas in qualitative research: Public knowledge and private lives* (pp. 119–46). Thousand Oaks, CA: Sage.

Mayall, B. (2001). Understanding childhoods: A London study. In L. Alanen & B. Mayall (Eds.), *Conceptualising child–adult relations* (pp. 114–28). London: Routledge-Falmer.

Ministry of Social Development. (2001). *New Zealand's agenda for children.* Wellington: Ministry of Social Development.

Ministry of Social Development. (2002). *The Youth Development Strategy.* Wellington: Ministry of Social Development.

Morison Dore, M. (1993). Family preservation and poor families: When 'homebuilding' is not enough. *Families in Society, 74*(9), 545–56.

Munford, R., & Sanders, J. (1999). *Supporting families.* Palmerston North, NZ: Dunmore.

Munford, R., & Sanders, J. (2005). Working with families: Strengths-based approaches. In M. Nash, R. Munford, & K. O'Donoghue (Eds.), *Social work theories in action* (pp. 158–73). London: Jessica Kingsley.

Phillips, B. (2004). Re-generation games: The politics of childhood in urban renewal. *Community Development Journal, 39*(2), 166–76.

Roth, J. (2004). Youth development programs. *The Prevention Researcher, 11*(2), 3–7.

Saleebey, D. (Ed.). (1997). *The strengths perspective in social work practice* (2nd ed.). New York: Longman.

Saleebey, D. (2002). *The strengths perspective in social work.* White Plains, NY: Longman.

Saleebey, D. (2006). A paradigm shift in developmental perspectives? The self in context. In A. Lightburn & P. Sessions (Eds.), *Handbook of community-based clinical practice* (pp. 3–18). New York: Oxford University Press.

Sanders, J. (2004). *Subject child.* Unpublished doctoral dissertation, Massey University, Palmerston North, NZ.

Sanders, J., & Munford, R. (2005). Authentic relationships: Possibilities for social work to make a difference for children and young people. *Childrenz Issues, 9*(1), 22–7.

Sanders, J., & Munford, R. (2006). Community centre practice: Potential and possibilities for creating change. *Journal of Social Work Practice, 20*(1), 39–50.

Scott, D., & O'Neill, D. (1996). *Beyond child rescue: Developing family-centred practice at St Luke's.* Sydney: Allen and Unwin.

Ungar, M. (2001). The social construction of resilience among 'problem' youth in out-of-home placement: A study of health-enhancing deviance. *Child and Youth Care Forum, 30,* 137–54.

Ungar, M. (2004). *Nurturing hidden resilience in troubled youth.* Toronto: University of Toronto Press.

Ungar, M. (Ed.). (2005). *Handbook for working with children and youth: Pathways to resilience across cultures and contexts.* Thousand Oaks, CA: Sage.

Valentine, G. (1996). Angels and devils: Moral landscapes of childhood. *Environment and Planning D: Society and Space, 14,* 581–99.

# 16 Policy Responses to Youth in Adversity: An Integrated, Strengths-Based Approach

E. ANNE MARSHALL AND BONNIE J. LEADBEATER

The number of children and youth experiencing adversity is a major concern to service providers, researchers, and policy makers alike. Limited and seemingly shrinking capacities to intervene on their behalf have exacerbated this concern. Why, despite good intentions and deployment of resources, are we still falling short of providing the basic services that all youth need in order to lead productive and fulfilling lives? Research-based conceptual models, behavioural interventions, and theoretical approaches all have implications for the implementation of policy decisions for youth in adversity, yet they frequently go unnoticed. Moreover, while these decisions can have a profound effect on them, children and youth themselves are seldom considered or consulted in policy development or implementation.

Policy exists to advance public goals and welfare as well as private good. Kingdon (1995) describes three broad influences related to public-sector reform: the problem stream, the policy stream, and the politics stream. The problem stream includes events and indicators at local, national, and global levels. The policy stream represents ideas and decisions advocated by specialists in academe, research institutes, and the private sector. Politicians, the general public, and special interest groups comprise the politics stream. All three streams attempt to influence government agendas and priorities; furthermore, each affects and is affected by the other two.

In Canada, recent attention to and support for progressive approaches to policy decisions have resulted in an attempt to involve a number of stakeholders (British Columbia Office of the Provincial Health Officer and Child and Youth Officer, 2006). The plight of children and youth, recent emphasis on cross-disciplinary approaches, and increased support for knowledge transfer across many kinds of 'borders' has fostered a new spirit of communication and collaboration among researchers, policy makers, and service providers (Perkins, Borden, & Villarruel, 2001; Schoon & Bynner, 2003). Such a move emerges from a contrasting historical context. Evaluation, for example, the final stage of policy development, is often left out or ignored in this process due to lack of time, changes in government, public response to media reports, and other factors. Furthermore, academic researchers and frontline practitioners have usually not concerned themselves with policy. Likewise, policy makers have usually operated within their own spheres. This move is therefore timely, given multiple and complex national and global threats to the health and well-being of youth.

Adversities experienced throughout childhood are neither static nor one-dimensional; they can become self-perpetuating, being affected by and simultaneously affecting ongoing processes of children's development (Leadbeater, Dodgen, & Solarz, 2005). Severe crises notwithstanding, many children do not manifest the expected negative stereotypical outcomes of hardship, remaining relatively unaffected, or even growing stronger in the face of adversity. This response has become known as *resilience*. Although several definitions of resilience have been proposed, a consistent thread is successful adaptation despite extreme adversity or trauma (Schoon & Bynner, 2003; Small & Memmo, 2004). The concept of resilience also provides evidence that negative outcomes are preventable, and it is in the best interest of society to support resilience in children at a young age.

We contend that achieving resilience requires, amongst various other approaches and acts, a shift in policy development and implementation, one that corresponds to the transformation we have recently witnessed in community-based research and strengths-based practice. We begin with our theoretical orientation and a brief description of our work within an interdisciplinary university research centre. We then identify several issues embedded in the cultural and family contexts of children's lives that affect efforts to align policy and research development and implementation. These challenges include cultural and contextual differences, an emphasis on risks, moving from a separate to a shared focus, methodological imbalance, and graduate-level training. Promoting resilience in children and youth requires responses to these challenges and potential solutions to address them. Examples from our own experience across several community-based research projects will be used to illustrate challenges as well as potential responses and solutions.

## Theoretical Framework

Our theoretical framework encompasses a lifespan, process-oriented, and contextually based approach to the study of children and youth (Leadbeater, Schellenbach, Maton, & Dogden, 2004; Marshall, 2002). This approach recognizes the continuous process of building individual, family, and community competencies and capacities in ever-changing social contexts. As life experiences evolve, new and changing barriers and supports arise, necessitating a reworking of understandings and responses. An important aspect of our social constructionist orientation is what several researchers and scholars have termed *positive youth development* (Cargo, Grams, Ottoson, Ward, & Green, 2003; Lerner, Almerigi, Theokas, & Lerner, 2005; Perkins et al., 2001). Positive youth development has its origins in academic research, in the voices of youth serving workers, and in health promotion policies and initiatives. This perspective focuses on what children and youth need to sustain trajectories of optimal development, rather than on fixing problems as they occur. Children are seen as both active collaborators in their own positive development and as responsive to opportunities in their environments.

Our own research context is the Centre for Youth and Society at the University of Victoria in British Columbia (see http://www.youth .society.uvic.ca). Established in 1998, Youth and Society is an interdisciplinary research centre that links researchers from several academic areas with community representatives, service agencies, all levels of government, youth, and media. Members have extensive experience in basic research, community action research, and direct service to youth. Core activities include research, advocacy, and training. Faculty and community partners affiliated with the centre are from diverse disciplines, including psychology, nursing, sociology, education, child and youth care, social work, medicine, and health promotion. Projects address a host of topics related to health, education, and development in children and youth.

A university–community alliance for health research emerged from the work of the centre to specifically address issues related to preventing child and youth injuries (Healthy Youth in a Healthy Society: A Community Alliance for Reducing Risks for Injuries in Children and

Adolescents – see http://www.youth.society.uvic.ca/activities/research/cahr/research.html). The 'Healthy Youth' project united researchers, practitioners, and policy makers in common research goals to answer questions derived from both research and practice. In the course of the research we have also learned a great deal about the challenges of integrating research with policy and practice and about practical responses to these challenges. We turn next to explicating both these challenges and the potential responses and solutions.

## Challenge: Cultural and Contextual Differences

Huang, et al. (2005) contend that the problem of unmet needs is particularly severe for children from racially and ethnically diverse backgrounds. Economic and power disadvantages are often evident in these cultural minority contexts. This is particularly true, for example, in Canadian aboriginal communities. It has been suggested that past policy decisions mandating residential school attendance for aboriginal children reflected a power imbalance rooted in colonial views and practices (Piquemal, 2001). Currently, aboriginal children and youth comprise about half of all the children in care (British Columbia Office of the Provincial Health Officer and Child and Youth Officer, 2006). This proportion is many times their representation in the general pop ulation. Researchers coming to aboriginal settings have also been criticized· exploitation, community damage, and misleading data have been identified as major concerns stemming from research conducted in native communities (Ponterotto & Casas, 1993).

Young people themselves constitute a cultural group that has also been disenfranchised and marginalized. Parents, caregivers, researchers, and policy makers all agree that young people have capabilities and potential, yet they are rarely involved in the policy process in any meaningful way. We know little about the pathways that children and youth navigate through the various structures and systems mandated to provide for their needs, and even less about the capabilities and attributes they utilize to negotiate those pathways (Ungar, 2005).

Policy recommendations and service provision for children and youth are often not designed for the particular contextual needs of individuals, families, and communities. This can result in what Ommer and team (2007) have termed a 'mismatch of scale' – a lack of fit that diminishes the effectiveness of policy and practice decisions.

Spatial scale mismatches occur when activities appropriate to one location are applied without considering the different properties of other locations, or when decisions are made at one level that pertain to another, without consultation. Mental health policy, for example, may be directed at the individual when the family is the more appropriate target, or approaches developed with urban populations may be implemented in rural environments. Organizational scale mismatches occur across sectors, when, for example, programmatic activities appropriate for a local agency are applied to government or national organizations. Misdirected flows of resources or benefits resulting from mismatched scale decisions can lead to implementation imbalances that are very difficult to correct after the fact. Given the diversity that exists within communities and regions, let alone within countries, the all-too-frequent practice of dismissing contextual, cultural, and community relevance and choosing a so-called universal 'best practice' is highly questionable (Pittman, Diversi, & Ferber, 2002; Schoon & Bynner, 2003).

Against the variety of contexts in which youth live, are the variety of contexts from which professionals interacting with youth lives emerge. In this regard, adopting a broad view of culture, Pedersen (1991) maintains that every interaction is to some extent a cross-cultural one. World view, values, language, and behaviours differ between and among cultures, compounded by degrees of acculturation. More obvious cultural differences in nationality or language are usually recognized, yet working across age groups, academic disciplines, communities, and institutional departments are also examples of cross-cultural encounters, as each group has its own sets of terminology, practices, goals, and so forth. Cultural differences mean that accurate and appropriate communication is vital when working across research, policy, and practice cultures, in attempts to minimize inaccuracies, assumptions, misconceptions, and disrespectful practices that also can be the product of engagement.

### Response: Building Relationships across Cultures and Contexts

A continued focus on building shared understanding through relationships is the single most important factor for communicating across cultures. Whether the differences are those of ethnicity, gender, discipline, institution, or rank, creating the conditions for mutually respectful working relationships needs to be first and foremost. Meeting community partners in their home territory, reading a journal article from another discipline, purchasing products through youth fundraising programs, or attending a government ministry briefing session are examples of the varied activities that foster relationships. These processes take time; however, investing the time needed to build relationships at the beginning of the process invariably saves time later on when there are concerns and problems to be managed.

Building trust is essential for positive, long-term productive relationships across multiple contexts (Marshall & Batten, 2004). Interpersonal trust is more likely to develop when members are aware of personal biases and perspectives, open to multiple perspectives, tolerant of complexity and unpredictability, and willing to share power. Communication processes must promote the free exchange of information and acceptance of dissenting voices.

Although most research and policy development has focused on individuals and families, Wolkow and Ferguson (2001) point out that the role of community vis-à-vis risks and protective factors has received little attention. The impact of community factors is especially salient in cultural contexts with a more collectivist orientation and extended family structures (McCormick, 1997), such as aboriginal communities. Furthermore, peers and community relationships are increasingly important influences as young people enter adolescence. Blum and Ellen (2002) attest that addressing 'community factors may be the best means for programs to protect at-risk youth because the influence of families fades with the transition from childhood to adulthood' (p. 289).

Youth engagement is critical; they need to be included in advocacy and developmental process decisions in order to promote optimal outcomes (Maton, 2005). One of the key recommendations in a recent Canadian joint governmental report on children's mental health outcomes is to engage adolescents in planning how to access services and supports needed to assist them in successfully navigating the transition to adulthood (British Columbia Office of the Provincial Health Officer and Child and Youth Officer, 2006).

Given the aforementioned concerns, Pittman et al. (2002) propose a set of seven 'framing questions' aimed at helping to tailor youth policies to the particulars of a given cultural and community context. The questions address the who, what, when, where, why, and how of youth development – the questions that are usually *answered* in policy decisions but not always fully *discussed* beforehand.

In this regard, knowledge translation and education are also required in order to communicate effectively across cultures. Policy makers, researchers, and practitioners need to know more about each other's roles, priorities, and constraints. Wilcox, Weisz, and Miller (2005) suggest that practitioners in the child policy arena, rather than adopting only an advocacy approach, can sometimes be more effective by 'focusing their efforts on educating policymakers on the relevance of their work to policy issues in a nonpartisan, nonadversarial manner' (p. 638).

Furthermore, the use of research evidence in policy making could be enhanced if researchers learned about competing influences on the policy process and engaged in public debates about important problems such as child antisocial behaviour (Waddell et al., 2005). Understanding each other's perspectives will enable the players to develop more realistic expectations and form creative research–policy partnerships.

## Challenge: Emphasis on Risks and Problems

Until recently, the dominant paradigm for improving child and adolescent welfare has been to identify risks and problems with the aim of reducing them (Cargo et al., 2003; Leadbeater et al., 2004). In this tertiary approach to youth policy and intervention, adolescents have been particularly stigmatized as being laden with risks and problems. Research has focused on their deficits and difficulties. Recommendations for policy and practice target the reduction of risks such as poverty, family violence, school drop-out rates, and so on. Although policy decisions stemming from this risk/deficit approach have demonstrated some positive results (Lerner et al., 2005), addressing the individual, family, and environmental factors needed to halt these widespread social ills appears to be a monumental challenge. Family mobility and constantly changing commitments and contexts can render specific programs out of date before they are even disseminated. Moreover, focusing on problem reduction does not necessarily generate constructive replacement alternatives.

Vulnerable youth populations are more prone to marginalization, often furthering their sense of alienation from community and support services (Simeonsson & Covington, 1994; Ungar, 2005). Fragmentary child welfare, juvenile justice, educational, and traditional medical services for these young people have proved insufficient to halt the social, cultural, economic, educational, and behavioural risks that threaten their healthy transitions to young adulthood. Services offered through provider-client relationships and standard educational programs are often unsuccessful in reaching them. Instability in the lives of some youth – frequently due to alienation from families, schools, and communities – makes it even less likely that they will access existing services and more likely that their problems will become complex and severe before they are addressed.

### Response: Focus on Positive and Strengths-Based Approaches

New approaches to youth health services that proactively engage and support vulnerable youth action on their own behalf are sorely needed. Positive youth development emphasizes supporting conditions that contribute to healthy youth development for all children (Lerner et al., 2005; Perkins et al., 2001). A similar perspective is the Development Assets approach espoused by scholars and researchers at academic institutions and at the Search Institute (Murphey, Lamonda, Carney, & Duncan, 2004). This approach focuses on the presence or absence of resources in communities that support healthy development in children and youth. Research conducted by Murphey and colleagues demonstrates that possessing even one asset can have a positive impact on reported behavioural outcomes for high-school students. Every additional asset increases the students' odds of engaging in healthy behaviours and decreases their odds of engaging in risk-taking behaviours.

According to Lerner et al. (2005), the key to supporting the positive development of youth is generating research-based policies that strengthen the capacities of families in diverse communities to raise healthy youth. These policies should be strengths focused, developmental in nature, and aimed at enhancing the relationships between youth and the assets located in their own communities. Implementation should begin with very young children; however, children and youth of all ages can benefit from positive efforts to support their development. Lerner and his colleagues argue that the built-in 'plasticity' of human development allows for positive changes at any age.

From the foundations of positive youth development and resilience concepts, Perkins et al. (2001) created the Community Development Model, a framework for looking at youth and policy response to youth in adversity. The model emphasizes assisting youth to overcome risks and become active partners in their own as well as their community's development. A community youth development approach engages youth in the interpretation of research results and in the development and implementation of solutions. From a policy perspective, it involves youth in identifying issues, generating solutions, and even writing legislation.

Our own community-based research at the Centre for Youth and Society underscores the importance of connecting in positive and meaningful ways with youth in order to address their sense of alienation and increase their engagement. We have listened to their suggestions in designing surveys and interviews, involved them in data collection, and stepped back when they were planning youth events (see Leadbeater, et al., 2006). Vulnerable youth are understandably wary of adults; they relate better to their peers. In the 'Risky Business' study within the Healthy Youth research project (Benoit, Jansson, Millar, & Phillips, 2005), street youth were trained to recruit and interview other youth about health needs. In addition to providing data and findings, these research experiences initiated relationships and opportunities that helped some at-risk youth access services and supports to improve their health status.

## Challenge: Moving from a Separate to a Shared Focus

Misalignment among policy, research, and practice arenas stems from differences in settings, goals, priorities, orientations, methods, and time schedules. Leadbeater et al. (2005) argue that these gaps are institutionalized, with the major players segregated into separate spheres of practice (universities versus government agencies), utilizing different sources of information, and developing divergent sets of terminology. Policy makers face decisions that have immediate effects on such things as the distribution of tax dollars in ways intended to advance public welfare or serve a particular constituency. The plight of individuals, bottom lines, popular opinion, and economic concerns weigh heavily in policy decision-making processes. Policy dialogue takes the form of verbal debates, often among strongly held views and competing interests. Conversely, researchers are entrenched in slower moving scientific processes related to the generation of knowledge or the evaluation of interventions. These efforts are subject to rules of scientific validity and to peer review at many levels, including funding decisions and publications – adding to the time needed to produce valid findings and to the unwillingness to base action on preliminary findings. Practitioners and service providers, in contrast, are involved in frontline interventions and service delivery to individuals and families. Their primary responsibility is to their clients.

The disadvantages of traditional 'separate silos' practice are well documented, and include institutional traditions and barriers, the difficulty of 'cross-cultural' communication, philosophical and value differences, difficulties in sharing leadership and establishing priorities, power differences, funding limitations, and time (Huang et al., 2005; Marshall, Shepard, & Leadbeater, 2006; Nissani, 1997). The multiple and complex differences between and among government departments, researchers, service providers, and community partners present a very real hurdle. Problems in creating an integrated approach are further exacerbated by the disparate nature of the terminology and concepts used throughout the research literature. Even the term 'resilience' represents differing concepts for policy, research, and practice (Small & Memmo, 2004). Moreover, the degree to which resilience exists in a given population is directly related to how 'successful' functioning is defined. Similarly, if adversity has a broader definition in one study than another, then more children will be found to be resilient. The current lack of agreement in defining high risk and successful adaptation is a methodological problem that needs to be addressed.

### Response: Interdisciplinary and Collaborative Approaches

There is increasing recognition of the importance of an interdisciplinary approach in policy, research, and practice settings (Lattuca, 2002; Perkins et al., 2001). Incorporating knowledge and skills from multiple perspectives adds substance and credibility to decision processes. Investigators, practitioners, and policy makers benefit from the combined expertise available. Benefits include greater project flexibility, ability to address complex issues and questions, creative solutions and fresh insights, provision of multiple perspectives, bridging gaps between or among sectors, and enrichment of individuals' lives.

Elsewhere, we have described a number of community-based collaborations fostered by universities, communities, and funding agencies (Leadbeater et al., 2006). We have adopted this approach at the Centre for Youth and Society, bringing together professionals from the many different settings, disciplines, and methodologies needed to understand between- and within-group differences and resilience processes. Research findings are irrelevant without the integration of policy and research. Thus, despite differing dogmas, it is crucial that researchers and policy makers work together for effective policy to be created. In our experience, this has meant becoming more versed in knowledge translation – translating research into terms and concepts more easily taken up by policy makers.

Experienced professionals are challenged when moving from a familiar model fostering disciplinary expertise, individualism, and competitiveness to one of interdisciplinary collaboration and reciprocity. This requires constant negotiating of roles and responsibilities. At the beginning of our Healthy Youth project, for example, individuals tended to focus more on the differences among disciplines and attempted to guide the direction of the project to fit with their own disciplinary frames of reference. Working together with a commitment to joint goals, however, we were able to view differences as opportunities for growth and for strengthening the project. Over time, and through many different opportunities designed to facilitate ongoing collaborations and joint presentations of our work (including monthly meetings, shared data, joint conference presentations and publications, and shared student supervision), researchers and community partners have become more familiar with each other's discourses and conceptualizations. Through open and respectful dialogue within the context of relationship building, we have worked to express ideas and questions more freely and to modify, expand, and reframe concepts and practice as we creatively solve problems and negotiate understandings. Roles and responsibilities have evolved over the course of the project. Overall decisions such as a youth survey and publication authorship guidelines (see www.youth.society.uvic.ca) were achieved through discussion and consensus. Smaller subgroups were also formed to work on specific activities, such as a community workshop or a conference presentation.

The WITS Primary Program is a specific example of an integrated community, family, and school violence prevention program developed by Bonnie Leadbeater and community partners in Greater Victoria School District Number 61 and the Rock Solid Foundation. WITS is aimed at enhancing social competencies and reducing peer victimization through creating responsive communities with a shared language (see program manual at www.youth.society.uvic.ca). The WITS acronym stands for Walk away, Ignore the bully, Talk it out, and Seek help. The overall goal of this collaboratively developed program is to create school, classroom, and family environments that speak with a uniform voice in responding to children's requests for help in dealing with bullying. Its success can be attributed to the common language and strategies used throughout the program, the user-friendly manual and classroom resources, and the sustained support from community partners.

On a cautionary note, a shared focus and cross-contextual approach make it imperative to monitor the occurrence of overlapping roles. It is not uncommon these days to have professional clinicians and service providers who are also participating in research or program evaluation. Such multiple perspectives are beneficial when working to improve the lives of children and youth. However, it is important to thoroughly discuss the implications, in order to avoid role-related confusion stemming from these overlapping responsibilities, priorities, and loyalties (Moretti, Leadbeater, & Marshall, 2006).

Opportunities for more open avenues of communication and discussion among researchers and policy makers are essential to both evidence-based policy and policy-relevant research. Regular information exchanges, joint conferences, and networking among policy makers, lobby groups, and academics should be established and funded. Websites can provide accessible links among these groups, but funding for monitoring and maintaining specific sites is rarely available in academic centres and seldom initiated by policy makers. In addition, acknowledging the importance of policy-relevant language, resources are required for the preparation and distribution of readable policy briefs from relevant research.

## Challenge: Methodological Imbalance

Knowledge used to inform youth health and welfare policy has been dominated by large-scale quantitative research investigations and the 'gold standard' of randomized control trials (RCT) methodology. While obtaining generalizable data comprises an important contribution to policy development, this methodology has typically favoured samples from large urban populations that provide a picture of the 'average' child or youth that, in reality, only exists on paper. When these research data are used to generate policy and service plans, the result can be universal or 'one size fits all' recommendations that are either inappropriate for local contexts or need to be extensively adapted (Huang et al., 2005). The complexities and particular combinations of attributes, ecological factors, and experiences that make up individual lives are lost. Services and interventions that are seen as irrelevant or inappropriate are less likely to be used, and this constitutes a waste of precious and sometimes scarce resources.

Qualitative and descriptive data have been criticized as being anecdotal and thus of little relevance to evidence-based practice priorities. However, well-conducted rigorous qualitative and small sample-studies that provide in-depth portrayals are extremely relevant to clinical practitioners and policy makers interested in the contextualized experiences of real individuals and groups. In addition, these types of investigations are the only way to acquire relevant information about the needs of children and youth in rural and small communities.

### Response: Multiple Methodologies

A variety of designs and approaches are not only consistent with the variety of individuals, families, and communities to be served, they also make the best use of the varied backgrounds and skills of policy makers, researchers, and practitioners serving them. Qualitative, quantitative, program evaluation, and mixed methods are needed. Huang et al. (2005) also contend that we need to broaden the concept of evidence-based interventions to include evidence-based *processes* that may cut across a number of clinical interventions, such as relationship building or skill building.

Researchers need to utilize both 'searchlight' and 'spotlight' approaches – the broader searchlight approach to indicate population characteristics and trends, and the more focused spotlight approach to identify contextually and locally relevant attributes and interventions. Cycles of large and smaller-scale investigations can be adapted to respond to the rapidly changing face of communities in society. Integration is also necessary, as no single policy or practice decision or intervention is likely to be successful across contexts (Richman & Fraser, 2001).

### Challenge: Graduate-Level Training

The fragmented and discipline-specific approaches with which professionals wrestle are equally problematic in training settings. As Borden and Perkins (2006) point out, there is a lack of educational opportunities available for youth development trainees that reflect the more current cross-cultural and contextually based approaches in the field. Traditional content and methods of university research training have been rooted in a view of science that emphasizes separateness and impartiality, with typically close-ended and static procedures. Post-secondary training for mental health practitioners and service providers tends to emphasize identification of pathology and problems together with subsequent interventions to eliminate or correct such problems. Textbooks and policy manuals typically present an objective, step-by-step approach to problem solving that rarely addresses the complex interrelationships that constitute multidisciplinary community services. These approaches are out of step with the emphasis espoused here on strengths-oriented and community-focused policies and actions.

When addressed in university programs, cultural differences tend to be limited to ethnic and racial differences. While attending to these is extremely important, focusing solely on racial or language differences can blind students to the need to consider the broad range of cultural perspectives. A further challenge is the tendency to assume that members of a culture hold similar values and views. There can be as much, if not more, diversity within a culture as between cultures (Marshall & Batten, 2004; Pedersen, 1991).

The major focus in most educational programs aimed at child and youth policy, practice, or research is on the recipients or clients. However, learning the steps of the policy process and developing skills to communicate with future colleagues are also important for timely and effective knowledge uptake. In addition, traditional discipline-bound training approaches are often proving to be too narrow in scope to effectively address the diversity and complexity of the issues facing young people today.

### Response: An Interdisciplinary Approach to Graduate Student Training

We have argued earlier in this chapter for a cultural and contextually relevant interdisciplinary approach among professionals in research, practice, and policy arenas; the same is needed for graduate student training and education. Again, building relationships and participating in a broad range of cross-cultural experiences are the means to achieve this goal.

Training needs to focus more on how to work with culturally diverse clients and their families (Huang et al., 2005). An emphasis on understanding and accepting the multiplicity of world views, values, and practices must go hand in hand with skill development and cross-cultural competencies. Culturally sensitive texts, training materials, and practical experiences in the field are integral elements to be included. In aboriginal contexts, for example, issues of protocol as well as ownership of data and resources need to be acknowledged and agreed upon at the time of entry into the community, if not before (Marshall & Batten, 2004).

One very successful training opportunity initiated within our Healthy Youth research project was a monthly graduate student colloquium (see http://www.youth.society.uvic.ca/activities/training .html). Graduate students being supervised by project faculty members participated in a monthly colloquium experience that further extended the interdisciplinary training several were receiving on individual collaborative projects. Students took the lead in facilitating the colloquia in consultation with faculty researchers and mentored by an 'elder' with extensive experience in academic research and administration. The seminars offered an interdisciplinary forum for students to interact with one another, to enhance research training, and to allow students to work collaboratively across the various faculty research projects (Slatkoff, Phillips, Corrin, Rozeck-Allen, & Strong-Wilson, 2006). Students discussed their research responsibilities, methodological orientations, academic interests, and past research experiences. The colloquia have provided a particularly valuable forum for graduate student researchers to explore the ethical challenges involved in community-based research with vulnerable populations. The student colloquia have continued after the completion of the Healthy Youth project, incorporating new students and new topics. We believe the key to the success of the colloquium, now going into its sixth year, is the joint student-faculty organizing, the inclusion of community partners, and the integration of research, practice, and policy topics such as children in care and dissemination to varied audiences.

Ethics education is especially critical for students. They need to become comfortable with the ambiguity and ever-changing nature of working with children, youth, and families in real-life situations. The potential for overlapping roles is an area that requires ongoing reflection and discussion. An ethics training model developed as part of our Healthy Youth research project includes four interrelated aspects: (1)

clarifying interests, assumptions, and developing relationships, (2) monitoring structures and procedures, (3) ensuring ethicality of research procedures, and (4) managing impacts and dissemination (Moretti et al., 2006). Although developed in a research context, the principles are broadly applicable to a multiplicity of settings.

## Implications and Recommendations

It is time to embrace the twenty-first century notion of collaborative governance and partnerships to support the well-being of children and youth. Many promising and positive youth-serving initiatives are not linked to or well supported by existing policy-generating structures. We believe it is vital that cross-cultural, cross-contextual, and interdisciplinary approaches and solutions be considered. A framework for local, regional, national, and international policy is needed that provides coordination, funding, and administrative support. A commitment to the concept of resilience is required, along with greater attention to community–institutional interrelationships.

The integrated, strengths-based process described here suggests a number of recommendations that may be applied to policy development and implementation in a range of contexts. First and foremost is taking the time needed to build strong and mutually collaborative partnerships. This requires resisting short-term political change and reacts to isolated events. Secondly, and related to the concept of mutual relationships, policy development and implementation must be firmly embedded in cultural and local contexts. A willingness to respect cultural and contextual values and world views, along with openness to making adjustments, is essential. One size does not fit all – different settings, communities, and cultures need different combinations of solutions. A third recommendation is to make strengths-based capacity building an integral part of the policy-planning process. Fourth, we must include the voices and actions of children and youth themselves. They arguably have the greatest stake in future outcomes. A further suggestion is to make full use of the variety of methods and strategies that are available to us across disciplines and methodologies. Finally, post-secondary educational programs need to keep pace with the changing landscape of child and youth development. Policy implications should be integrated into research and clinical practice training.

An integrated, strengths-oriented, and comprehensive approach is required to create and implement policy to improve the lives of children and youth in adversity. This goal is in accordance with Christians' (2003) conditions of communitarian ethics – the inclusion of multiple voices, the enhancement of moral discernment, and the promotion of social transformation. While there are numerous challenges along the way, the top priority for all researchers, practitioners, and policy makers should be working together to promote a healthy and fulfilling life for all children and youth.

## REFERENCES

Benoit, C., Jansson, M., Millar, A., & Phillips, R. (2005). Community-academic research on hard-to-reach populations: Benefits and challenges. *Qualitative Health Research, 15*(2), 263–82.

Blum, R.W., & Ellen, J. (2002). Work group V: Increasing the capacity of schools neighborhoods, and communities to improve adolescent health outcomes. *Journal of Adolescent Health, 31*, 288–92.

Borden, L.M., & Perkins, D.F. (2006). Community youth development professionals: Providing the necessary supports in the United States. *Child and Youth Care Forum, 35*(2), 101–58.

British Columbia Office of the Provincial Health Officer & Child and Youth Officer. (2006). *Joint Special Report. Health and well-being of children in care in British Columbia. Report 1 on health services utilization and mortality.* Retrieved 29 August 2006 from http://www.gov.bc.ca/cyo/down/complete_joint_special_report.pdf.

Cargo, M., Grams, G., Ottoson, J., Ward, P., & Green, L. (2003). Empowerment as fostering positive youth development and citizenship. *American Journal of Health Behavior, 27*, 66–79.

Christians, C. (2003). Ethics & politics in qualitative research. In N. Denzin & Y. Lincoln (Eds.), *Collecting & interpreting qualitative materials* (2nd ed., pp. 208–43). Thousand Oaks, CA: Sage.

Huang, L., Stroul, B., Friedman, R., Mrazek, P., Friesen, B., Pires, S., & Mayberg, S. (2005). Transforming mental health care for children and their families. *American Psychologist, 60*(6), 615–27.

Kingdon, J. (1995). *Agendas, alternatives, and public policies* (2nd ed.). New York: Harper Collins.

Lattuca, L.R. (2002). Learning interdisciplinarity: Sociocultural perspectives on academic work. *Journal of Higher Education, 73*(6), 711–39.

Leadbeater, B., Banister, E., Benoit, C., Jansson, M., Marshall, A., & Riecken,

T. (2006). *Ethical issues in community-based research with children and youth.* Toronto: University of Toronto Press.

Leadbeater, B., Dodgen, D., & Solarz, A. (2005). The resilience revolution: A paradigm shift for research and policy? In R.D. Peters, R.J. McMahon, & B. Leadbeater (Eds.), *Resilience in children, families, and communities: Linking context to practice and policy* (pp. 47–61). New York: Kluwer Academic/Plenum.

Leadbeater, B., Schellenbach, C., Maton, K., & Dogden, D. (2004). Research and policy for building strengths: Processes and contexts of individual, family, and community development. In K. Maton, C. Schellenbach, B. Leadbeater, & A. Solarz (Eds.), *Investing in children, youth, families, and communities: Strengths-based research and policy* (pp. 13–30). Washington, DC: American Psychological Foundation.

Lerner, R., Almerigi, J., Theokas, C., & Lerner, J. (2005). Positive youth development: A view of the issues. *Journal of Early Adolescence, 25*(1), 10–16.

Marshall, A. (2002). Life-career counselling issues for youth in coastal and rural communities. The impact of economic, social and environmental restructuring. *International Journal for the Advancement of Counselling, 24*(1), 69–87.

Marshall, A., & Batten, S. (2004). Researching across cultures: Issues of ethics and power. *Qualitative Social Research, 5*(3), Art. 39. Retrieved 2 September 2006, from http://www.qualitative-research.net/fqs-texte/3-04/04-3-39-e.pdf.

Marshall, A., Shepard, B., & Leadbeater, B. (2006). Interdisciplinary research: Charting new directions collaboratively. *International Journal of the Humanities, 2*(2), 953–60.

Maton, K.I. (2005). The social transformation of environments and the promotion of resilience in children. In R. Peters, B.J. Leadbeater, & R. McMahon (Eds.), *Resilience in children, families and communities: Linking context to intervention and policy* (pp. 119–36). New York: Kluwer Academic/Plenum.

McCormick, R. (1997). Healing through interdependence: The role of connecting in First Nations healing practices. *Canadian Journal of Counselling, 31*(3), 172–84.

Moretti, M., Leadbeater, B., & Marshall, A. (2006). Stepping into community-based research: Preparing students to meet new ethical and professional challenges. In B. Leadbeater, E. Banister, C. Benoit, M. Jansson, A. Marshall, & T. Riecken (Eds.), *Ethical issues in community-based research with children and youth* (pp. 232–47). Toronto: University of Toronto Press.

Murphey, D.A., Lamonda, K.H., Carney, J.K., & Duncan, P. (2004). Relationships of a brief measure of youth assets to health-promoting and risk behaviors. *Journal of Adolescent Health, 34*(3), 184–91.

Nissani, M. (1997). Ten cheers for interdisciplinarity: The case for interdisciplinary knowledge and research. *Social Sciences Journal, 34*(2), 201–17.

Ommer, R.E. & Coasts Under Stress research project team. (2007). *Coasts Under Stress: Restructuring and social-ecological health*. Montreal: McGill-Queen's University Press.

Pedersen, P. (1991). Multiculturalism as a generic approach to counseling. *Journal of Counseling and Development, 70*, 6–12.

Perkins, D.F., Borden, L.M., & Villarruel, F.A. (2001). Community youth development: A partnership for action. *School Community Journal, 11*(20), 7–26.

Piquemal, N. (2001). Free and informed consent in research involving Native American communities. *American Indian Culture and Research Journal, 25*(1), 65–79.

Pittman, K., Diversi, M., & Ferber, T. (2002). Social policy supports for adolescents in the twenty-first century: Framing questions. *Journal of Research on Adolescence, 12*(1), 149–58.

Ponterotto, J.G., & Casas, J.M. (1993). *Handbook of ethnic/racial minority counseling research*. Springfield, IL: Charles C. Thomas.

Richman, J.M., & Fraser, M.W. (2001). Resilience: Implications for evidence-based practice. In J.M. Richman & M.W. Fraser (Eds.), *The context of youth violence: Resilience, risk, and protection* (pp. 187–97). Westport, CT: Greenwood.

Schoon, I., & Bynner, J. (2003). Risk and resilience in the life course: Implications for interventions and social policies. *Journal of Youth Studies, 6*(1), 21–31.

Simeonsson, R.J., & Covington, M. (1994). Policy and practice: Implications of a primary prevention agenda. In R.J. Simeonsson (Ed.), *Risk, resilience and prevention: Promoting the well-being of all children* (pp. 299–320). Baltimore: Paul Brooks.

Slatkoff, J., Phillips, R., Corrin, S., Rozeck-Allen, T., & Strong-Wilson, T. (2006). Unique roles, unique challenges: Graduate students' involvement in community-academic research. In B. Leadbeater, E. Banister, C. Benoit, M. Jansson, A. Marshall, & T. Riecken (eds.), *Ethical issues in community-based research with children and youth* (pp. 221–31). Toronto: University of Toronto Press.

Small, S., & Memmo, M. (2004). Contemporary models of youth development and problem prevention: Toward an integration of terms, concepts, and models. *Family Relations, 53*(1), 3–11.

Ungar, M. (2005). Pathways to resilience among children in child welfare, corrections, mental health and educational settings: Navigation and negotiation. *Child and Youth Care Forum, 34*(6), 423–44.

Waddell, C., Lavis, J.N., Abelson, J., Lomas, J., Shepherd, C.A., Bird-Gayson, T., Giacomini, M., & Offord, D.R. (2005). Research use in children's mental health policy in Canada: Maintaining vigilance amid ambiguity. *Social Science and Medicine, 61,* 1649–57.

Wilcox, B.L., Weisz, P.V., & Miller, M.K. (2005). Practical guidelines for educating policymakers: The Family Impact Seminar as an approach to advancing the interests and children and families in the policy arena. *Journal of Clinical Child and Adolescent Psychology, 34*(4), 638–45.

Wolkow, K.E. & Ferguson, H.B. (2001). Community factors in the development of resiliency: Considerations and future directions. *Community Mental Health Journal, 37*(6), 489–98.

# Contributors

**Kim M. Anderson,** PhD, is an assistant professor in the School of Social Work at the University of Missouri-Columbia, U.S.A., where she teaches clinical practice and evaluation courses at the graduate level. Dr. Anderson's scholarship bridges gaps between theory and practice by offering conceptual frameworks for survivors of family violence and mental health practitioners that allow for variation in individual expressions of trauma, trauma recovery and resilience. Specific populations of women that she studies (although not mutually exclusive) include survivors of childhood incest, adult children of battered women, and individuals formerly in a domestic violence relationship. Her research interests include assessment of risk and resiliency in trauma populations and implementation of strengths-based mental health practice. Throughout the past twenty years, Dr. Anderson has crossed the boundaries among the many roles that interest her – practitioner, researcher, educator, and advocate – to help survivors of family violence and the practitioners who serve them.

**Betty Bastien,** PhD, is a member of the Piikani First Nation and associate professor at the University of Calgary, Faculty of Social Work. Her doctoral work, *Blackfoot Ways of Knowing*, laid the foundation for dissemination of Aboriginal knowledge and ways of knowing, including optimum approaches for the dissemination of this knowledge. This research began her traditional learning path, allowing Betty to become a member of Brave Dog Society and partner to a Thunder Pipe. Consequently, she continues to work in this area, publishing on trauma and violence associated with colonization and cultural genocide of indigenous peoples, and reparation of indigenous knowledge systems. This interest is also reflected in Betty's contribution to curriculum design, teaching, and research on indigenous social work practice, pedagogy, and epistemology with Red Crow Community College on the Blood Tribe; Native American Studies, University of Lethbridge; and International Indigenous Studies, University of Calgary.

Born and raised in Israel, **Roni Berger** holds a BSW, MSW, and PhD from the Hebrew University of Jerusalem and a diploma in psychotherapy from Tel Aviv Medical School. She is a professor at Adelphi University, consultant to the Jewish Board of Families and Children Services and other organizations, and holds a private practice. Her fields of expertise include families, specifically stepfamilies, immigrants, post-traumatic growth qualitative research, and direct practice. She has published and presented extensively nationally and internationally. Prior to her emigration to the United States, she worked in Israel in academia, direct practice, supervisory and administrative positions in diverse settings, and as a consultant to various organizations.

**Ralph C. Bodor,** PhD, RSW, has extensive experience in the delivery of human services and social work education in rural, remote, and First Nation communities in Alberta. In addition, he has completed a number of research projects employing hermeneutic concepts to explore a variety of social work practice issues in rural, remote, and First Nations and Métis communities. Dr Bodor is assistant professor at the Faculty of Social Work, University of Calgary, where he has been primarily involved in developing and delivering accredited social work courses to rural, remote, and First Nations communities throughout Alberta. Dr Bodor lives by a lake in rural Alberta with his family and his codependent cat, Max.

**Normand Carrey,** MD, is a child and adolescent psychiatrist specializing in developmental psychopharmacology, neuroimaging in disruptive behaviour disorders, and family therapy. His research interests include spectroscopy of ADHD and effects of stimulants on gene expression in brain development, and he is a co-investigator of the International Resilience Project. He holds several research grants from CIHR (Canadian Institute of Health Research). Recently he co-authored (with Michael Ungar) a monograph on resilience (*Child and*

*Adolescent Psychiatric Clinics of North America*, vol. 16, *no.2*). His current clinical position is medical director, Children's Response Program, IWK Health Centre, Halifax, Nova Scotia, a long-term residential program specializing in children with attachment/disruptive behaviour difficulties. He also enjoys writing poetry.

**Lynne Cohen,** PhD, is an associate professor and is undergraduate coordinator in the School of Psychology at Edith Cowan University (ECU). Her research focuses on issues in higher education and has resulted in many publications and presentations on learning and teaching in higher education. She is the current editor of the community psychology journal *The Australian Community Psychologist*. Lynne is also a community psychologist in the area of sense of belonging and its relationship to successful outcomes for students, and has extensive experience in working with children with learning difficulties. She has also been involved in the design and implementation of research projects in different areas such as cognitive interpretations of depression, social attribution theory, and evaluation of crime prevention programs. Lynne has undertaken numerous evaluation projects for government and non-government organizations over the past ten years, incorporating different methodologies, reflecting her interest in combining qualitative and quantitative methodologies.

**Sandra J. Drower,** PhD, is professor at the University of Winchester, Hampshire, England, and immediate past Chair of Social Work, University of the Witwatersrand, Johannesburg, South Africa. She has held senior positions in social work practice and social work education in South Africa and in England. While her initial specialization was psychiatric social work, she has written and conducted research in the areas of social work with groups, social work ethics and values, and social work education. She has a particular interest in the interface between the process of social work education, the development of resilience in young people, and the cultural context.

**Nancy Heath,** PhD, is associate professor of educational and counselling psychology at McGill University in Montreal, Canada. She is director of the Inclusive Education and Special Populations Programs, as well as being cross-appointed in School/Applied Child Psychology. Dr Heath has worked with youth at risk for close to twenty years. Her research program explores resilience and adaptive functioning in youth at risk, and her most recent work has focused on the understanding of self-injury in the schools. In 2001 she was elected as fellow in the International Academy of Research on Learning Disabilities and is currently the editor of the academy's newsletter. Dr. Heath is a founding member of the International Society for the Study of Self-Injury (ISSS) and the developer of the International Self-Injury in Youth Research Network. In 2004 she was awarded the William Dawson Scholar Award at McGill for outstanding research and future promise.

**Krista Hungler,** MSc, continues to work at the Social Support Research Program as a research associate. Krista was the project coordinator in phase 2 of the Support Intervention for Homeless Youth Project, which involved the implementation of the intervention and data collection and analysis of information collected from youth and other intervention participants. She now is involved with writing for this past project and in ongoing research examining the outcomes of social support interventions with vulnerable populations. Currently, data analysis is in progress for a support intervention project for women living in low-income situations who smoke. Krista is conducting the quantitative portion of the analysis.

**Jean Lafrance,** MSW, PhD, has been involved in child welfare work for over forty-two years, beginning as frontline social worker in northern Alberta in 1964 and serving in various leadership roles in northern, central, and southern Alberta as well as in Edmonton and Calgary. He has also worked in staff development, policy and program development, and strategic planning as an assistant deputy minister, capping his thirty-three years in government as Alberta's Provincial Children's Advocate. He earned an MSW at Carleton University in 1970 and a PhD in social work from the University of Southern California in 1993. He joined the Faculty of Social Work with the University of Calgary in 1997, where he is now an associate professor with a keen interest in child welfare work with aboriginal communities.

**Julie Anne Laser,** MSW, PhD, has a BA in political science focusing on international relations and studies in religion (University of Michigan, 1985), an MSW (University of Michigan, 1987), and a PhD from Michigan State University in family and child ecology (2003). Laser has worked in Mexico, Switzerland, Japan, China, and various American urban and rural settings. She has over twenty years of clinical social work experience and is particularly interested in school social work. Dr Laser's research focus is adolescent resilience, particularly the relevance of internal and ecological protective and risk factors by culture and gender. She recently completed a large study of Japanese youth and is presently investigating resilience in Korean, Chinese, and Senegalese youth. She also is involved in a collaborative evaluation of a new charter high school for homeless youth. Laser coordinates and teaches at the University of Denver Graduate School of Social Work.

**Bonnie J. Leadbeater,** PhD, is professor of psychology at the University of Victoria, which she joined in 1997 after nine years as faculty at Yale University. She is director of the Centre for Youth and Society's research and programs promoting youth health and resilience through community–university research partnerships (www.youth.society.uvic). She is also co-director of the BC Child and Youth Health Research Network (www.cyhrnet.ca), funded by the Michael Smith Foundation for Health Research. This network provides funds to enable community–university research partnerships. Dr Leadbeater's areas of research expertise include depression in adolescence, resilience among high-risk youth, and prevention of peer victimization. She is co-editor of several books, including *Resilience in Children, Families and Communities: Linking Context to Intervention and Policy* (with Ray Peters and Robert McMahon [New York: Kluwer]) and a recent interdisciplinary volume *Ethical Issues in Community-Based Research with Children and Youth* (with Elizabeth Banister, Cecilia Benoit, Mikael Jansson, Anne Marshall, and Ted Riecken [University of Toronto Press, 2006]).

**Francis Wing-lin Lee,** PhD, in criminology, is an associate professor in the Department of Social Work and Social Administration, University of Hong Kong, and has been involved in social work education for over twenty years. With his undergraduate and master training in social work, he is a registered social worker (RSW) with the Hong Kong Social Workers' Registration Board. He has taught in the Hong Kong Baptist University, City University of Hong Kong, Chinese University of Hong Kong, and is now with the University of Hong Kong. He has conducted research and published locally, regionally, and internationally in his areas of specialty, which include understanding and working with young people, youth at risk, and young offenders; youth services; causes of juvenile delinquency; treatment programs for young offenders; policing; and criminology.

**Mah-Ngee Lee** holds a PhD, from the National Institute of Education, Nanyang Technological University, Singapore. After teaching English and Malay at Sam Tet Secondary School, Perak, Malaysia, from 1987 to 2002, Lee was appointed head of Malay Language Department (1994 to 1997) and school counsellor (1997 to 2002). She also planned and organized the school mentor-mentee system and reported on students' truancies and illiteracy to the Perak State Education Department. In recognition of her dedication, she was awarded the Excellent Service Teacher Award in 1994 by the Ministry of Education, Malaysia. Lee has resumed her career as a school counsellor in Sam Tet Secondary School after completing her doctoral program in June 2006.

**Nicole Letourneau,** PhD, RN, is full professor in the Faculty of Nursing at the University of New Brunswick. She holds a Peter Lougheed New Investigator award from the Canadian Institutes for Health Research and a Tier 2 Canada Research Chair in Healthy Child Development. Her research program, entitled 'Child Health Intervention and Longitudinal Development' (CHILD; http://www.unbf.ca/nursing/child/index.html) Studies Program, focuses on developing and testing interventions to support vulnerable children's development. Since collaborating on the social support project for homeless youth, she has established a program of research aimed at children's early caregiving environment. Currently she is conducting studies examining (1) the impact of interventions for mothers with postpartum depression on maternal-infant relationships, maternal mental health, and infant health; (2) social support needs and preferences of mothers of infants exposed to domestic violence; and (3) support needs and intervention preferences of male partners of women with postpartum depression.

**Kathryn Levine**, PhD, is currently an assistant professor with the Faculty of Social Work at the University of Manitoba. Her practice and research interests focus on family violence issues, child and adolescent mental health, and the promotion of resilience in at-risk youth. She has extensive experience as a clinical social worker and has provided a wide range of therapeutic and clinical services to individuals, families, and groups within the child welfare, child and adolescent mental health, and public school systems. Her current research projects include examining the cumulative impact of violence exposure on adolescent girls and exploring factors that promote family involvement in the career development processes for children.

**Linda Liebenberg,** PhD, director of research for the Pathways to Resilience Project at Dalhousie University, is a methodologist with an interest in both image-based methods and mixed-methods designs. Her research examines the use of both visual methods and mixed-method research designs and how these facilitate an understanding of women and children in developing contexts, in particular South Africa. She has previously managed a number of programs pertaining to these interests, including the International Resilience Project, Dalhousie University. Other projects she has coordinated relate to out-of-school youth in informal settlements surrounding Cape Town (Department of Educational Psychology and Specialised Education, Stellenbosch University, South Africa) and research with women on farms in the Winelands region of South Africa (Department of Psychology, Stellenbosch University).

**E. Anne Marshall,** PhD, RPsych, is a professor of counselling psychology and former chair of the Department of Educational Psychology and Leadership Studies at the University of Victoria. She is a founding member of the Centre for Youth and Society and has been training counsellors to work with youth and families since 1980. Dr. Marshall's research interests include adolescent mental health, youth transition and resilience, cultural identity, career development, and ethical research practice. She has been a visiting scholar in Thailand and The People's Republic of China, working with colleagues in the area of youth career transition. Dr Marshall is currently involved in research projects investigating transition processes in aboriginal and non-aboriginal youth. She is co-editor of a recent interdisciplinary book entitled *Ethical Issues in Community-Based Research with Children and Youth* (University of Toronto Press).

**Robyn Munford,** PhD, is a professor of social work, Massey University, Palmerston North, New Zealand. She has qualifications in social work, sociology, and disability studies. She lectures in social and community work, disability studies, and research methods. A key focus of her academic work is the supervision of master's and doctoral theses and research projects. Of particular interest is the mentoring of emerging researchers in social science and in social work practice research.

Robyn has extensive experience in disability and family research and has worked for the past decade on family well-being research, including research on young people. This program utilizes participatory and action research methodologies. She has published widely on social work theory and practice, community development, bicultural frameworks for social and community work practice, social service interventions, and family well-being.

**Kennedy Kwong-hung Ng,** MSocSc, is a trained social worker specialized in youth service. He has his concentration on preventive and remedial programs, including the Understanding Adolescent Project (UAP), Youth-Pre-employment-Training-Program, and wilderness and adventure counselling groups for substance abusers. Kennedy is an MSW graduate from the Department of Social Work of the Chinese University of Hong Kong. He is also a registered social worker (RSW) with the Hong Kong Social Workers' Registration Board. He has various after-job involvements, such as being a senior volunteer of Breakthrough Limited, which was responsible for the running of the UAP. He is also the training director of Challenge Course Association of Hong Kong, PRC, from 2006 to 2008.

**Lisbeth Pike,** PhD, is associate professor in the School of Psychology at Edith Cowan University in Perth, Western Australia. She holds two specialist psychologist titles: clinical psychologist and educational and developmental psychologist. Her teaching and research has focused on life-span developmental psychology and family issues, most notably the effects of parental separation and divorce on children's growth and development and how families adjust and evolve as new family forms post-divorce. Study in the United States and her ongoing research in Australia have focused on the experience of children and adults with the family court system and the role and impact of community agencies on separating and divorcing families. Dr Pike has managed research projects as chief investigator for a range of public, not-for-profit, University, and industry collaborative projects. She has also been involved as a consultant to a range of national and international government and training organizations.

**Julie Ann Pooley,** PhD, is a senior lecturer in the School of Psychology at Edith Cowan University. She is involved in teaching in both the undergraduate and postgraduate psychology programs and has recently been awarded a National Teaching Award by the Australian University Teaching Committee (2003). Her current research focuses on communities facing natural disasters, to determine what enables communities to become resilient to impending threats. She is also interested in the area of environmental education and attitudes towards the environment. Dr Pooley is a community psychologist who teaches and conducts research in the area of applied social and community psychology. She has been involved in and directed many community-based research consultancies, projects, and workshops. Much of her work has been written for and presented to community groups and organizations as well as at international conference presentations.

**Linda Reutter,** RN, PhD, is professor in the Faculty of Nursing, University of Alberta. Her research program focuses on inequities resulting from socio-economic status. Study populations include low-income people, professionals, the public, and those who influence and effect poverty-related policies. She has investigated public understandings of poverty and its effects, public support for poverty-related policies, social exclusion and isolation among low-income populations, and nursing student attitudes and beliefs about poverty and health. She is currently an investigator in a large randomized control trial to determine effective support interventions to link low-income families to community services. Dr Reutter's clinical expertise and teaching experience is in public health nursing. She has written several book chapters in Canadian nursing textbooks related to health and wellness, primary health care, and socio economic determinants of health and has published articles on incorporating policy content in graduate and undergraduate nursing curricula.

**Jackie Sanders,** PhD, is a senior researcher and the director of the Children, Youth and Families Research Project, School of Sociology, Social Policy and Social Work, Massey University, Palmerston North, New Zealand. This research program focuses on identifying changing patterns of family life and the different ways in which parents and children/young people respond to change. Jackie has twenty years of experience in health and social service planning and management. Her interests are the study of children and families, evaluation and planning for social service delivery, and the development of new models of practice. She maintains an active research practice program through ongoing relationships with a number of key social service providers in

New Zealand, and is a member of the International Association for Outcome-Based Evaluation and Research in Child and Family Services. She is an editor and reviewer for a number of key social work journals.

**Linda Smith** completed her undergraduate training at the University of Stellenbosch in 1980. She completed her Masters of Social Science with distinction at Rhodes University in 1990 and earned her honours degree in psychology from the University of South Africa (UNISA). She is currently completing her PhD at the University of the Witwatersrand in the area of anti-oppressive social work practice. She worked as a social worker in the area of community development and child and family welfare between 1981 and 2000 and has been lecturing at the University of the Witwatersrand since then. Her fields of interest include oppression and social justice; anti-oppressive practice; human rights; child and family welfare; Freirian methodology; culture and spirituality; environment and development; post-colonial discourse; and indigenous practice. She is also a consulting social worker in the areas of relationship counseling, play therapy with children, youth work, and organizational development.

**Miriam Stewart,** PhD, is a professor in the Faculties of Nursing and Medicine at the University of Alberta. She is a Health Senior Scholar, Alberta Heritage Foundation for Medical Research and a former Medical Research Council of Canada and National Health Research Development Program (MRC/NHRDP) Scholar. Dr Stewart is principal investigator of the Social Support Research Program and has devoted many years to research on social support as a determinant of life-long health. She has developed and tested social support interventions for many populations, including chronically ill children and adults, immigrant and multicultural communities, and health professionals. Dr Stewart is also the principal investigator of studies of resilience at individual and community levels. She is scientific director of the Canadian Institutes of Health Research, Institute of Gender and Health.

**Dawn Sutherland,** PhD, is currently the Canada Research Chair in Indigenous Science Education and teaches science methods courses at the University of Winnipeg. Her research program is guided by the desire to examine the impact of culturally inclusive science teaching on students and develop science programs that are inclusive and engaging for all students. Dr Sutherland finds the resilience framework useful when looking at educational settings with students who are often labelled as educationally at risk, especially in the sciences, where culture has previously been identified as a barrier to science learning. Using the resilience framework to examine how culture can enhance and sustain science learning is one of Dr Sutherland's interests.

**Siew-Luan Tay-Koay,** (BA Hons DipEd University of Malaya, MEd [guidance and counselling] University of Philippines, MEd MA [psychology] Columbia University, PhD [psychology] University of Oregon) is an associate professor in the Psychological Studies Academic Group and former vice-dean at the National Institute of Education (1994–7), Nanyang Technological University, Singapore. She received the Penang State Scholarship for her undergraduate studies in the University of Malaya and the American Association of University Women International Fellowship, Altrusa International Fellowship, and the Singapore Government Scholarship for her graduate studies in psychology. Prior to joining Nanyang Technological University, she was a lecturer in Science Universiti Sains Malaysia, Penang, Malaysia. Her area of specialization is in psychometrics, and her areas of research include personality and personal development. Dr Tay-Koay is a full member of the American Psychological Association.

**Linda C. Theron,** DEd, is a practising educational psychologist and associate professor in educational psychology at the North-West University of South Africa (Vaal Triangle Campus). She obtained her doctoral degree in educational psychology in 2000 and joined the university in the same year. Her research interests include resilience in youth living in South African townships or with learning difficulties. Currently, Linda holds a National Research Foundation grant to research how educators affected by the HIV and AIDS pandemic can be empowered towards resilience. She serves as an executive committee member in the Division of Research and Methodology of the Psychological Association of South Africa (PsySSA).

**Jessica R. Toste,** BEd, MA, is a doctoral student in the educational psychology program in the Department of Educational and Counselling Psychology at McGill University. Jessica has been involved in community-based educational programs for many years and has worked extensively in schools with youth at risk. She has been the recipient of provincial and national research fellowships. Additionally, her research contributions have been recognized through McGill's Stansfield Award for School-Based Classroom Research and the Learning Disabilities Association of Canada's Doreen Kronick Scholarship for future promise in the field of learning disabilities. Jessica's research interests focus on resilient functioning and educational outcomes of youth at risk. Specifically, she is interested in factors that contribute to the classroom resilience of students with learning disabilities and in conducting research that will have direct implications for educational practice.

**Michael Ungar**, PhD, is both a social worker and marriage and family therapist with experience working directly with children and adults in child welfare, mental health, and educational and correctional settings. Now a professor at the School of Social Work, Dalhousie University, Halifax, Canada, Dr Ungar conducts research internationally on resilience-related themes relevant to the treatment and study of at-risk youth and families, including the study he currently leads, titled 'Methodological and Contextual Challenges Researching Childhood Resilience: An International Collaboration.' In addition to his research and teaching interests Dr Ungar maintains a family therapy practice in association with Phoenix Youth Programs, a prevention program for street youth and their families.

**Lana C. Zinck**, PhD, is a school psychologist and a graduate of the School/Applied Child Psychology program at McGill University, Department of Educational and Counselling Psychology. She worked closely with Dr Nancy Heath throughout the duration of her graduate studies. Lana has experience working with children and youth in recreational, educational, and clinical settings. Lana's research interests are focused on the family relationship factors that support positive adjustment in youth at risk, particularly youth with learning disabilities (LD). Her doctoral dissertation examined whether youth perceptions of maternal control, involvement, and communication are associated with various domains of adjustment in youth with and without LD. She has been awarded provincial and national research fellowships for her research and has presented her work in local and national forums. Lana's continuing interest in collaborating on clinical research of this nature stems from a commitment to improve the quality of life for youth and families.